AF668211

World Clinics

Dermatology

Fungal Infections of the Skin

World Clinics

Dermatology

Fungal Infections of the Skin

Editor-in-Chief
Rashmi Sarkar MD MNAMS

Guest Editor
Seemal R Desai MD FAAD

December 2016 Volume 3 Number 1

JAYPEE *The Health Sciences Publisher*

New Delhi | London | Panama

Jaypee Brothers Medical Publishers (P) Ltd

Headquarters

Jaypee Brothers Medical Publishers (P) Ltd
4838/24, Ansari Road, Daryaganj
New Delhi 110 002, India
Phone: +91-11-43574357
Fax: +91-11-43574314
Email: jaypee@jaypeebrothers.com

Overseas Offices

J.P. Medical Ltd
83 Victoria Street, London
SW1H 0HW (UK)
Phone: +44-2031708910
Fax: +02-03-0086180
Email: info@jpmedpub.com

Jaypee-Highlights Medical Publishers Inc
City of Knowledge, Bld. 235, 2nd Floor, Clayton
Panama City, Panama
Phone: +1 507-301-0496
Fax: +1 507-301-0499
Email: cservice@jphmedical.com

Jaypee Brothers Medical Publishers (P) Ltd
17/1-B Babar Road, Block-B, Shaymali
Mohammadpur, Dhaka-1207
Bangladesh
Mobile: +08801912003485
Email: jaypeedhaka@gmail.com

Jaypee Brothers Medical Publishers (P) Ltd
Bhotahity, Kathmandu, Nepal
Phone: +977-9741283608
Email: Kathmandu@jaypeebrothers.com

Website: www.jaypeebrothers.com
Website: www.jaypeedigital.com

© 2016, Jaypee Brothers Medical Publishers

All rights reserved. No part of this issue may be reproduced in any form or by any means without the prior permission of the publisher.

Inquiries for bulk sales may be solicited at: jaypee@jaypeebrothers.com

This issue has been published in good faith that the contents provided by contributors contained herein are original, and is intended for educational purposes only. While every effort is made to ensure the accuracy of information, the publisher and the editors specifically disclaim any damage, liability, or loss incurred, directly or indirectly, from the use or application of any of the contents of this work. If not specifically stated, all figures and tables are courtesy of the contributing authors. Where appropriate, the readers should consult with a specialist or contact the manufacturer of the drug or device.

Cover images: (*Left*) Tinea manum: A well defined annular plaque with erythema and scaling on ventral surface of left hand. *Courtesy:* Sumit Sethi, Surabhi Sinha. (*Middle*) Numerous yeast cells of *Histoplasma capsulatum* are visualized in histology sections from skin biopsy (H&E, x400). *Courtesy:* Vikram K Mahajan. (*Right*) Mother with resistant tinea. *Courtesy:* Yogesh S Marfatia, Sheethal K Jose.

WORLD CLINICS DERMATOLOGY: Fungal Infections of the Skin

December 2016, Volume 3, Number 1

ISSN: 2347-7156

ISBN: 978-93-86322-10-4

Printed in India

Contributors

Editor-in-Chief

Rashmi Sarkar MD MNAMS
Professor, Department of Dermatology
Maulana Azad Medical College and Lok Nayak Hospital
New Delhi, India

Guest Editor

Seemal R Desai MD FAAD
Clinical Assistant Professor, Department of Dermatology
University of Texas Southwestern Medical Centre
Dallas, Texas, USA

Contributing Authors

Theresa N Canavan MD
Resident, Department of Dermatology
University of Alabama
Birmingham, Alabama, USA

Malini R Capoor MD
Professor, Department of Microbiology
Vardhman Mahavir Medical College and Safdarjung Hospital
New Delhi, India

Tania F Cestari MD PhD
Professor, Department of Dermatology
Hospital de Clínicas de Porto Alegre
Porto Alegre, Rio Grande do Sul, Brazil

Janaki Chellam MD DD MAMS
Consultant, Billroth Hospitals
Professor (Retd.)
Department of Dermatology
Madras Medical College
Chennai, Tamil Nadu, India

Boni E Elewski MD
Professor, Department of Dermatology
University of Alabama
Birmingham, Alabama, USA

Sentamilselvi Ganapati MD DD PhD FAMS
Professor and Head (Retd.), Department of Dermatology
Madras Medical College
Chennai, Tamil Nadu, India

Aditya K Gupta MD PhD
Professor, Department of Medicine
University of Toronto
Toronto, Ontario, Canada

Tanvi Gupta MD DNB
Senior Resident, Department of Dermatology,
Leprology, and Venereology
Maulana Azad Medical College
New Delhi, India

Sheethal K Jose MBBS
Postgraduate Student, Department of Skin-VD
Medical College Baroda
Vadodara, Gujarat, India

Pradnya R Joshi MD DVL
Lecturer, Department of Dermatology
Rajiv Gandhi Medical College and Chatrapati Shivaji Maharaj Hospital
Thane, Maharashtra, India

Larissa R Leopoldo MD
Post Graduate Student, Department of Dermatology
Hospital de Clínicas de Porto Alegre
Porto Alegre, Rio Grande do Sul, Brazil

R Madhu MD DCH
Senior Assistant Professor, Department of Dermatology
Madras Medical College
Chennai, Tamil Nadu, India

Vikram K Mahajan MD
Professor
Department of Dermatology, Venereology, and Leprosy
Dr R.P. Government Medical College
Kangra, Himachal Pradesh, India

Yogesh S Marfatia MD
Professor, Department of Skin-VD
Medical College Baroda
Vadodara, Gujarat, India

Malathi Munisamy MD DNB
Assistant Professor, Department of Dermatology and STD
Jawaharlal Institute of Postgraduate Medical Education and Research
Puducherry, India

Brijesh Nair MD
Consultant, Department of Dermatology
INHS Sanjivani
Kochi, Kerala, India

Allen SW Oak BS
Medical Student, Department of Dermatology
University of Alabama
Birmingham, Alabama, USA

Poonam Puri MD
Professor and Consultant, Department of Dermatology,
Venereology, and Leprosy
Vardhman Mahavir Medical College and Safdarjung Hospital
New Delhi, India

Sumit Sethi MD DNB
Consultant, Genesis Centre for Dermatology
Skin Allure Aesthetic Clinic
New Delhi, India

Surabhi Sinha MD DNB
Specialist, Department of Dermatology and Leprosy
Dr Ram Manohar Lohia Hospital and Post Graduate Institute of Medical Education and Research
New Delhi, India

Devinder M Thappa MD DHA FRCP FAMS FIMSA
Professor and Head, Department of Dermatology and STD
Jawaharlal Institute of Postgraduate Medical Education and Research
Puducherry, India

Sarah G Versteeg MSc PhD
Medical Research Associate, Mediprobe Research Inc
London, Ontario, Canada

Vishalakshi Viswanath MD DNB DDV
Professor and Head
Department of Dermatology
Rajiv Gandhi Medical College and
Chatrapati Shivaji Maharaj Hospital
Thane, Maharashtra, India

Casey L Wang MD
Clinical Research Fellow
Department of Dermatology
University of Alabama
Birmingham, Alabama, USA

Contents

World Clin Dermatol. 2016;3(1):xi-xii.

Editorial

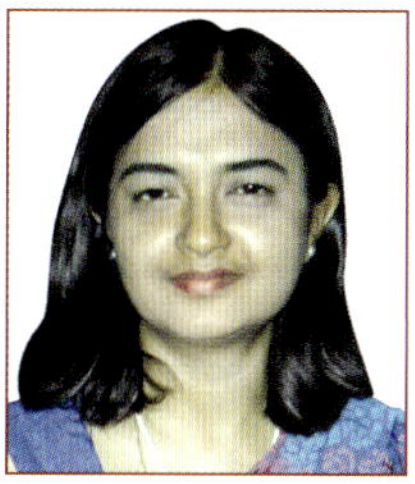

Rashmi Sarkar MD MNAMS
Editor-in-Chief

Fungal diseases are common dermatologic complaints in medical practice and definitely one of the commonest skin infections seen worldwide. In fact, a lifetime risk of acquiring dermatophytosis is said to be 10–15%. What has been surprising and alarming recently, is the rising incidence of recalcitrant dermatophytosis and the failure of superficial fungal infections of the skin to respond to conventional doses of antifungals. It was appropriate and timely to bring out a World Clinics of Dermatology issue devoted to fungal infections of the skin with Dr Seemal R Desai.

Dermatologists and mycologists have been brought together to provide rich insights into classification, taxonomy, clinical features, laboratory diagnosis, and management of superficial, subcutaneous, and systemic mycoses. Although superficial fungal infections have still received attention, subcutaneous and systemic mycoses have received less attention. Global experts in these subjects have provided perspectives from their own vast publications from India, United States, and South America. A chapter has been devoted to Tinea incognito, which is very pertinent in a country like India and Asia where topical steroid abuse is rampant. Dermato-mycologists have also provided perspectives on changing and rising incidence of fungal infections, causes of resistance and topical, systemic, and physical therapies for fungal infections.

I would like to thank Jaypee Brothers Medical Publishers (P) Ltd., especially Dr Neeraj Choudhary for getting me on board and Ms Barkha Arora for collaborating as Editorial Co-ordinator, and to all our wonderful authors for their invaluable contributions. I would also like to thank Dr Sneha Ghunawat, Dr Pallavi Ailawadi, Dr Tanvi Gupta, Dr Jaspriya Sandhu, Dr Isha Narang, Dr Shankila Mittal for their inputs and copyediting help.

© 2016 Jaypee Brothers Medical Publishers. All rights reserved.

I hope this edition would be equally helpful to practitioners, dermatology departments, and students of dermatology, all over the world.

Rashmi Sarkar MD MNAMS
Professor, Department of Dermatology
Maulana Azad Medical College and Lok Nayak Hospital
New Delhi, India

Email: rashmisarkar@gmail.com

Abbreviations

ABC	Adenosine triphosphate-binding cassette
AEs	Adverse effects
AGEP	acute generalized exanthematous pustulosis
AIDS	Acquired immunodeficiency syndrome
BATT	Boosted antifungal topical treatment
BID	Twice a day
BOAT	Boosted oral antifungal treatment
CBC	Complete blood count
CC	Complete cure
CHF	Congestive heart failure
CI	Confidence interval
CT	Computerized tomography
CYP450	Cytochrome P450
DLSO	Distal and lateral subungual onychomycoses
DNA	Deoxyribonucleic acid
DOPA	3,4-dihydroxyphenylalanine
DRESS	Drug reaction with eosinophilia and systemic symptoms
ELISA	Enzyme-linked immunosorbent assay
ERG	Ergosterol
FDA	Food and Drug Administration
GGI	Granuloma gluteale infantum
GI	Gastrointestinal
GMS	Gomori methenamine silver
GU	Genitourinary
H and E	Hematoxylin and eosin stain
HAART	Highly active antiretroviral therapy
HIV	Human immunodeficiency virus
HLA	Human leukocyte antigen
Hsp	Heat shock protein
IADVL	Indian Association of Dermatologists, Venereologists and Leprologists
ICBN	International Code of Botanical Nomenclature
IgG	Immunoglobulin G
IgM	Immunoglobulin M
IL	Interleukin
ITATSA	Task Force Against Topical Steroid Abuse
IV	Intravenous
KOH	Potassium hydroxide
LCB	Lactophenol cotton blue
LFT	Liver function test
LION study	Lamisil vs. Itraconazole in Onychomycosis study
MB	Methylene blue
MC	Mycologic cure
MF	Major facilitator
MIC	Minimum inhibitory concentration
mRNA	Messenger ribonucleic acid
NAC	Non-albicans Candida
NCCLS	National Committee for Clinical Laboratory Standards
NDMs	Nondermatophyte molds
OTC	Over-the-counter
PAS	Periodic acid-Schiff
PCR	Polymerase chain reaction
PDT	Photodynamic therapy
PSO	Proximal subungual onychomycoses
R	Resistant
RR	Risk ratio
rRNA	Ribosomal ribonucleic acid
S	Susceptible
SAP	Secreted aspartic proteinases
SCLE	Subacute cutaneous lupus erythematosus
SDA	Sabouraud's dextrose agar
SDD	Susceptible dependent upon dose
SJS	Stevens-Johnson syndrome
SLN	Solid lipid nanoparticles

SSKI	Saturated solution of potassium iodide
SWO	Superficial white onychomycoses
TCs	Topical corticosteroids
TDO	Total dystrophic onychomycoses
Th	T helper
TID	Three times a day
tRNA	Transfer ribonucleic acid
UV	Ultraviolet
VIS-NIR	Visible to near-infrared

World Clin Dermatol. 2016;3(1):1-2.

Fungal Diseases

[1,*]Seemal R Desai MD FAAD, [2]Rashmi Sarkar MD MNAMS

Department of Dermatology, University of Texas Southwestern Medical Centre
Dallas, Texas, USA
[2]Department of Dermatology, Maulana Azad Medical College and Lok Nayak Hospital
New Delhi, India

INTRODUCTION

Fungal diseases are common dermatologic complaint in medical practice. Because these conditions can manifest in many different ways, it is important to get a clear understanding of the classification, characteristics, and treatment options for these often complex disorders.

In general, common cutaneous fungal infections can be divided into broad categories; specifically, superficial fungal infections, subcutaneous fungal infections, and systemic fungal infections. It is important to note that systemic fungal infections are often referred to as "deep" infections.[1]

Superficial fungal infections[2,3] commonly invade the stratum corneum, and include conditions such as pityriasis versicolor, tinea nigra, black piedra, white piedra, tinea capitis, tinea corporis, tines cruris, tinea manuum, tinea faciei, tinea pedis,[4] and cutaneous candidiasis.

Subcutaneous fungal infections tend to result from inoculation or implantation of the causative organism. Conversely, systemic fungal infections most commonly occur from direct extension of the organism into the surrounding structures or hematogenous spread.

Of the three broad categories listed above, dermatophyte infections are some of the most common skin fungal infections seen in dermatology and non-dermatology practices. It is well-known that the most common dermatophyte infection worldwide is *Trichophyton rubrum*. Humans typically get infected with dermatophyte infections through human contact and would be referred to as antropophilic fungal infections, or if acquired from animal to human would

*Corresponding author
Email: seemald@yahoo.com

© 2016 Jaypee Brothers Medical Publishers. All rights reserved.

be referred to as zoophilic. A less common category is geophilic dermatophyte infections which occur from soil contact to human or animal. There are several known risk factors for the development of dermatophyte infections including household contact, sebum production, physiologic factors, and sex. In general, men more commonly get tinea pedis and tinea cruris, and postpubertal men are typically more affected by onychomycosis than women. Dermatophyte infections can have various clinical presentations, and have been known to mimic other dermatologic conditions, e.g., tinea corporis can often be mistaken for various eczematous dermatitides like nummular, atopic, and even contact dermatitis. Psoriasis, impetigo, pityriasis versicolor, and erythema annulare centrifugum are just examples of other papulosquamous conditions that can commonly be in the differential diagnosis of cutaneous fungal infections. Conversely, tinea capitis can often be mistaken for alopecia areata, trichotillomania, folliculitis, pyoderma, seborrheic dermatitis, and if extensive even scarring alopecia.

Because of the complexity and nuances in the diagnosis and management of cutaneous fungal infections, the articles and topics included in this text have been designed with the hope that clinicians will find practical pearls to better aid in the treatment of their patients.[5]

REFERENCES

1. Elewski BE, Sobera J. Fungal disease. *Dermatology.* 2008;1:1135-63.
2. Assaf RR, Weil ML. The superficial mycoses. *Dermatol Clin.* 1996;14:57-67.
3. Elewski BE, Hazen PG. The superficial mycoses and the dermatophytes. *J Am Acad Dermatol.* 1989;21:655-73.
4. Leyden JJ, Aly R. Tinea pedis. *Semin Dermatol.* 1993;12:280-4.
5. Smith EB. The treatment of dermatophytosis: safety considerations. *J Am Acad Dermatol.* 2000;43:S113-19.

World Clin Dermatol. 2016;3(1):3-13.

Classification of Fungal Infections and Fungi

*,[1]Malini R Capoor MD, [2]Poonam Puri MD

[1]Department of Microbiology, [2]Dermatology, Venerology, and Leprosy
Vardhman Mahavir Medical College and Safdarjung Hospital,
New Delhi, India

ABSTRACT

Fungal identification and interpretation of laboratory reports on fungi can be challenging and frustating because of the importance placed on the morphological characteristics of the organism. Therefore, investing time to learn the basic clinical classification, basic structures, taxonomy, mycological classification and nomenclature can result in ability to interpret the laboratory reports and identify them correctly. This article explores the same.

INTRODUCTION

There is an increase in incidence of fungal infections over the past three decades owing to increase in number of immunocompromised states. The knowledge of clinical classification, principles of taxonomy, mycological classification has important implications on patient management owing to targeted antifungal therapy after correct interpretation of laboratory report.

CLINICAL CLASSIFICATION OF FUNGAL INFECTIONS OF SKIN

The common cutaneous fungal skin infections are divided into three major subgroups:

1. Superficial fungal infections

*Corresponding author
Email: rajeevmalini@rediffmail.com

© 2016 Jaypee Brothers Medical Publishers. All rights reserved.

2. Deep fungal infections: This is further divided into subcutaneous and systemic infections
3. Opportunistic infections.

Classification of cutaneous mycoses is given in table 1.

Superficial Fungal Infections of Skin

Superficial fungal infections are caused by numerous fungi that are capable of superficially invading the epidermis, hair follicles, nail apparatus. They can be further subdivided into two types—those that induce minimal inflammatory response and those that causes substantial inflammatory response.[1]

Classification of Superficial Fungal Infections of Skin

- Those provoking significant inflammatory response
  - Dermatophytoses
  - Candidiasis
- Those not provoking significant inflammatory response
  - *Malassezia* infections
  - Tinea nigra
  - *Trichosporon* infections.

Superficial Fungal Infections Invoking Significant Inflammatory Response

1. Dermatophytoses

Dermatophytoses are a unique group of fungus that affect the nonviable keratinized stratum corneum of skin, hair, and nails[2] and include the three genera (i) *Trichophyton,* (ii) *Microsporum*, and (iii) *Epidermophyton*.[3]

Site of infection of various dermatophytes based on genera has been shown in table 2.

Dermatophytes are further divided into three species: (1) geophilic, (2) zoophilic, and (3) anthropophilic depending on their habitat (Table 3). Classification of dermatophytoses:

Table 1: Cutaneous Mycoses Classification	
Superficial	Involves stratum corneum, hair, and nails
Subcutaneous	Involves dermis and subcutaneous tissue. Often due to implantation
Systemic	Involves dermis and subcutaneous tissue. Skin involvement is usually due to extension from underlying structures or by hematogenous spread
Opportunistic	Primary or secondary lesions in immunocompromised hosts

Table 2: Site of Infection of Various Dermatophytes Based on Genera

Dermatophytes	Skin	Hair	Nails
Epidermophyton	+	-	+
Microsporum	-	+	+
Trichophyton	+	+	+

Table 3: Dermatophytes and Their Habitats

Geophilic species	Zoophilic species	Anthropophilic species
Grow in soil	Found in animals	Restricted to human host
Sporadically infect humans	Sporadically infect humans	Transmitted from one person to other
Produce marked inflammatory lesions	Produce highly inflammatory lesions	Produce mild but chronic lesions
Microsporum gypseum	*Microsporum canis, Trichophyton mentagrophytes, T. verrucosum*	*T. rubrum, T. tonsurans, T. violaceum, T. schoenleinii, E. floccosum*

1. Dermatophytoses of keratinized epidermis
    - Tinea corporis
    - Tinea cruris
    - Tinea pedis
    - Tinea faciei
    - Tinea manuum
    - Tinea incognito
2. Dermatophytoses of hair
    - Tinea capitis
    - Tinea barbae
    - Dermatophytic folliculitis
    - Majocchi's granuloma
3. Dermatophytoses of nails (onychomycosis): Onychomycosis is a term used for all fungal infections of the nail and includes those due to dermatophytes as well as nondermatophytes.

Tinea corporis is most commonly caused by *T. rubrum;* however, the inflammatory type is caused by *T. verrucosum, T. mentagrophytes, M. canis, and M. gypseum.* The most common causative agents for tinea cruris, tinea pedis, and tinea manuum are *E. floccosum, T. rubrum, and T. mentagrophytes.*[1]

A large retrospective study of tinea incognito in children showed *T. mentagrophytes* (Figure 1) was the most common organism.[3]

The four clinical types of tinea pedis are:

1. Interdigital
2. Moccasin
3. Vesicular (inflammatory)
4. Ulcerative.

The five clinical patterns of tinea capitis are:

1. Seborrheic pattern
2. Black dot pattern
3. Grey patch
4. Kerion
5. Favus.

The two types of invasion of hair in tinea capitis are (i) endothrix and (ii) ectothrix. Endothrix infections are produced by fungi which invade the hair shaft from inside and are composed of fungal arthroconidia and hyphae. The organisms causing endothrix are *T. tonsurans*, *T. violaceum*, and *T. soudanense*. Ectothrix infections are produced by fungi that primarily invade the shaft from outside and these fungi cause fluorescence. The organisms causing ectothrix are *M. audouinii* and *M. canis*.

Trichophyton tonsurans is the most common cause of tinea capitis in the United States and *M. canis* is the second most common etiology. However, studies from India by Grover et al. and Singal et al. have consistently shown *T. violaceum* and *M. audouinii* to be the most common species causing tinea capitis.[4,5]

Favus is caused by *T. schoenleinii* infection.

Majocchi's granuloma is caused by *T. rubrum* and *T. tonsurans*.

The five clinical presentations of onychomycosis are:

1. Distal subungual
2. Proximal subungual
3. Superficial white
4. Total dystrophic
5. Endonyx.

The causative organisms are commonly *T. rubrum*, *T. mentagrophytes* (Figure 1), and *E. floccosum*. The nondermatophyte molds that can cause onychomycosis are *Fusarium* spp., *Aspergillus* spp., *Acremonium* spp., *Scopulariopsis brevicaulis*, and *Scytalidium hyalinum*.

2. Candidiasis:

The various clinical presentations are:

- Cutaneous candidiasis
- Oropharyngeal candidiasis
- Genital candidiasis (vulvovaginitis and balanoposthitis)

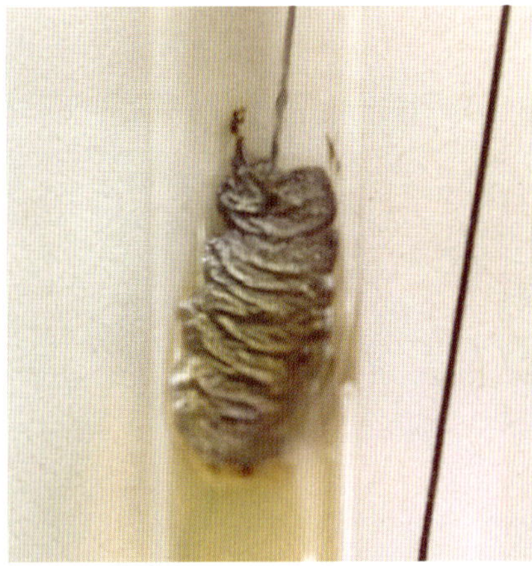

Figure 1: Thin septate hyphae and spiral hyphae of dermatophyte *Trichophyton mentagrophytes*.

- Candidial onychomycosis and paronychia
- Chronic mucocutaneous candidiasis.

Candidiasis is most commonly caused by the yeast *Candida albicans* and less often by *Candida* spp. that include *C. tropicalis*, *C. parapsilosis*, *C. krusei*, and *C. glabrata*.

Superficial Fungal Infections Not Provoking Significant Inflammatory Response

1. *Malassezia infections* are of two types:
   a. Pityriasis versicolor
   b. Pityrosporum folliculitis.
   Pityriasis versicolor is caused by *Malassezia* species. *Malassezia globosa* is the organism most frequently associated with pityriasis versicolor. The various other forms include *M. furfur* and *M. sympodialis*. *Malassezia dermatis* is specifically associated with atopic dermatitis.[6] Pityrosporum folliculitis is due to excessive growth of *M. furfur* and *M. globosa* within the hair follicle.
2. *Tinea nigra* is due to infection by *Phaeoannellomyces werneckii* which is a dematiaceous fungus.
3. *Trichosporon infections* are of three types:
   a. White piedra
   b. Black piedra
   c. Disseminated trichosporonosis.

White piedra is caused by *T. beigelii* whereas black piedra is caused by *Piedraia hortae*.

Deep Fungal Infections of Skin

Deep fungal infections are divided into two major subgroups:

1. Subcutaneous mycosis
2. Systemic mycosis.

Subcutaneous Mycosis

These are heterogeneous group of fungal infections which involve the dermis or subcutaneous tissue and develop after cutaneous inoculation at the site of trauma.

Classification of Subcutaneous Mycosis

These are subdivided into four types:

1. Mycetoma
2. Chromomycosis
3. Sporotrichosis
4. Subcutaneous phaeohyphomycosis.

Eumycetoma is caused by *M. mycetomatis, M. grisea, Pseudallescheria boydii, Phialophora jeanselmei.*

Chromomycosis is mainy caused by dematiaceous fungus such as *Fonsecaea pedrosoi* and also by *F. compacta, Phialophora verrucosa*, and *Cladosporium carrionii.*

Sporothrix schenckii, a dimorphous fungus is the etiological agent for sporotrichosis.

Several species of *Exophiala* (Figure 2), *Cladosporium*, and *Alternaria* have been recognized as agents of subcutaneous phaeohyphomycosis.

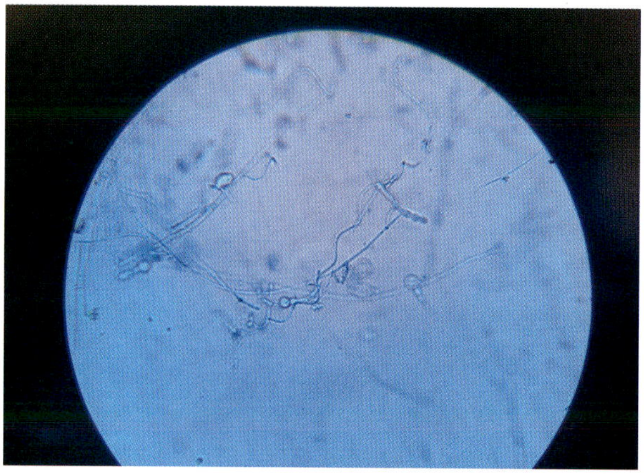

Figure 2: *Exophiala jeanselmei* (dematiaceous fungus) on Sabouraud's dextrose agar.

Systemic Fungal Infections

These are fungal infections affecting internal organs. In these infections, dissemination to skin most commonly occurs in immunocompromised individuals.

Classification of Systemic Fungal Infections[1]

These are subdivided into the following types:

- Cryptococcosis
- Histoplasmosis
- Coccidioidomycosis
- Paracoccidioidomycosis
- Penicilliosis
- Acute candidemia and disseminated candidiasis
- North American blastomycosis
- Lobomycosis
- Subcutaneous zygomycosis (Entomophthoromycosis).

Cryptococcus neoformans (serotypes A, B, C, and D) causes cryptococcosis. Serotypes A and D are designated as *C. neoformans* var. *neoformans*. Serotypes B and C are designated as *C. neoformans* var. *gattii*.

Histoplasmosis is caused by *Histoplasma capsulatum* var. *capsulatum*. In Africa, *H. capsulatum* var. *duboisii* is common.

Etiologic agent for blastomycosis is *Blastomyces dermatitidis*.

Coccidioides is the etiologic agent for coccidioidomycosis (Figure 3).

Etiologic agent for penicilliosis is *Penicillium marneffei*, a dimorphous fungus.

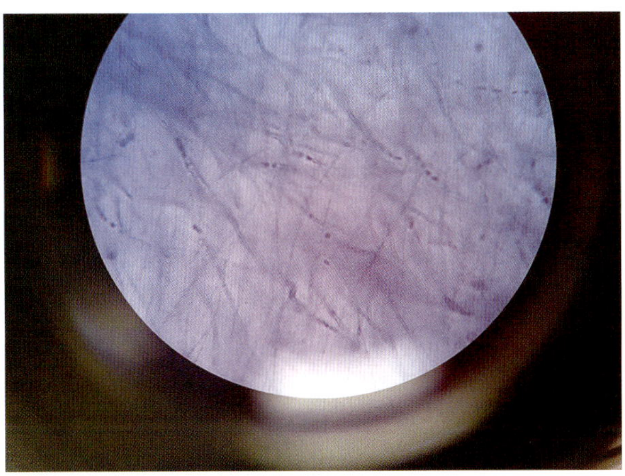

Figure 3: Arthroconidia with disjunctor cells of *Coccidioides immitis* (dimorphic fungus).

Acute candidemia and disseminated candidiasis is caused by *C. albicans* and non-*C. albicans* species.

Lobomycosis is caused by *Lacazia loboi,* whereas *Basidiobolus ranarum* causes subcutaneous zygomycosis.

Opportunistic Infections of Skin

Opportunistic infections are infections occurring in patients of primary or secondary immunodeficiencies. They include the following:

- Aspergillosis
- Mucormycosis
- Fusariosis
- Cryptococcosis.

The most common fungal infections in human immunodeficiency virus-infected patients are *Candida* and *Cryptococcus* species. The other fungal pathogens with clinical presentations are listed in table 4.

TAXONOMY OF FUNGI

The scientific names of fungi are subject to the International Code of Botanical Nomenclature (ICBN), an old convention. The rules of ICBN must be followed when proposing the name for a new fungal species. The essential requirements for valid name are that the name must be in Latin binomial form, the publication must contain a concise description of the essential and differential characteristics of the fungus in Latin and a living culture of the specimen on which the author

Table 4: Fungal Pathogens in Human Immunodeficiency Virus Infection

Organism	Clinical features
Candida albicans	Thrush, vaginal, and esophageal candidiasis
Cryptococcus neoformans	Pulmonary and disseminated disease
Histoplasma capsulatum	Disseminated disease with fever and weight loss
Coccidioides immitis	Disseminated and pulmonary disease
Blastomyces dermatitidis	Disseminated and pulmonary disease
Aspergillus fumigatus	Disseminated and pulmonary disease
Penicillium marneffei	Disseminated and pulmonary disease with fever, weight loss, and anemia
Sporotrichosis schenckii	Disseminated disease

based his original description of the species must be preserved. Many fungi have an asexual stage (or anamorph), characterized by the production of asexual conidia and a sexual stage (or teleomorph) characterized by sexual spores (ascospores and basidiospores). Mycologists give separate names to the asexual and sexual stages. The code of the teleomorph takes precedence and covers both stages, the name given to an anamorph may be used as appropriate. The anamorph stage is encountered in culture (e.g., *Blastomyces dermatitidis*) and it remains the name in some fungi, i.e., most widely recognized and used.

Taxonomy and Classification

The kingdom fungi is one of the six kingdoms of life. It has a hierarchy, each rank being named by a particular ending: phylum, -mycota; subphylum, -mycotina; class, -mycetes; order, -ales; and family, -aceae. Each family is composed of a number of genera and these are divided into species. The kingdom fungi is currently divided into seven phyla, which include the Ascomycota, Basidiomycota, Glomeromycota. The phylum Zygomycota is no longer accepted due to its polyphyletic nature. The organisms which were in the Zygomycota are now divided among the phylum Glomeromycota and four subphyla incertae sedis. The subphylum Mucoromycotina has been proposed to accommodate the Mucorales, while the subphylum Entomophthoromycotina has been created for the Entomophthorales.[7-12]

Kingdom Fungi

Subphyla Mucoromycotina and Entomophthoromycotina (Formerly Zygomycotina)

In this group of lower fungi, the thallus is aseptate and consists of wide, hyaline (colorless) branched hyphal elements. The asexual spores (termed sporangiospores) are nonmotile and are produced inside a closed sac called sporangium. Sexual reproduction leads to the formation of zygospores. The subphylum Mucoromycotina contains the order Mucorales and includes the genera *Lichtheimia (Absidia), Mucor, Rhizomucor*, and *Rhizopus*. The subphylum Entomophthorales includes the genera *Basidiobolus* and *Conidiobolus*, agents of subcutaneous mycoses.

Phylum Basidiomycota

These are a group of higher fungi have a septate, filamentous thallus, but some are typical yeasts. Sexual reproduction leads to the formation of haploid basidiospores on the outside of a generative cell known as basidium. The important members are *Cryptococcus*, *Malassezia*, *Trichosporon*, and *Schizophyllum commune* (Figure 4).

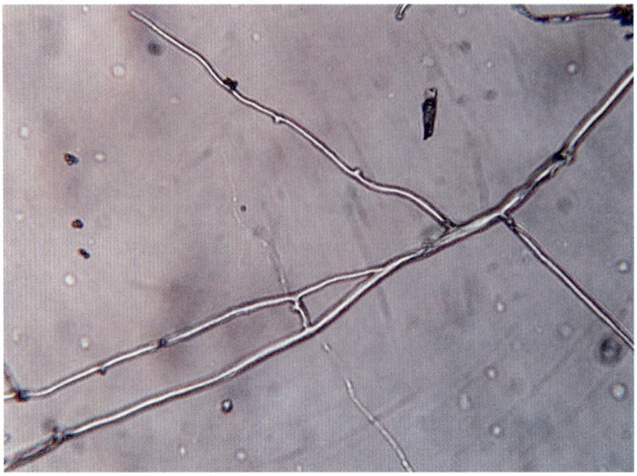

Figure 4: Hyaline hyphae of *Schizophyllum commune* (Basidiomycetes).

Phylum Ascomycota

The large phylum Ascomycota contains almost 50% of all named fungal species and accounts for around 80% of fungi of medical importance. Sexual reproduction leads to the development of haploid spores, termed ascospores, which are produced in a sac-like structures termed as ascus. The phylum Ascomycota includes four classes of medical importance: (i) the Pneumocystidomycetes (*Pneumocystis*), (ii) Saccharomycetes (anamorphic stage to *Candida* spp., *Pichia, Clavispora, Debaryomyces*, etc.), (iii) Eurotiomycetes [*Histoplasma capsulatum, Blastomyces dermatitidis* and Eurotiales (teleomorphs of *Aspergillus* and *Penicillium* and melanized fungi)], and (iv) Sordariomycetes (*Fusarium*, teleomorphs of melanized fungi).

CONCLUSION

There is a need to learn the basic clinical classification, basic structures, taxonomy, mycological classification and nomenclature as this results in better ability to interpret the laboratory reports and identify the fungi correctly. Fungal classification and identification has important implications on patient management owing to targeted antifungal therapy after the aetiological diagnosis.

Editor's Comment

The authors have written a very elaborate and detailed classification of the dermatologically significant fungi. The tables are informative and precise. The taxonomy provided in the end is quite helpful. This is a particular segment we are very ignorant about as dermatologists. Together, Dr Malini Capoor and Dr Poonam Puri, have worked as an able team of a microbiologist and dermatologist to provide a very useful article.

Rashmi Sarkar, Seemal R Desai

REFERENCES

1. Elewski BE, Hughey LC, Sobera JO, Hay R. Fungal diseases. In: Bolognia JL, Jorizzo JL, Schaffer JV, editors. Dermatology. 3rd ed. Philadelphia: Elsevier Saunders; 2012. pp. 1251-84.
2. Weitzman I, Summerbell RC. The dermatophytes. *Clin Microbiol Rev.* 1995;8:240-59.
3. Moriarty B, Hay R, Morris-Jones R. Diagnosis and management of tinea. *BMJ.* 2012;344:e4380.
4. Grover C, Arora P, Manchanda V. Tinea capitis in the pediatric population: a study from North India. *Indian J Dermatol Venereol Leprol.* 2010;76(5):527-32.
5. Singal A, Rawat S, Bhattacharya SN, Mohanty S, Baruah MC. Clinico-myocological profile of tinea capitis in North India and response to griseofulvin. *J Dermatol.* 2001;28(1):22-6.
6. Prohic A, Ozegovie L. Malassezia species isolated from lesional and non-lesional skin in patients with pityriasis versicolor. *Mycoses.* 2007;50:58-63.
7. Brandt M, Warnock D. Taxonomy and classification of fungi. In: Jorgensen J, Pfaller M, Carroll K, Funke G, Landry M, Richter S, Warnock D, editors. Manual of Clinical Microbiology. 11th ed. Washington, DC: ASM Press; 2015. pp. 1935-43.
8. Buckley M. (2008). The Fungal Kingdom: diverse and essential roles in earth's ecosystem. American Academy of Microbiology, Washington, DC. [online] Available from: http://academy.asm.org/images/stories/documents/fungalkingdom.pdf. [Accessed December, 2016].
9. Guarro J, Gené J, Stchigel AM. Developments in fungal taxonomy. *Clin Microbiol Rev.* 1999;12:454-500.
10. Hawksworth DL. A new dawn for the naming of fungi: impacts of the decisions made in Melbourne in July 2011 on the future publication and regulation of fungal names. *IMA Fungus.* 2011;2(2):155-62.
11. Hibbett DS, Binder M, Bischoff JF, Blackwell M, Cannon PF, Eriksson OE, et al. A higher-level phylogenetic classification of the fungi. *Mycol Res.* 2007;111:509-47.
12. Adl SM, Simpson AG, Lane CE, Lukes J, Bass D, Bowser SS, et al. The revised classification of eukaryotes. *J Eukaryot Microbiol.* 2012;59:429-93.

World Clin Dermatol. 2016;3(1):14-40.

Superficial Fungal Infections: Dermatophytes

*,[1]Sumit Sethi MD DNB, [2]Surabhi Sinha MD DNB

[1]Consultant, Genesis Centre for Dermatology,
Skin Allure Aesthetic Clinic
New Delhi, India
[2]Department of Dermatology and Leprosy, Dr Ram Manohar Lohia Hospital
and Post Graduate Institute of Medical Education and Research
New Delhi, India

ABSTRACT

Dermatophytes are multicellular filaments (hyphae) which reproduce by the formation of spores while yeasts are unicellular and multiply by budding. They include three genera of fungi that have the unique ability to invade and multiply within keratinized tissue (hair, skin and nails) namely *Microsporum, Trichophyton* and Epidermophyton. The infection that results from these dermatophytes is known as Tinea. The location of the tinea on cutaneous surface defines the disease e.g., Tinea pedis (feet), T. mannum (hands), T. corporis (body), T. cruris (inguinal folds), T. capitis (scalp), T. barbae (beard) and T. faciei (face). T. pedis is the most common variant in developed nations while T. corporis and T. capitis is more common in developing countries.

INTRODUCTION

Superficial fungal infections arise from a pathogen that is restricted to the stratum corneum, hair, or nails with or without tissue reaction. They are further subdivided into those that induce minimal cutaneous inflammation (piedras and pityriasis versicolor), and those that lead to more substantial inflammation (dermatophytes and candidiasis). Dermatophytes are classified according to the genera (*Trichophyton, Microsporum, Epidermophyton*), the ecology (anthropophilic, geophilic, or zoophilic), and site of involvement (e.g., tinea pedis, tinea corporis).

*Corresponding author
Email: sethi1587@gmail.com

© 2016 Jaypee Brothers Medical Publishers. All rights reserved.

They have the unique ability to invade and multiply within keratinized tissue (hair, skin, and nails). In naming clinical infections due to dermatophytes, "tinea" precedes the Latin name for the involved body site. Dermatophytic infections have names starting from generic term "tinea" followed by a qualifying term that denotes the location of infection. The only exception is "tinea versicolor", which was a misnomer as it is not caused by a dermatophytic infection and is now called pityriasis versicolor.[1-4]

EPIDEMIOLOGY

Dermatophyte infections are common at all ages, in both sexes, and they have a worldwide distribution. Increased incidence is seen in postpubertal hosts, exception is tinea capitis (dermatophytosis of the scalp), which occurs primarily in children. Tinea pedis, tinea cruris, and tinea unguium are more common in men than women. Socioeconomic status, occupation, and the use of footwear are important epidemiologic factors that determine prevalence.[5,6]

ETIOPATHOGENESIS

The transmission of infection is through arthrospores shed by the infected host in skin scales and transferred by human to human, soil to human, or animal to human contact. Occupational and recreational exposure, occlusive clothing, warm humid climate, immunosuppression, and contact with contaminated materials predispose to infection. Most common predisposing factor in adults is excessive perspiration contributed by occlusive clothing which provides an environment for the dermatophytes to thrive. Individuals participating in contact sports, such as football, wrestling, or rugby, are at increased risk of acquiring a tinea infection. Autoinoculation by dermatophytes elsewhere in the body, especially the foot or groin, is also causative.

Free fatty acids, transferring globulins, and surface moisture are all local factors that can determine host susceptibility and whether infection will take place. The epidermal immune response to infection is via Langerhans cells and increased cell proliferation, seen clinically as scaling, to get the skin rid of dermatophytes.[3,4,7]

CLINICAL FEATURES

Tinea Pedis

Introduction

Synonyms: Ringworm of the foot athlete's foot.

Tinea pedis also known as athlete's foot affects 10% of the world population at any given time. It is more prevalent among men than women, and uncommon in children. The lateral toes are most often affected, particularly in the web space between the fourth and fifth toes.

Etiopathogenesis

Trichophyton rubrum is the most common causal organism of tinea pedis; however, *Trichophyton mentagrophytes* and *Epidermophyton floccosum* are also frequent causes of infection. Contact with infected people, animals, or fomites: living in a warm or moist climate, occlusive footwear, excessive sweating, community showers or swimming pools, poor foot hygiene, and health conditions or medications that suppress the immune system are sources of fungal transmission.

Clinical Features

Dermatophyte infection of the soles and interdigital web spaces of the feet is termed tinea pedis. Involvement of the dorsal aspect of the foot is considered tinea corporis. Four distinct clinical presentations have been described: (i) chronic interdigital, (ii) inflammatory (vesicular), (iii) chronic scaly hyperkeratotic (moccasin), and (iv) ulcerative.

Interdigital Tinea Pedis

Interdigital toe web infections are a result of complex interplay between dermatophytes, bacteria, and, rarely, *Candida* species. There are two variants (i) dermatophytosis simplex—uncomplicated fungal infection associated with scaling, fissuring and (ii) dermatophytosis complex, a highly macerated, often malodorous leukokeratotic symptomatic process caused by an overgrowth of a variety of bacterial species. The causative fungal species include *T. rubrum* and *T. mentagrophytes* and the bacterial species include *Staphylococcus aureus*, *Micrococcus sedantarius*, *Brevibacterium epidermidis*, *Corynebacterium minutissimum*, and Gram-negative species like *Pseudomonas* and *Proteus*.

Plantar Moccasin-type Infection

Mocassin foot can present as a chronic mild dry, hyperkeratotic presentation or the moderate to severe variant with cracked and inflamed skin, erythema, and odor, and in some instances progress to onychomycosis. The scales are silvery fine and more prominent on the creases of the foot with underlying pink to red skin. Many patients have an atopic history and nail involvement is common. In some

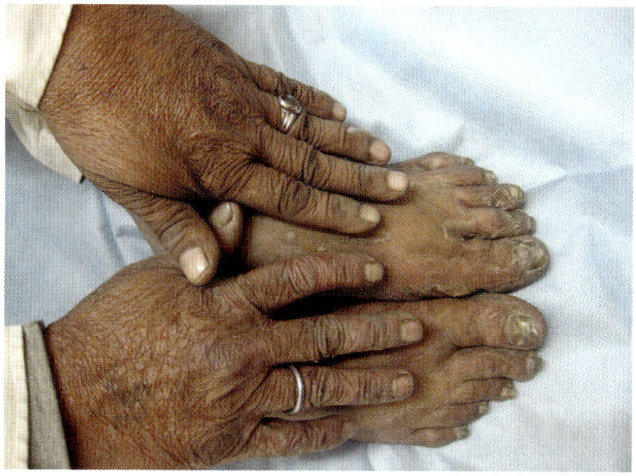

Figure 1: One hand two feet distribution: Erythema and scaling of the dorsum of bilateral feet and right hand associated with distal/ lateral subungual onychomycosis, typical of *T. rubrum* infection.

instances, the individual may exhibit the "two foot one hand" pattern, with the hand that is used to scratch being the one more commonly involved (Figure 1). The fungal organisms that cause tinea pedis may also be responsible for tinea manuum, with *T. rubrum* being the most frequent etiologic agent. When tinea manuum is present, it is prudent to observe for tinea pedis; however, most individuals with tinea pedis do not have tinea manuum.

Vesiculobullous Tinea Pedis

Vesicobullous tinea pedis is the least common form commonly caused by *T. mentagrophytes*. It starts with the development of small, isolated vesicles filled with clear fluid particularly on the arch and side of the foot. The vesicular reaction is a result of T cell-mediated hypersensitivity against the fungal antigen. Patients with recurrent episodes often have low grade scaling between bouts of acute inflammation. If infection is allowed to progress, the vesicles may coalesce into large, acute, pruritic, spreading, ulcerative lesions which may become secondarily infected. Complications such as cellulitis, lymphangitis, lymphadenopathy, and fever may result.

Differential Diagnosis

Contact dermatitis, atopic dermatitis psoriasis, erythrasma, juvenile plantar dermatosis, or a bacterial infection.

Management

General Measures

Compresses and topical steroids in conjunction with antifungal agents are used with acute attacks. Acute episodes especially interdigital can be treated with open wet compresses (Burrow's solution 1:80) or potassium permanganate (1:4,000), aluminum chloride, Castellani's paint, and Gentian violet. Keeping the feet dry wearing cotton socks and use of lightweight-ventilated footwear will help prevent relapses and can be achieved with open footwear or absorbent socks/antifungal foot powder. Tinea pedis can cause pompholyx of the hands and the feet should always be examined when a patient presents with pompholyx.

Course and Prognosis

Tinea pedis is difficult to treat and tends to be chronic and prone to recurrence in hot weather or with exercise. Macerated skin may get secondarily infected leading to lymphangitis or cellulitis.[1-4,7-10]

Tinea Manuum

Introduction

Tinea manuum is a chronic dermatophytosis of the hand(s), mostly unilateral, and commonly involving the dominant hand.

Etiopathogenesis

Tinea manuum is almost invariably associated with preexisting tinea pedis or tinea unguium.

T. rubrum, T. mentagrophytes, and E. floccosum, the organisms responsible for tinea pedis, also cause tinea of the hands.

Clinical Features

Tinea manuum is similar to tinea pedis but less common and interdigital form is not seen. Tinea of the dorsal aspect of the hand exhibits a classical ringworm appearance while palmer involvement has the appearance of dry, diffuse, hyperkeratotis with fine white scales, emphasizing the normal lines of the hand (Figure 2). The dry keratotic form can be asymptomatic and is often attributed by patients to hard physical labor rather than infection. The asymmetric pattern of involvement involving 1 foot and 2 hands or 2 feet and 1 hand, referred to as "one hand-two feet syndrome" is typical for tinea. The hand that is used to scratch the foot with the rash is typically affected.

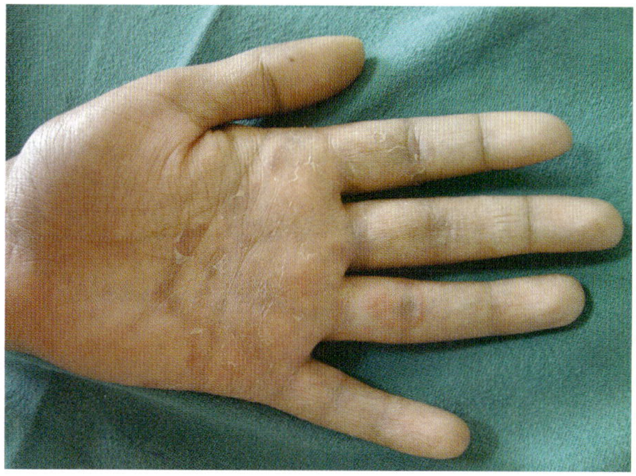

Figure 2: Tinea manum: A well defined annular plaque with erythema and scaling on ventral surface of left hand. *Courtesy:* Dr Shankila Mittal, Junior resident, Dermatology, Maulana Azad Medical College.

Differential Diagnosis

Contact dermatitis, palmar psoriasis, dyshidrosis, or dryness of the hand. Always consider tinea in cases of unilateral "hand dermatitis" and if a patient's eczema is not responding to steroids.

Course and Prognosis

Like tinea pedis, it tends to have a chronic and relapsing course.[1,3,4,7,10]

Tinea Corporis

Synonyms: Ringworm, tinea glabrosa, and tinea circinata.

Introduction

Tinea corporis, ringworm of the body, includes dermatophyte infection of the trunk and extremities excluding scalp, face, nails, groins, beard, hands, and feet.

Epidemiology

It has a worldwide distribution but is more commonly found in hot, humid tropical climates. It occurs both in children and adults, with equal sex distribution.

Etiopathogenesis

T. rubrum, *T. mentagrophytes*, and *M. canis* are frequently responsible for this form of tinea. *Trichophyton tonsurans* is the main culprit of tinea corporis in wrestlers and in family member of children with tinea capitis. The transmission of infection is through arthrospores shed by the infected host in skin scales and transferred by human to human, soil to human, or animal to human contact. Occupational and recreational exposure, immunosuppression, obesity, diabetes, stress, and contact with contaminated clothing predispose to infection.

Clinical Features

One to three weeks after inoculation, the infection spreads centrifugally resulting in annular scaly plaques of various shapes and sizes with pustules at the active border (Figure 3). Lesions start as erythematous flat, scaly spots and then develop a raised border that expands slowly in all directions with healing in the center, giving the classical "ring-like" appearance. The symptoms, extent of inflammation and response to treatment depend on the causative organism and the immune response of the host (Table 1). The lesions may self-resolve or multiple lesions may coalesce together to involve large areas of body. Systemic involvement is not seen.

Differential Diagnosis

Impetigo, nummular eczema, pityriasis rosea, annular erythemas, psoriasis, contact dermatitis, seborrhea, granuloma annulare, or subacute cutaneous lupus erythematosus.

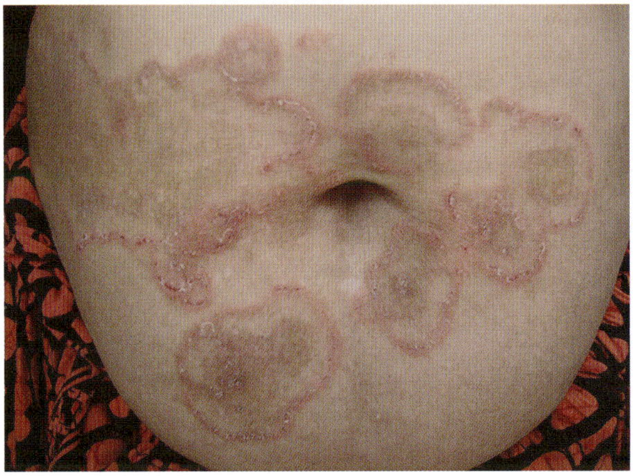

Figure 3: Tinea corporis: Multiple sharply marginated erythematous annular plaques on trunk with active margins and pigmentation in the centre. *Courtesy:* Dr Shankila Mittal, Junior resident, Dermatology, Maulana Azad Medical College.

Table 1: Clinical Variants of Tinea Corporis

Type	Organism	Clinical features
Tinea profunda	*T. verrucosum*	An intense inflammatory reaction against zoophilic fungi can result in large pustular lesions or a kerion with a red, boggy, pustular surface. The follicular pustules represent the deep invasion of organism into hair follicle
Majocchi's granuloma (dermatophytic granuloma)	*T. rubrum*	Women with tinea pedis or onychomycosis who shave their legs, get perifollicular papulopustules or granulamatous nodules. This dermatophytic folliculitis represents a foreign body granulomatous reaction in response to fungal elements in dermis after follicle rupture
Tinea imbricate	*T. concentricum*	Plaque with erythematous concentric annular rings
Bullous tinea corporis	*T. rubrum*	Intense inflammatory response causes vesicles at the margins

Management

General Measures

Excessive heat and moisture promote the spread of tinea so patients should be advised to wear loose fitting cotton clothes. Discouraging close contact with infected individuals and avoiding sharing of fomites (clothing, towel, and combs) may help in reducing infection. Affected members of the household should be treated simultaneously. It is recommended to continue the topical medication for 1 more week after clinical clearing to ensure clinical cure.

Course and Prognosis

The prognosis for localized tinea corporis is excellent after correct diagnosis and treatment; however, recurrences are common. Hair follicles serve as reservoirs of infection especially *T. rubrum* and thus, areas of body with more hair follicles are resistant to treatment.[1-4,7,10-15]

Tinea Cruris

Introduction

Synonyms: Jock itch, gym itch, ringworm of the groin eczema marginatum.

Tinea cruris (or "jock itch") is an extremely pruritic infection of the groin and surrounding pubic area, perineal, and perianal skin. The promoting factor is the presence of a warm, moist environment.

Epidemiology

It is the second most common dermatophytosis in the world after tinea pedis. It is common in men than women and in adults more than children.

Etiopathogenesis

Heat, humidity, excessive perspiration, obesity, and wet clothing (tight occlusive clothes, exercise outfits, bathing suits) predispose to this infection. The common causative organisms are *T. rubrum*, *T. mentagrophytes*, and *E. floccosum*. Most cases of tinea cruris are due to autoinfection from tinea of the foot which typically precedes the groin infection. The arthrospores spread when underclothes are dragged over the infected feet up to the groin area.

Clinical Features

Tinea cruris is the dermatophytic infection involving the inguinal region with extension to surrounding area. The eruption starts from crural fold, is unilateral and asymmetrical in beginning, with a well-defined leading edge. A half-moon shaped plaque forms in the crural fold region, and the border advances out extending to the thighs, buttocks, and gluteal cleft area (Figure 4). The skin inside the border may display clearing or turns red-brown, as a manifestation of immune response of the host against the infecting organism. Older lesions can have a leathery, lichenified appearance. In contrast to candidal infection of the groin; the scrotum and penis are not involved.

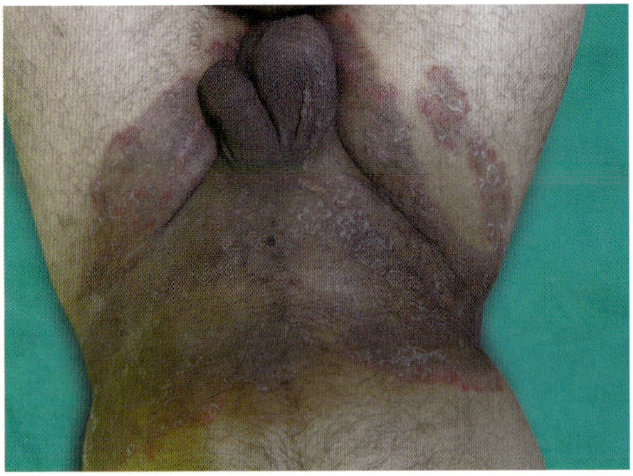

Figure 4: Tinea cruris: Confluent, erythematous, scaling plaques involving the medial thighs, inguinal folds, and pubic area extending to anterior abdomen.

Differential Diagnosis

Candidiasis, erythrasma, intertrigo, inverse psoriasis, seborrheic dermatitis, contact dermatitis.

Complication

Secondary infection by *Candida* or bacteria, chronic fungal infection may cause lichenification of the area.

Management

General Measures

Measures to prevent tinea cruris include weight reduction (if obese), wearing less occlusive clothing, drying thoroughly after bathing, using topical antifungal powders, laundering contaminated clothing, and treating concomitant onychomycosis or tinea pedis if present. To prevent autoinoculation, socks should be put on before underwear to avoid transfer of fungal elements from the floor or infected feet up to their groin area.

Course and Prognosis

Prognosis is excellent with correct diagnosis and treatment. Recurrence is common. Chronic fungal infection with associated pruritus results in lichenification of crural area. Secondary bacterial or *Candida* infection or even contact dermatitis may develop due to topically applied medication including steroids.[1-4,7,10,12-15]

Tinea Unguium (Tinea of the Nails)

Synonyms: Ringworm of the nail and dermatophytic onychomycosis.

Introduction

Onychomycosis (fungal infection of the nail) is the most common nail disease, representing up to half of all onychopathies. It is referred to as tinea unguium when caused by a dermatophytic pathogen.

Epidemiology

It has a worldwide distribution and is more prevalent in urban than in rural areas (associated with wearing occlusive footwear). It is more common in men and incidence increases with advancing age.

Etiology

Dermatophytes are the causative agents in more than 90% of all cases of onychomycosis, while yeasts (*Candida* spp.) and other nondermatophyte molds are recovered as primary pathogens much less frequently. Tinea unguium is most often caused by *T. rubrum, T. mentagrophytes,* or *E. floccosum,* similar to agents of tinea pedis.

- Distal and lateral subungual onychomycosis: *T. rubrum, T. mentagrophytes*
- Proximal subungual onychomycosis: *T. rubrum*
- Superficial white onychomycosis: *T. mentagrophytes.*

Pathophysiology

Predisposing host factors include atopic dermatitis, human immunodeficiency virus (HIV), diabetes, and occlusive footwear. Defective vascular supply leads to increased probability of nail invasion by fungi (i.e., with increasing age, chronic venous insufficiency, peripheral arterial disease), in post-traumatic states (lower leg fractures), or disturbance of innervation (e.g., injury to brachial plexus trauma of spine). Increased propensity of first and fifth toenails probably occurs secondary to damage to these nails by footwear. Infection of toenails is more common than fingernails due to their slow growth.

Clinical Features

The onset is slow and insidious. The characteristic yellow-white thickening and crumbling of the nail is caused by a proliferative response of the stratum corneum under the nail plate in response to fungal infection. This subungual hyperkeratosis results in separation of the nail from the bed, and thickening of the nail results. Usually, a few nails are infected, toenails more commonly than fingernails. There is no paronychia as seen in infections due to *Candida.*

Classification by Anatomic Site Involved

Distal and Lateral Subungual Onychomycosis

Fungal invasion begins in stratum corneum of hyponychial area, extending subungually, and progressively involves the nail. Nail bed produces soft keratin in response to infection that accumulates subungually, raising the nail plate and altering the color of nail from transparent to creamy-yellow (Figure 5). Matrix and dense keratin of nail is usually not involved, and normal production of nail plate remains unimpaired. With progressive infection and subungual accumulation of hyperkeratotic debris, the nail becomes raised, opaque, thickened cracked, and friable.

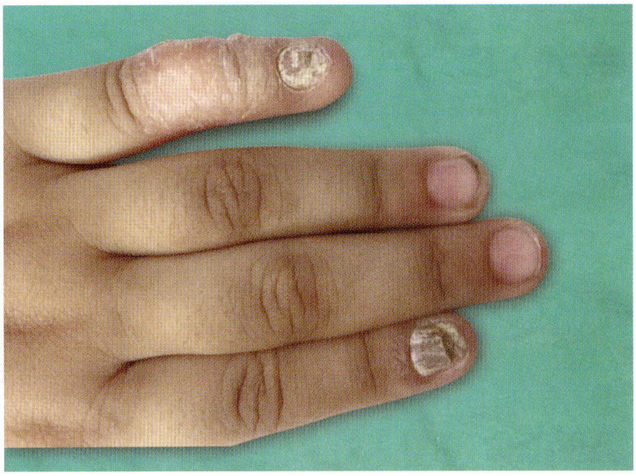

Figure 5: Distal lateral subungual onychomycois: Distal subungual hyperkeratosis and onycholysis involving most of the nail bed of index and little finger of left hand. Nail plate discolouration and thickening is also seen.

Superficial White Onychomycosis

A white chalky plaque is seen on the proximal nail plate, which may become eroded with loss of the nail plate. The organism directly invades the dorsal nail plate.

Proximal Subungual Onychomycosis

Fungal organism enters from proximal nail fold-cuticle area and then progresses to involve the matrix and finally the whole nail plate (Figure 6). It occurs commonly in persons with HIV disease or other immunocompromised states.

Secondary Tinea Unguium

Superinfection occurs in already diseased nail apparatus, such as psoriatic or traumatized nail. Tinea of the toenail usually follows tinea pedis and fingernail involvement is usually associated with tinea manuum, tinea corporis, or tinea capitis.

Differential Diagnosis

Nail psoriasis, eczema, chronic onycholysis, lichen planus, Reiter's syndrome, chronic paronychia, traumatic or chemical injury to nail, onychogryphosis, aging, pincer nails, and congenital nail dystrophies all may cause nail changes.

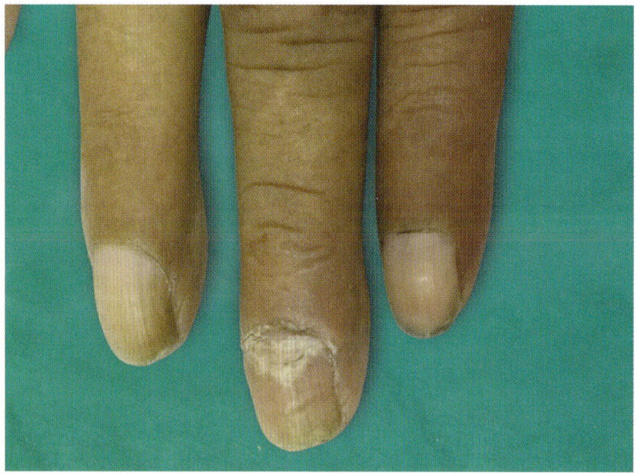

Figure 6: Proximal sunungual onychomycosis: Chalky white discolouration of proximal nail plate due to invasion from the undersurface of the nail matrix.

Complications

Bacterial superinfection, ulceration, cellulitis, osteomyelitis, necrosis, and amputation.

Management

General Measures

Discard old shoes, wear proper footwear, cotton socks, absorbent powders on feet, and weekly debridement of nails may be helpful. Benzoyl peroxide soap should be used for washing feet when bathing.

Indications for Topical Therapy

Indications for topical monotherapy include:

- Involvement limited to distal 50% of nail plate, 3 or 4 nails involvement
- No matrix area involvement
- Superficial white onychomycosis
- In children with thin and fast growing nails
- As prophylaxis after treatment in patients at risk of recurrence
- Patients where oral therapy cannot be given.

Indications for Systemic Therapy

Indications for systemic therapy include:

- Involvement of more than 50% of distal nail plate/multiple nail involvement more than 4 nails
- Involvement of nail matrix
- Topical drug penetration is expected to be suboptimal, e.g., dermatophytoma formation, very thick nail plate.[16]

Course and Prognosis

Without effective therapy, onychomycosis does not resolve spontaneously; progressive involvement of multiple toenails is the rule. Mycologic cultures may be positive without any clinically apparent disease. Prognosis is better in younger, healthier individuals than in older individuals with more extensive involvement and associated comorbidities. Causes of relapse/reinfection uncertain: reinfection, immunologic incompetence, persistent trauma, unknown causes.[1,2,7,16-19]

Tinea Capitis

Synonyms: Ringworm of the scalp/hair, tinea tonsurans, and herpes tonsurans.

Introduction

Tinea capitis (scalp ringworm) is a common childhood infection of the scalp caused by dermatophytes; the predominant age range affected is between 3 and 7 years of age.

Epidemiology

The epidemiology of tinea capitis varies throughout the world and high prevalence is associated with poor hygiene, overcrowding, and low socioeconomic standards (Table 2). Tinea capitis is common in children; adults are protected by their sebaceous secretion, which is fungistatic.

Table 2: Changing Epidemiology of Tinea Capitis after Introduction of Griseofulvin

Predominant etiologic agents of tinea capitis	Western and Mediterranean Europe	Eastern Europe	United States
Late 19th and early 20th centuries	*M. audouinii* and *M. canis*	T. schoenleinii	*M. audouinii* and *M. canis*
Current	*T. tonsurans*	*T. violaceum*	*T. tonsurans*

Etiopathogenesis

The six species which are most frequently encountered in tinea capitis are *M. canis, M. gypseum*, *T. tonsurans*, *T. mentagrophytes*, *T. violaceum*, and *T. verrucosum*. *E. floccosum* and *T. concentricum* are the two species that never invade scalp hair.

Clinical Features

Its clinical manifestations range from mild scaling with little hair loss to large inflammatory and pustular plaques with extensive alopecia (Table 3). Cervical or occipital adenopathy is almost always associated with tinea capitis. Despite being the most prevalent dermatophytic infection worldwide, tinea capitis due to *T. rubrum* is uncommon.

Differential Diagnosis

Atopic dermatitis, alopecia areata, psoriasis, bacterial infection, trichotillomania, Langerhans' cell histiocytosis, pityriasis amiantacea, and seborrheic dermatitis. Kerion should be differentiated from a boil or carbuncle. These bacterial infections are painful and tender, and will not have hair loss.

Complications

Tinea corporis, bacterial pyoderma, "Id" reaction, lymphadenitis, scarring alopecia, secondary bacterial infection.

Asymptomatic Carrier State

Asymptomatic carrier is a person with no signs or symptoms of tinea capitis but from whom positive scalp cultures are obtained. The anthropophilic organisms, *T. tonsurans* or *T. violaceum* have high rates of asymptomatic carriage. Clinically, they produce a seborrheic dermatitis-like tinea capitis with only a mild or absent host inflammatory response. Asymptomatic family members should be evaluated, particularly in cases of persistent or recurrent infection, because of high carrier rates in adult family members.[1-3,7,13-15,20-23]

Tinea Barbae

Synonyms: Ringworm of the beard and barber's itch.

Introduction

Tinea barbae is a dermatophytic trichomycosis involving the bearded areas of the face and neck, with invasion of the hair shaft.

Table 3: Characteristics Type and Features of Tinea Capitis

Morphological pattern clinical presentation	Predominant species	Microscopic examination/types of hair invasion	Pathophysiology	Wood's light
Noninflammatory—epidemic tinea capitis/gray patch: Scaly areas with or without hair loss with hair shafts breaking 2–3 mm or more above the scalp level (Figure 7)	*M. audouinii* or *M. ferrugineum* Seborrheic variant commonly due to *T. tonsurans*	Ectothrix hair colonization, with dermatophytic arthroconidia both within and surrounding the hair shaft giving the appearance of a sheath	Hyphae invade the hair shaft at mid follicle, then grow out of the follicle destroying the hair cuticle and cover the hair surface	Bright green fluorescence under filtered ultraviolet or Wood's light in ectothrix caused by microsporum species
Noninflammatory—"Black dot" tinea capitis: Hairs often break at scalp level leaving swollen hair stubs within the follicles (Figure 8)	*T. tonsurans, T. violaceum, T. soudanese*	Endothrix colonization, hyphae within the hair are converted to arthroconidia (spores)	Hyphae grow down the hair follicle and then penetrate the hair shaft. The cuticle surface of the hair remains intact	Nonfluorescent under Wood's light
Infammatory tinea capitis/kerion: painful and boggy swelling, manifests as a confluent oozing mass with pustules, loose hair, sinus tracts, and discharge of pus Fever and lymphadenopathy may be associated (Figure 9)	*M. canis* or *M. gypseum.*, *T. verrucosum*	Ectothrix colonization of the hair shaft	Microscopy may be negative due to intense delayed type hypersensitivity to fungal organism	Fluorescence may be seen when kerion is due to microsporum species, but is often negative because the inflammation obscures the presence of the fungus
Favus: yellow, cup-shaped keratotic crusts around the hair shafts called scutula	*T. schoenleinii*	*Favic*	Hyphae are produced parallel to the long axis of hair shaft and when they degenerate air spaces are left behind	Dull green fluorescence under wood's light

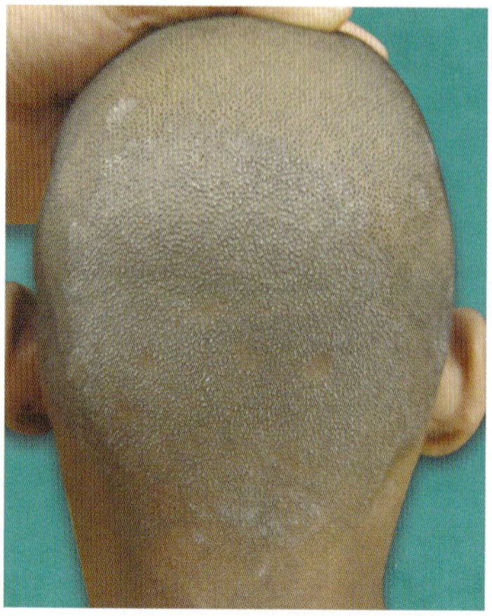

Figure 7: Grey patch tinea capitis: A well defined scaly plaque due to fungal hyphae and spores surrounding broken off hair shafts. Some areas of alopecia are also seen between the patch.

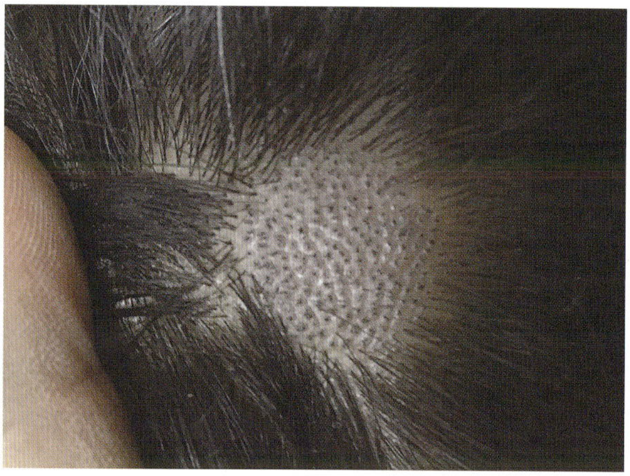

Figure 8: 'Black dot' tinea capitis: Asymptomatic patch of alopecia with broken off hairs at the scalp surface.

Epidemiology

Tinea barbae occurs almost exclusively in older adolescent and adult males. It was initially acquired by contaminated barber's razors; however, with the increased use of disinfectants and disposable razors, the infection from this source has greatly decreased. Nowadays, it is more commonly contacted from animals, is more common in farmers or ranchers and those with infected pets in household.

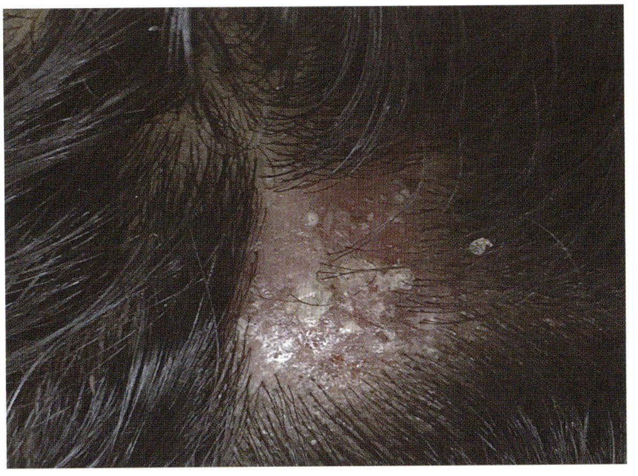

Figure 9: Kerion: Erythematous boggy swelling on scalp of child with pus discharge and easily dislodged hairs.

Etiopathogenesis

The causative organisms are typically zoophilic dermatophytes, namely *T. mentagrophytes* var. *mentagrophytes* and *T. verrucosum* contracted through occupational exposure to animals. *T. rubrum* can occasionally cause tinea barbae.

Clinical Features

Tinea barbae is classically unilateral and involves the beard area more commonly than the moustache or upper lip. Three clinical forms are recognized (Table 4).

Table 4: Clinical Types of Tinea Barbae

Clinical type	Organism	Clinical features
Deep inflammatory	Zoophilic organisms like *T. mentagrophytes* var. *mentagrophytes* and *T. verrucosum*	The clinical presentation is severe with intense inflammation and multiple follicular pustules resembling kerion (Figure 10). Hairs are loose or broken, and depilation is easy and painless. Constitutional symptoms such as malaise, fever, and lymphadenopathy may be present; scarring alopecia may develop
Superficial	Anthropophilic, *T. violaceum*	Resembles bacterial folliculitis with mild diffuse erythema with perifollicular papules and pustules, often with exudation and crusting
Circinate	*T. rubrum*	Dry scaly erythematous lesions with active border and central clearing resembling tinea corporis. Hairs are usually spared

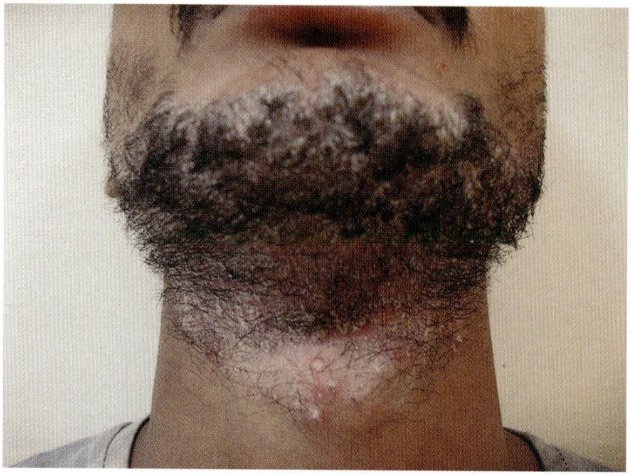

Figure 10: Tinea barbae: Erythematous plaque on the beard area of adolescent with follicular pustules and scarring hair loss. *Courtesy:* Dr Shankila Mittal, Junior resident, Dermatology, Maulana Azad Medical College.

Differential Diagnosis

Bacterial folliculitis, viral infections (herpes simplex or zoster), acne vulgaris, rosacea, cervicofacial actinomycosis, and a dental sinus tract.

Management

General Measures

Diagnosis of tinea barbae requires suspicion based on appropriate exposure. Pets should be examined for any focus of fungal infection. Treatment should be taken for tinea pedis or onychomycosis.

Course and Prognosis

Spontaneous resolution may occur in inflammatory variant if all of the infected hairs fall out; however, if untreated, scarring alopecia may result. Noninflammatory lesions are more likely to be chronic and may not resolve spontaneously. In superficial chronic tinea barbae, alopecia may occur in the center of the lesions; however, this is not common.[1,3,13-15,23]

Tinea Faciei

Introduction

Tinea faciei is dermatophytosis of the glabrous facial skin, presenting with both inflammatory and noninflammatory lesions.

Epidemiology

Tinea faciei occurs worldwide. It is more common in females than males and in children than adults.

Etiopathogenesis

It is more common in children, sometimes associated autoinoculation from tinea capitis or spread from their parents. Animal exposure and topical application of steroids and tinea at other site in body are predisposing factors. *T. tonsurans, T. mentagrophytes,* and *T. rubrum* are commonly involved organisms.

Clinical Features

Tinea faciei is the most commonly misdiagnosed type of cutaneous dermatophytic infection. Lesions may be well circumscribed, variable sized, macules, or plaques, with active elevated margins and central regression, resembling corporis variant (Figure 11). Lesions are almost always pruritic, and may be sometimes associated with photosensitivity. Any area of face may be involved but usually not symmetric. The most commonly involved locations are the cheeks, followed by the nose, periorbital area, chin, and forehead. Atypical presentation may also occur with asymptomatic lesions and minimal scaling. Anthropophilic species may present with less inflammatory and produce larger facial patches, while zoophilic fungi produce more inflammatory and have smaller patches. The atypical clinical features and incognito presentations separate this entity from tinea corporis.

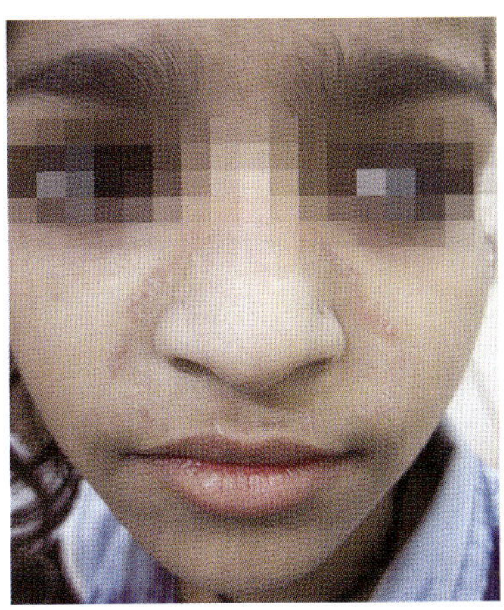

Figure 11: Tinea faciei: Erythematous sharply marginated annular plaque on face with mild scaling.

Differential Diagnosis

Cutaneous lupus erythematosis, seborrheic dermatitis, rosacea, contact dermatitis, or polymorphous light eruption.

Course and Prognosis

Prognosis if good after correct diagnosis and appropriate treatment.[1,4,10,13-15,24]

Tinea Incognito

Epidermal dermatophyte infection altered (masked or exacerbated) by application of steroids is known as tinea incognito. Topical steroids available over the counter are a commonly abused household therapy for many cutaneous infections. Lesions can be asymptomatic with absence of inflammation and scaling or very pruritic and painful associated with dermatophytic folliculitis (Figure 12). The typical annular pattern is usually absent; masked lesions may present as diffuse erythema, or diffuse scaling, without a well defined margins although an expanding border may still be present. Steroid application may also lead to exaggerated features of epidermal dermatophytoses with deep red/violaceous follicular papules or pustules. Epidermal atrophy caused by chronic application of glucocorticoid is seen on surrounding skin. Always rule out a dermatophyte infection if a patient's eczema is not responding to steroids.[1,3,13-15]

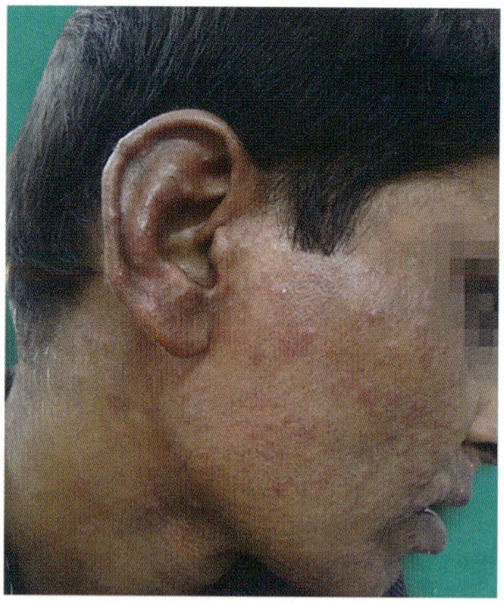

Figure 12: Tinea incognito: Erythematous plaque on right side of face with well defined lower margin on neck and follicular papules on face. The upper margin is not defined as the lesion has been modified by application of local steroids.

Tinea Indecisiva

Long-term alternating use of antifungals with topical steroids may produce a clinical picture mimicking the classical lesions of tinea imbricata caued by *T. concentricum*. The rash of tinea indecisiva consists of widespread annular concentric erythematous rings produced as a result of cyclical immunosuppression produced by topical corticosteroids followed by reinfection due to early discontinuation of topical antifungals.[25]

Recalcitrant and Recurrent Tinea Infection

Refractory and recalcitrant dermatophyte infections may occur in immunologically intact individuals. They are often caused due to *T. rubrurn* invading beyond the stratum corneum into the follicles, resulting in chronic inflammatory lesions. Once this organism becomes established, it tends to spread and become chronic with a recurrence rate of 60 to 70% after initial clearance. Recurrence is more common than re-infection in chronic dermatophytic infection and is primarily due to under-treatment because patients frequently stop treatment when their symptoms improve. Prolonged therapy with systemic and topical agents for 2 to 3 months or longer is required to cure infection.[7,26]

Dermatophytid

Widespread dermatophytid (Id) reaction may occur after starting antifungal therapy treatment in inflammatory tinea, as a result of cell mediated immune response. The id reaction is a nonfungal, generally pruritic, papular, or vesicular eruption that typically begins on the face, then spreads to the trunk and extremities. The eruption is usually follicular, lichenoid, or papulosquamous, rarely morbilliform or scarlatiniform. The most common type is seen on the hands and sides of the fingers associated with tinea of the feet. These lesions are mostly vesicular, extremely pruritic, and tender. Secondary bacterial infection may occur.

Topical steroids may be tried for symptomatic relief, although they are commonly refractory to them. The histologic picture is characterized by spongiotic vesicles and a superficial, perivascular, predominantly lymphohistiocytic infiltrate. Diagnosis is dependent on the demonstration of fungal hyphae at a site distant from the dermatophytid, the absence of organism in the id lesion, and resolution of the eruption as the fungal infection subsides.[27]

Laboratory Diagnosis

Diagnoses of dermatophytic infection can be made by patient's history, physical examination, use of a Wood's lamp, skin scrapings for microscopic examination, and fungal cultures (Table 5).

Table 5: Laboratory Diagnosis of Dermatophytic Infections[13-15]

	Specimen	Direct microscopy	Culture	Histology
Tinea corporis/ cruris/faciei	• Scales from active margins	• KOH examination with addition of chlorazol black E/dimethyl sulfoxide and/or Parker Quink blue-black ink to highlight hyphae • Calcofluor white stain for examination with fluorescent microscope • Species identification is usually not possible by microscopy, but, in most cases, yeasts can be differentiated from dermatophytes by morphology	• Samples of scales/ hair/nails are inoculated onto Sabouraud's agar. Selective media include Mycosel and dermatophyte test medium containing chloramphenicol and cycloheximide	• Spongiosis, parakeratosis, and pustules are often seen in cutaneous dermatophytic infections • In onychomycosis, hyphae and arthroconidia may be visible in the nail plate and nail bed with PAS staining, and little to no inflammation is generally present • Biopsy specimens of tinea capitis, Majocchi's granuloma and tinea barbae demonstrate hyphae or arthroconidia within hair shafts • PAS or methenamine silver stains are used in histopathological specimen to demonstrate fungal hyphae to demonstrate fungal organisms • Most reliable technique for diagnosing onychomycosis
Tinea manuum/ Tinea pedis	• Scales from active margins or • Scraping from roof of vesicles			
Tinea capitis	• Scales or epilate broken hairs			
Tinea unguium	• For DLSO: distal portion of involved nail bed; SWO: involved nail surface; PSO: punch biopsy through nail plate to involved nail bed			

DLSO, Distal and lateral subungual onychomycosis; PSO, Proximal subungual onychomycosis; SWO, Superficial white onychomycosis; PAS, periodic acid–Schiff.

The scrapings should be taken from the active scaly margins of a skin lesion. Positive results from nail scrapings are difficult to get as the active border is at the proximal end of the nail. Culture takes about 3 weeks. The broken hair should be epilated for the diagnosis of tinea capitis.

Wood's lamp examination is a useful screening method for examination in schoolchildren. A green fluorescence is present in mycosporum species and in *T. schoenleinii*, while the black dot variety does not fluoresce.

Management

General Measures

Good personal hygiene and compliance to therapy is an important adjunct to antifungal therapy. Decisions regarding a patient's therapy must take into account the extent and location of the infection, the benefits and risks of each of the treatments, and cost. Tinea corporis, tinea faciei, and tinea cruris are treated by topical antifungal preparations, while tinea of the scalp, nails, palms, and soles require systemic treatment. The thick stratum corneum in these sites makes the penetration of topical medicines difficult. The patient is advised to use the antifungal preparations until the infection disappears and then to apply them for further 1–2 weeks to prevent recurrence.

Treatment of uncomplicated dermatophytic infection has been shown in table 6.

Quality Of Life

Dermatophytosis affects the quality of life because significant symptoms of pruritus and pain generally occur with infection. Chronic and recurrent dermatophytic infections cause distress to the patients socially, emotionally, and financially.

CONCLUSION

Dermatophyte infections are common with a worldwide distribution, caused by *Epidermophyton*, *Trichophyton*, and *Microsporum* genera infecting the skin, hair, and nails. The clinical manifestations include tinea pedis, tinea manuum, tinea capitis, tinea corporis, tinea cruris, and tinea barbae. An inaccurate diagnosis can result in inappropriate treatment, such as with topical corticosteroids, which worsen the clinical picture resulting in tinea incognito. A potassium hydroxide preparation can be used to confirm the diagnosis, whenever in doubt. Most topical therapies are effective in cutaneous infection and safe systemic therapy is required in resistant or advanced cases with involvement of hair or nails. It is essential for primary care

Table 6: Treatment of Dermatophytic Infections[13-15,28,29]

Dermatophytic infection	Drug	Dose	Duration	Topical and adjunctive therapy
Tinea capitis	Griseofulvin (drug of choice)	10–20 mg/kg/day	6–8 weeks or longer until fungal cultures are negative	• Avoid sharing of hairbrushes • Add ketoconazole shampoo to reduce transmission
	Terbinafine	10–20 kg—62.5 mg 20–40 kg—125 mg >40 kg—250 mg or 4–5 mg/kg/day	*Trichophyton* spp.: 4–6 weeks *Microsporum* spp.: 8–12 weeks	
	Itraconazole	Capsules: 5 mg/kg/day Oral solution: 3 mg/kg/day	4–6 weeks	–
	Fluconazole	Daily dosing—5–6 mg/kg/day Weekly therapy—8 mg/kg/week	4–6 weeks	–
Tinea cruris/ corporis/faciei	Terbinafine Itraconazole Fluconazole Griseofulvin	250 mg OD 100 mg OD 150 mg/week 500 mg BD	1–2 weeks 1–2 weeks 2–4 weeks 4 weeks	Topical therapy preferred in localized involvement Topical terbinafine or imidazoles BD for 2 weeks Systemic therapy when multiple areas are affected, topical treatment has failed, hairy areas other than scalp and with excessive inflammatory reactions
Tine manuum/ pedis	Terbinafine Itraconazole	250 mg OD 200 mg BD	2 weeks 1–2 weeks	Topical therapy Terbinafine or imidazoles BD application for 4 weeks Glycolic acid, lactic acid, or urea may help to reduce the amount of hyperkeratosis
Tinea unguium	Terbinafine	250 mg OD	6 weeks—fingernails 12 weeks—toenails	Topical therapy like amorolfine nail lacquer and ciclopirox olamine nail lacquer may be added
	Itraconazole	100 mg BD	6 weeks—fingernails 12 weeks—toenails	
		200 mg BD (pulse- one week for each month)	2 pulses—fingernails 3 pulses—toenails	

OD, once daily; BD, twice daily.

providers to be aware of various presentations of dermatophyte infections and treatment options available to accurately care for their patients.

ACKNOWLEDGMENT

Dr Shankila Mittal, Junior resident, Dermatology, Maulana Azad Medical College, New Delhi, for contributing to images.

Editor's Comment

Dermatophytic infection of the skin, hair and nail is one the commonest conditions presenting in the dermatological OPD at least in Asia. A detailed account of the morphological types, common causative agents and treatment options is a useful aid for the treating physician.An increased interest is now therefor superficial infections in India and tropical countries as several are recalcitrant to treatment. Drs Sumit Sethi and Surabhi Sinha have attempted to delineate these very important superficial fungal infectioins as a ready reckoner to the practicing dernatologists.

Rashmi Sarkar, Seemal R Desai

REFERENCES

1. Zaidi Z, Lanigan SW. Superficial fungal infection. In: Zaidi Z, Lanigan SW, editors. Dermatology in Clinical Practice. London: Springer-Verlag; 2010. pp. 73-99.
2. Rezabek GH, Friedman AD. Superficial fungal infections of the skin. Diagnosis and current treatment recommendations. *Drugs.* 1992;43(5):674-82.
3. Kaushik N, Pujalte GG, Reese ST. Superficial fungal infections. *Prim Care.* 2015;42(4):501-16.
4. Rupke SJ. Fungal Skin Disorders Primary Care: Clinics in Office Practice. 2000. pp. 407-21.
5. Ameen M. Epidemiology of superficial fungal infections. *Clin Dermatol.* 2010;28(2):197-201.
6. Aly R. Ecology and epidemiology of dermatophyte infections. *J Am Acad Dermatol.* 1994;31(3 Pt 2):S21-5.
7. Odom R. Pathophysiology of dermatophyte infections. *J Am Acad Dermatol.* 1993;28(5 Pt 1):S2-S7.
8. Leyden JL. Tinea pedis pathophysiology and treatment. *J Am Acad Dermatol.* 1994;31(3 Pt 2):S31-3.
9. Masri-Fridling GD. Dermatophytosis of the feet. *Dermatol Clin.* 1996;14(1):33-40.
10. Drake LA, Dinehart SM, Farmer ER, Goltz RW, Graham GF, Hardinsky MK, et al. Guidelines of care for superficial mycotic infections of the skin: tinea corporis, tinea cruris, tinea faciei, tinea manuum, and tinea pedis. Guidelines/Outcomes Committee. American Academy of Dermatology. *J Am Acad Dermatol.* 1996;34(2 Pt 1):282-6.
11. Adams BB. Tinea corporis gladiatorum. *J Am Acad Dermatol.* 2002;47(2):286-90.
12. Gupta AK, Chaudhry M, Elewski B. Tinea corporis, tinea cruris, tinea nigra, and piedra. *Dermatol Clin.* 2003;21(3):395-400.
13. Hay RJ, Ashbee HR. Mycology. In: Burns T, Breathnach S, Cox N, Griffiths C, editors. Rook's Textbook of Dermatology, 8th edition. West Sussex: Wiley-Blackwell; 2010. pp. 36.1-36.93.
14. Elewski BE, Hughey LC, Sobera JO, Hay R. Fungal diseases. In: Bolognia JL, Jorizzo JL, Schaffer JV, editors. Dermatology. 3rd ed. Philadelphia, PA: Mosby Elsevier; 2012. pp. 1251-84.

15. Verma S, Heffernan MP. Superficial fungal infection: dermatophytosis, onychomycosis, tinea nigra, piedra. In: Wolff K, Goldsmith LA, Katz SI, Gilchrest BA, Paller AS, Leffell DJ, editors. Fitzpatrick's Dermatology in General Medicine. 7th ed. New York: McGraw-Hill; 2008. pp. 1807-21.
16. Singal A, Khanna D. Onychomycosis: diagnosis and management. *Indian J Dermatol Venereol Leprol.* 2011;77(6):659-72.
17. Drake LA, Dinehart SM, Farmer ER, Goltz RW, Graham GF, Hardinsky MK, et al. Guidelines of care for superficial mycotic infections of the skin: onychomycosis. Guidelines/Outcomes Committee. American Academy of Dermatology. *J Am Acad Dermatol.* 1996;34(1):116-21.
18. Gupta AK, Ryder JE, Summerbell RC. Onychomycosis: classification and diagnosis. *J Drugs Dermatol.* 2004;3(1):51-6.
19. Faergemann J, Baran R. Epidemiology, clinical presentation and diagnosis of onychomycosis. *Br J Dermatol.* 2003;149(Suppl 65):1-4.
20. Elewski BE. Tinea capitis: a current perspective. *J Am Acad Dermatol.* 2000;42(1 Pt 1):1-20; quiz 21-4.
21. Frieden IJ, Howard R. Tinea capitis: epidemiology, diagnosis, treatment, and control. *J Am Acad Dermatol.* 1994;31(3 Pt 2):S42-6.
22. Gupta AK, Summerbell RC. Tinea capitis. *Med Mycol.* 2000;38(4):255-87.
23. Drake LA, Dinehart SM, Farmer ER, Goltz RW, Graham GF, Hordinsky MK, et al .Guidelines of care for superficial mycotic infections of the skin: tinea capitis and tinea barbae. Guidelines/Outcomes Committee. American Academy of Dermatology. *J Am Acad Dermatol.* 1996;34(2 Pt 1):290-4.
24. Lin RL, Szepietowski JC, Schwartz RA. Tinea faciei, an often deceptive facial eruption. *Int J Dermatol.* 2004;43(6):437-40.
25. Batta K, Ramlogan D, Smith AG, Garrido MC, Moss C. Tinea indecisiva may mimic the concentric rings of tinea imbricata. *Br J Dermatol.* 2002;147(2):384.
26. Dogra S, Uprety S. The menace of chronic and recurrent dermatophytosis in India: Is the problem deeper than we perceive? *Indian Dermatol Online J.* 2016;7(2):73-6.
27. James WD, Berger TG, Elston DM. Diseases Resulting from Fungi and Yeasts In Andrews' Diseases of the Skin: Clinical Dermatology. 11th ed. Philadelphia, PA: Saunders Elsevier; 2011, p 287-321
28. Gupta AK, Cooper EA, Ryder JE, Nicol KA, Chow M, Chaudhry MM. Optimal management of fungal infections of the skin, hair, and nails. *Am J Clin Dermatol.* 2004;5:225-37.
29. Moossavi M, Bagheri B, Scher RK. Systemic antifungal therapy. *Dermatol Clin.* 2001;19:35-52.

World Clin Dermatol. 2016;3(1):41-59.

Other Superficial Fungal Infections: Piedra, Tinea Nigra, Cutaneous Candidiasis, and Pityriasis Versicolor

*,[1]Sumit Sethi MD DNB, [2]Tanvi Gupta MD DNB

[1]Genesis Centre for Dermatology,
Skin Allure Aesthetic Clinic
New Delhi, India
[2]Department of Dermatology, Leprology, and Venereology
Maulana Azad Medical College
New Delhi, India

ABSTRACT

Superficial fungal infections are caused by pathogens affecting stratum corneum and its adnexal structures with little or no tissue reaction. In this article, four types of infection will be covered: Piedra, tinea nigra, candidiasis and tinea versicolor. Black piedra is caused by *Piedraia hortae* and white piedra is due to pathogenic species of the *Trichosporon* genus. Tinea nigra is caused by *Hortaea werneckii* and presents with black scaly patches on palms. The yeast like fungus Candida produces skin, mucous membrane, and internal infections. C albicans is the most common species in human candidal infections, causing cutaneous infections even in otherwise healthy individuals, whereas other species manifest in setting of significant immunocompromised state. Tinea versicolor is a common infection worldwide, caused by *Malassezia* spp., which are human saprophytes that switch from commensal yeast to pathogenic mycelial form under influence of predisposing environment.

INTRODUCTION

Superficial fungal infections arise from a pathogen that is restricted to the stratum corneum, hair, or nails with or without tissue reaction. They are further subdivided

*Corresponding author
Email: sethi1587@gmail.com

© 2016 Jaypee Brothers Medical Publishers. All rights reserved.

into those that induce minimal cutaneous inflammation (piedras and pityriasis versicolor), and those that lead to more substantial inflammation (dermatophytes and candidiasis).

PIEDRA

Introduction

Piedra, meaning "stone" in Spanish, is a superficial fungal infection of scalp characterized by nodules formed by aggregation of fungal elements along hair shaft. There are two types of piedra: (i) black (trichomycosis nodularis) and (ii) white (trichosporosis nodosa), differentiated by clinical and microscopic examination.

Epidemiology

Black piedra occurs in humid wet tropical regions in the Americas and in Southeast Asia, and affects monkeys as well as humans. White piedra occurs in temperate climate zones of South America, Africa, central and eastern Europe, and Japan.

Etiology

Piedraia hortae causes black piedra. It is found in soil and water. Infection commences in subcuticular area and further growth of fungus may rupture the cuticle. The organism may then grow on the outside of the cuticle, completely surrounding the hair shaft. Because the fungus grows into the hair shaft, the hair may fracture easily at the site of nodules.

The causative agent of white piedra is the genus *Trichosporon* with *T. asahii, T. mucoides, T. inkin, T. ovoides,* and *T. cutaneum*, all being isolated from patients. The lesions may fluoresce when associated with corynebacteria. The fungus grows both within and outside the hair shaft, causing weakening and breakage of the hair. The incidence of white piedra is high in pubic hair of human immunodeficiency virus (HIV)-infected patients. In immunosuppressed patients, *T. beigelii* can cause trichosporosis, a serious systemic infection with fungemia, fever, pulmonary infiltrates, skin lesions (papulovesicular and purpuric, often with central necrosis), and renal disease.

Clinical Features

Clinical features, diagnosis, and treatment have been described in table 1.

Table 1: Clinical Features, Diagnosis, and Treatment of Piedra[4,9]

	White piedra	Black piedra
Organism	*T. beigelii* *T. inkin* *T. asahii* *T. ovoides* *T. asteroides* *T. cutaneum* *T. mucoides*	*Piedraia hortae*
Climatic preference	Temperate climates	Tropical climates
Anatomic involvement	Hair of the scalp, brows, lashes, or beard, axillae, groins	Scalp hair, rarely other sites
Characteristic of nodule	Soft, light yellow or beige-colored nodules loosely attached to the hair shaft with intrapilar extension	Dark, pigmented, gritty hard, well organized, firmly fixed nodules, sized up to a few millimeters, may be multiple, involved hair may be broken
Potassium hydroxide crushed preparation mount	Nondematiaceous closely packed hyphae form a sheath around hair shaft; loose septate hyphae, blastoconidia and arthroconidia aligned at the periphery-"pseudoparenchyma"	Compactly arranged dematiaceous hyphae held together to form a hard mass arranged perpendicularly to hair shaft; ascus with 8 ascospores are seen along with arthroconidia in thicker parts (sexual stage seen in humans)
Wood's lamp	May fluoresce due to coexistence of corynebacteria	Does not fluoresce
Culture	Grows rapidly on Sabouraud's dextrose agar without cycloheximide to form light-colored yeast-like colonies that resemble "butter cream frosting"; grows best at 28–30°C[10]	Growth not inhibited by cycloheximide, forms slow growing dark colored velvety colonies at 25°C[4]
Treatment	Shaving or cutting the affected hair is an effective treatment. Topical antifungals may be added. Among the systemic antifungals, terbinafine and itraconazole have shown good results	

Differential Diagnosis

Piedra needs to be differentiated from pediculosis (nits), hair casts, trichomycosis axillaris, and trichorrhexis nodosa. The nits of pediculosis are yellow brown and cover only a part of the circumference of the hair shaft. Hair casts can be easily moved along the hair shaft. All the conditions can be easily differentiated using dermoscopy and potassium hydroxide (KOH) mount. The concretions in trichomycosis axillaris are yellow/red/black and show the narrow rod-shaped bacteria. Trichorrhexis nodosa shows the classical "paintbrush appearance" of the hair end.

Course and Prognosis

Untreated, the infection may last for months or years. White piedra may recur.[1-11]

TINEA NIGRA

Synonyms: Keratomycosis nigricans palmaris, pityriasis nigra.

Introduction

Tinea nigra is a superficial cutaneous fungal infection affecting usually the skin of the palms and characterized by deeply pigmented, macular, and nonscaly patches.

Epidemiology

It is a disease of the tropical climate with major cases reported from Asia, and Central and South America. Patients of any age can be affected with cases described even in infants. A female predilection as seen by some of the early authors is not supported by more recent studies.

Etiology

Tinea nigra is caused by *Hortaea werneckii* (formerly termed *Phaeoannellomyces werneckii* and *Exophiala werneckii*). Another fungus *Stenella araguata* has been found in a few cases from Venezuela. The lesions develop following an incubation period of 2–7 weeks; traumatic inoculation onto the skin from contact with decaying vegetation, sewage, wood, or soil seems to be the form of acquisition. Hyperhidrosis may be a predisposing factor.

Clinical Features

The lesions are asymptomatic, flat, brown-black, and irregular; with no inflammation or scaling. Either of the palms is involved commonly, but it has been reported to occur on both palms and on unusual sites like wrists and soles. The color change is because of deposition of melanin-like substance in the fungus.

Differential Diagnosis

It can be commonly misdiagnosed as a chemical stain, nevus, melanoma, or palmar lesions of syphilis and dermoscopy has proved to be a useful tool in diagnosing this rare infection. On dermoscopy, tinea nigra shows a fine nonmelanocytic pigmented reticular pattern, not following the dermatoglyphics. Melanomas demonstrate a parallel-pigmented ridge pattern whereas "melanocytic nevi" have a parallel furrow pattern. The black color and the absence of scaling differentiate the condition from pityriasis versicolor.

Laboratory Diagnosis

Potassium hydroxide mount shows brownish septate thick hyphae with budding yeast cells.

Culture on Sabouraud's dextrose agar (SDA) with cycloheximide and chloramphenicol reveals brownish-black colonies in a week. On microscopic examination, typical two-celled yeast cells are seen.

Histopathological examination shows hyperkeratosis and acanthosis with periodic acid-Schiff (PAS) positive hyphae in the corneal layer. A mild lymphocytic infiltrate may be noted in the dermis.

Treatment

Various topical agents have been used with success in tinea nigra: topical imidazoles, ciclopirox olamine, Whitfield ointment, and terbinafine; applied topically for 2–4 weeks. Among the systemic agents, itraconazole has shown benefit but it is rarely required to give systemic therapy.

Course and Prognosis

Spontaneous cure is rare in cases of tinea nigra.[1-3,5,6,8,12-23]

CUTANEOUS CANDIDIASIS

Introduction

Cutaneous candidiasis refers to skin lesions caused by the fungi of genus *Candida*. These yeasts can cause infection of the skin, nails, mucosa of gastrointestinal (GI) and genitourinary (GU) tract, and systemic infections; however, we will restrict ourselves to cutaneous involvement. The major skin manifestation is in the form of intertrigo; others are diaper (intertriginous) dermatitis in children, candidal onychomycosis, and paronychia. Skin is also the major organ involved in congenital candidiasis.

Etiology

The genus *Candida* is a heterogeneous group encompassing various species. It can form the rounded yeast form, pseudohyphae, and budding yeast cells. It has been found to be a normal commensal of skin and the GI tract with as much as 30% of healthy infants demonstrating it in stools.[24] A common isolate from the mucous membranes, from the skin, it has only been isolated from the intertriginous sites. The most common species isolated from skin lesions is *C. albicans* followed by other species like *C. glabrata*, *C. topicalis*, and *C. parapsilosis*.[25]

Pathogenesis

Fungal Virulence

The agglutinin-like sequence has a major role in the adhesion of the fungus to the host cell. A shift from yeast to mycelial form has also been implicated in the causation of cutaneous manifestations, as the hyphal form is more penetrative. The fungus secretes proteases (secreted aspartic proteases) which may be responsible for the adhesion to the host cell as well as the penetration.[26] Invasion by *Candida* can be through endocytosis or active penetration and tissue damage is a result of either necrosis or apoptosis of the host cell.[26]

Biofilm formation has also been seen by *Candida* isolates leading to persistence and nonresponsiveness to therapy.[27]

Interaction with Bacteria

Candida has shown synergistic as well as antagonistic interactions with the bacteria. The synergistic interactions in the form of coaggregation that is forming combined biofilms with the oral bacteria or its synergistic relation with streptococci as seen in few cases of intertrigo (the streptococci secrete lactate to promote yeast growth which itself reduces the oxygen tension as suitable to the bacteria). Antagonism has been demonstrated by *Pseudomonas aeruginosa* which kills the fungal hyphae and also by *Lactobacillus* which inhibits the fungus by secreting hydrogen peroxide. *Candida-Staphylococcus* interactions may be dangerous in the way that biofilm formation may lead to fatal antimicrobial-resistant infections.[28]

Host Factors Predisposing to Infection

There are a lot of conditions which can predispose one to develop *Candida* infections. In the oral cavity, use of dental prostheses, xerostomia, and poor oral hygiene are implicated.[29] Underlying skin conditions, like psoriasis or atopic eczema and maceration, lead to increased fungal carriage.[30] Solid organ cancers and leukemia/lymphomas, immunosuppressive therapy, diabetes mellitus, steroid intake, parenteral nutrition, malnutrition, indwelling catheters, long-term antibiotic usage, primary immunodeficiencies, and extremes of age, all predispose to *Candida* infections.[31]

Human Immunodeficiency Virus/ Acquired Immunodeficiency Syndrome and Candida

Candidiasis is a common cutaneous manifestation of HIV/acquired immunodeficiency syndrome (AIDS). The Carriage of non-albicans Candida (NAC) is increased in HIV-positive individuals in the oral cavity. Low CD4 count is a major risk factor.[32] Non-albicans Candida predominates over *C. albicans* in cases of HIV/AIDS with as high as 61.5% of the isolates being NAC in a study from South India.[33] In the same study, oral candidiasis was the major mucocutaneous presentation. Also, oral candidiasis is an important marker of progression of HIV infection to AIDS.

Epidemiology

Candida accounts for 11–12.5% of superficial fungal skin infections.[25,34] Women and individuals more than 40 years of age are affected more.[34] It has been isolated from skin of 40–75% of infants having diaper dermatitis. *Candida* is the causative agent of onychomycosis in 37.9% patients, more so in the females and fingernails.[25]

Candidal Intertrigo

It is the most common form and mainly involves the groin and genital areas (Figure 1) followed by the web spaces of hands and feet (Figure 2); other flexural sites, like the inframammary area, may also be involved (Figure 3).[34] Erythema and maceration develops in the skin folds and a very fine scaling, pustules may be seen with peeling of superficial layers; satellite lesions is the classical finding. It needs to be differentiated from tinea, flexural psoriasis, Hailey-Hailey disease, and intertrigo. These diseases will lack the satellite pustules and KOH mount may be useful but a histopathological examination may be required in case of doubt.

Diaper Dermatitis

It is generally a secondary involvement in an already irritated skin more so after antibiotic therapy and infants having diarrhea with maceration of the area.[24] It involves the inguinal creases and perianal area with similar clinical presentation as intertrigo (Figure 4).

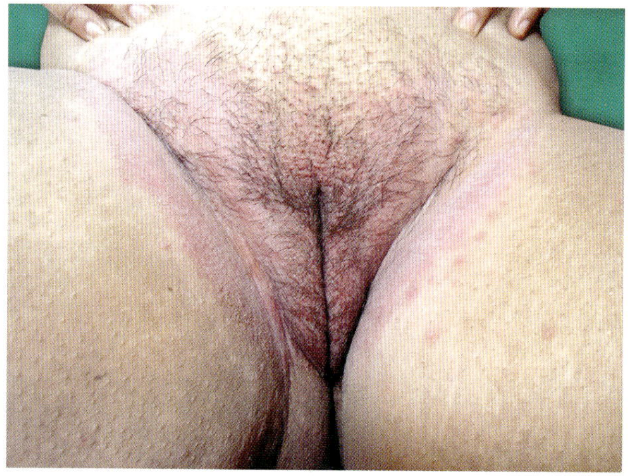

Figure 1: Erythematous plaques in the groin with satellite lesions.

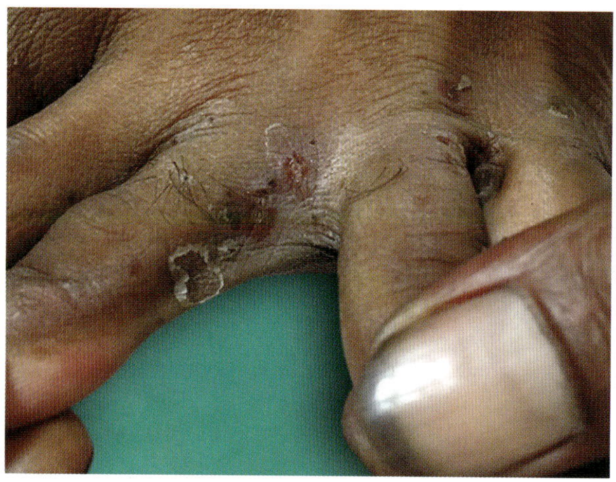

Figure 2: Erosion and pustule in the interdigital web space.

Granuloma gluteale infantum (GGI) is a form of diaper dermatitis which is implicated along with other factors like potent topical steroid usage and chronic irritation. Reddish-blue nodules are formed on the convexities of the diaper area.[35]

Paronychia and Onychomycosis

Seen in individuals whose fingers are immersed in water for long periods like housewives, salon workers, chefs, and household helps.[36] There is loss of cuticle and erythema of the nail fold along with pain and tenderness. Nails may show

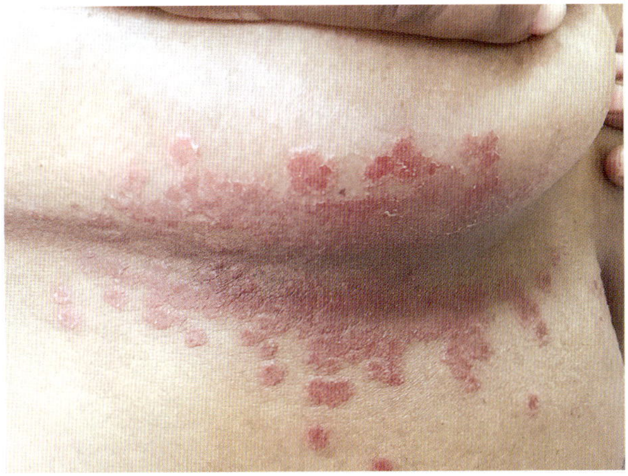

Figure 3: Erythematous papules and plaques with irregular scaly edge and satellite lesions in the inframammary area.

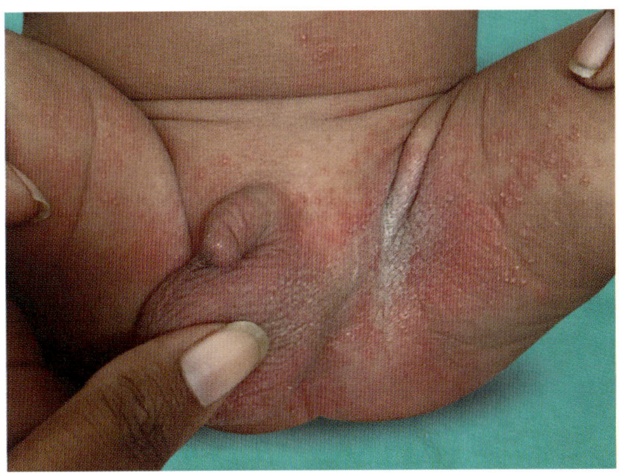

Figure 4: Candida diaper dermatitis in an infant. Satellite pustules can be clearly seen.

Beau's lines and discoloration. Pus may be formed. Infection of the nail may cause dystrophy, onycholysis, distal subungual hyperkeratosis, or nail plate thickening.

Congenital Cutaneous Candidiasis

It is generally acquired *in utero* and the major risk factor is the presence of an intrauterine device. Skin lesions are seen on day one of life but may be seen till day six. Widespread papulopustular eruption or diffuse erythema looking like a burn with erosions or exfoliation may be seen.[37]

Laboratory Diagnosis

KOH mount shows budding yeast cells with the pseudohyphae (Figure 5). Gram stain shows Gram-positive budding yeast cells (Figure 6).

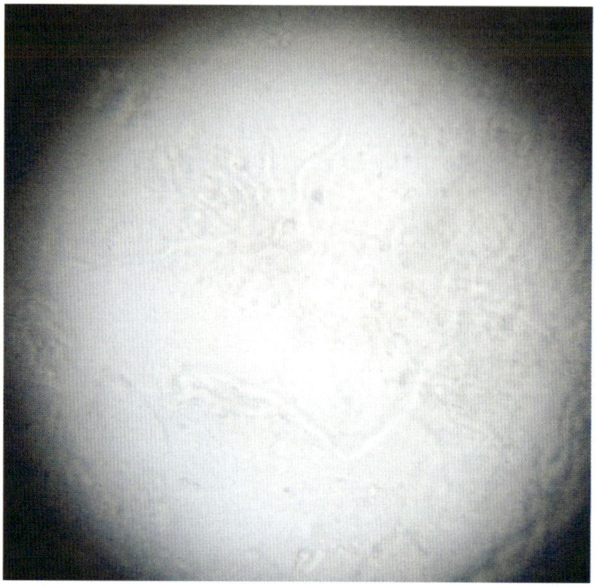

Figure 5: Potassium hydroxide mount showing the yeast cells and the pseudohyphae (400x magnification).

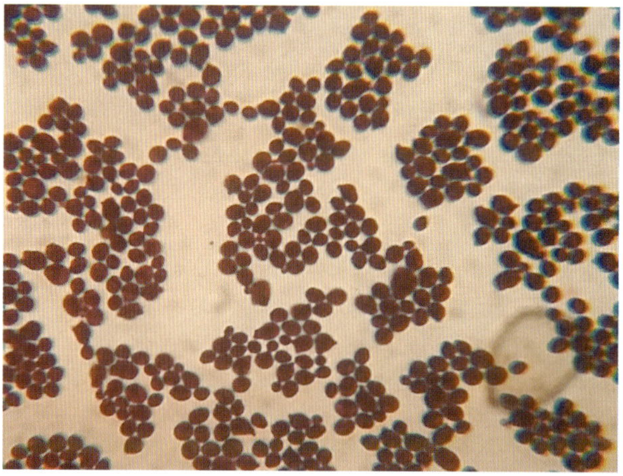

Figure 6: Gram stain shows the Gram-positive budding yeast cells (1,000x magnification).

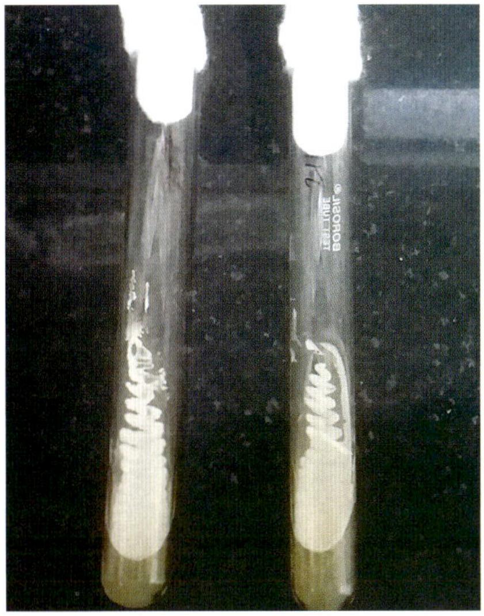

Figure 7: Growth of *Candida albicans* on Sabouraud's dextrose agar.

It grows within 2–5 days on SDA showing white colored colonies (Figure 7).

Histopathology shows the yeast in the stratum corneum and stained with PAS stain. Subcorneal pustules and neutrophilic microabscesses may be seen. In GGI, there is dense infiltrate of lymphocytes, plasma cells, eosinophils, and neutrophils in the dermis.

Treatment

General measures like maintaining local hygiene, keeping the area dry, open footwear, frequent change of diaper, avoidance of any irritants, and avoiding prolonged dipping of hands in water are very vital. Topical azoles applied for 1–2 weeks usually suffices.[38] Mild topical corticosteroid may sometimes be given in cases of diaper dermatitis and paronychia. In extensive involvement or with no improvement with topical therapy and in onychomycosis, systemic therapy with fluconazole or itraconazole is needed. Itraconazole and fluconazole are both effective in onychomycosis and given for 4–6 weeks for fingernail and 12 weeks for toenail. Itraconazole can be given 200 mg daily or as pulse therapy (400 mg daily for a week every month; 2–3 such pulses), and fluconazole to be given 150–300 mg/week.[39]

PITYRIASIS VERSICOLOR (*P. VERSICOLOR*)

Introduction

Pityriasis versicolor is a common chronic, fungal infection of skin caused by the dimorphic lipophilic *Malassezia* yeast. It is characterized by scaly patches of variable colors (pink, brown, or white), primarily affecting lipid-rich areas of the body, including the upper trunk, neck, or upper arms. It is usually asymptomatic; however, some patients may experience mild pruritus.

Epidemiology

Pityriasis versicolor is distributed worldwide; however, it is predominant in tropical climates. Disease can occur at any age, although it is more frequent in young adults and is equally distributed between men and women.

Etiopathogenesis

Both tinea versicolor and pityriasis versicolor have been used in the literature. Tinea "worm-like" is usually reserved for infections produced by dermatophytes, whereas pityriasis meaning "bran-like scaling", accurately describes the appearance of the lesions. *Malassezia* is part of normal skin flora and densely colonizes the areas of scalp, upper trunk, and flexures, where sebaceous activity is high. It lives within the stratum corneum and hair follicles where it feeds off free fatty acids and triglycerides. Currently, 14 species of *Malassezia* are known out of which six common ones are *M. globosa, M. sympodialis, M. slooffiae, M. furfur, M. obtusa,* and *M. restricta*. With the exception of *M. pachydermatis*, all species of this genus are lipophilic. *Malassezia globosa* and *M. sympoidalis* are reported to be the predominant species causing the disease.

Predisposing host factors implicated in the transformation of *Malassezia* from commensal yeast form to pathogenic mycelial phase are both endogenous and exogenous. The most important exogenous factors are high temperatures and high relative humidity which explains the high incidence in tropics. Other external factors include burns, application of oily preparations, and sunlight. Occlusion of the skin by either clothing or cosmetics results in increased local humidity, carbon dioxide concentration, an altered microflora, and an altered pH range, which help in transformation of fungus. The most important endogenous factors are greasy skin, hyperhidrosis, pregnancy, malnutrition, systemic steroids, hereditary predisposition, and immunodeficiency. Pityriasis versicolor is not contagious and not caused due to poor personal hygiene.

Various hypotheses have been put forward to explain pigmentary changes in pityriais versicolor. The fungi secrete dicarboxylic acids such as azelaic acid which inhibit tyrosinase and damage the melanocytes to induce hypopigmentation. Although the melanosomes are reduced in size and number, their number remains unchanged and the transfer of melanosomes to keratinocytes becomes defective. Secretion of tryptophan derivatives by the fungus interfering with the 3,4-dihydroxyphenylalanine (DOPA) reactions and a "pseudoleukoderma" because of the screening effect of pityriacitrine and pityrialactone has also been proposed. Hypopigmentation becomes more apparent in whites after the skin tans. Two theories have been proposed regarding pathogenesis of hyperpigmentation are: (i) increased thickness of the keratin layer; and (ii) pronounced inflammatory cell infiltrate acting as a stimulus to melanocytes, resulting in the production of more pigment. In hyperpigmented lesions, increase in the size of melanosomes has also been seen.

Other dermatologic conditions associated with these yeasts are seborrheic dermatitis, folliculitis, dandruff, atopic dermatitis, psoriasis, and less commonly confluent and reticulated papillomatosis, onychomycosis, and transient acantholytic dermatosis. In these cases, *Malassezia* spp. only appear in the yeast phase form.

Clinical Features

Tinea versicolor is characterized by the presence of fine scaly patches (pityriasis) or macules, which may be hypochromic or hyperchromic (versicolor). Commonly located on the upper aspects of the trunk, neck, and arms, lesions may involve the face, groin, and even thighs (Figure 8). In children, the face is frequently involved.

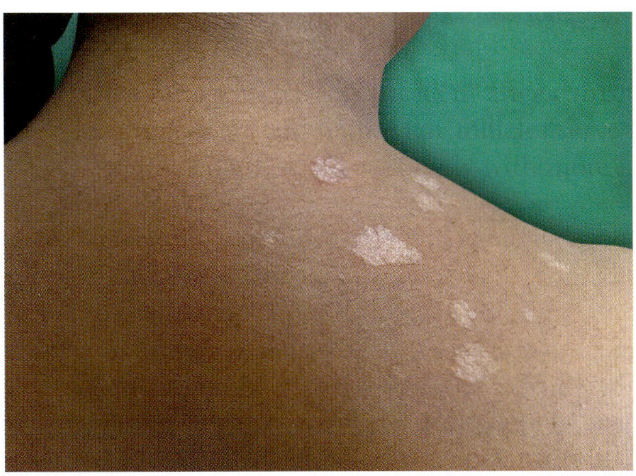

Figure 8: Hypopigmented scaly lesions of pityriasis versicolor on the back.

Inverse distribution of lesions is seen in immunocompromised individuals. The initial lesions are 3–5 mm diameter macules, round or oval-shaped which enlarge radially and coalesce with time to affect extensive areas of the body, taking irregular shapes. Eruption is insidious in onset and asymptomatic; pruritus only if lesions are inflammatory. Easy flaking of scales in characteristic sheets is observed when stroked by the edge of a glass slide, or fingernail, known as the *coup d'ongle* or "stroke of the nail" sign. Three variants are seen: (i) pink, (ii) atrophic, and (iii) trichrome. Lesions may be less visible in fair-complexioned individuals and most become aware when the involved areas do not tan.

Laboratory Diagnosis

The diagnosis is based on the typical clinical picture combined with direct microscopy and Wood's light examination.

Direct microscopy with KOH shows the typical "spaghetti and meatballs" appearance; rounded yeast cells in grape-like clusters intermixed with the nonbranching coarse short hyphae (Figure 9).

Wood's light examination accentuates pigment changes, and a yellow-green fluorescence of the lesions is seen due to pityriacitrine and pityrialactone (Figure 10). The fluorescence sign can be used to detect subclinical areas of involvement and in assessing cure after treatment; however, it is positive in just 50% of the patients in which infection is caused by fluorescent *M. furfur* species.

Histopathology with PAS or methenamine silver staining shows a thick basket weave stratum corneum with abundant short hyphae and round budding

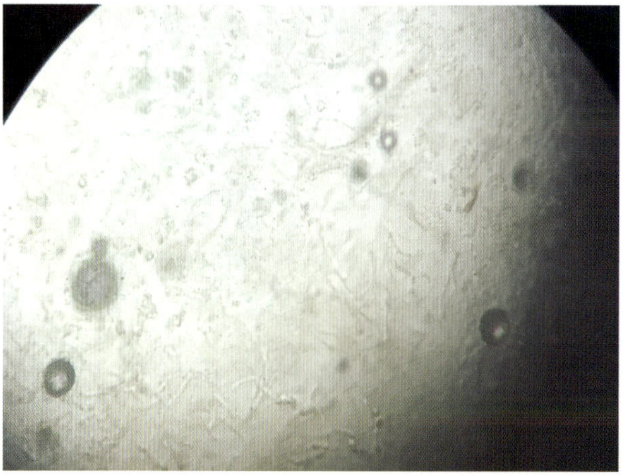

Figure 9: Yeast cells with branching short hyphae (400x magnification).

Figure 10: Wood's lamp examination of the lesions showing yellow-green fluorescence.

cellular fungal elements. Mild superficial, perivascular lymphocytic infiltrate without any pigment incontinence is observed in dermis. In the atrophic variant, epidermal colonization with hyphae and spores is accompanied by effacement of the rete ridges, subepidermal fibroplasia, pigment incontinence, and elastolysis.

Culture and polymerase chain reaction can be done to identify the species; however, since culture requires lipid enrichment of the media, it is rarely done to confirm diagnosis.

Differential Diagnosis

Pityriasis alba, pityriasis rosea, tinea corporis, seborrheic dermatitis, erythrasma, secondary syphilis, and vitiligo.

Management

General Measures

Predisposing factors should be avoided as much as possible, especially use of oily creams/lotions, sun exposure, heavy clothing, excessive heat, and humidity. Improving hygiene and reducing perspiration prevents recurrence. Discarding or boiling frequently worn garments, which retain fungal elements, also decrease the chance of relapse.

Treatment

The turnover time for sloughing of the stratum corneum, where the organism resides is 4 weeks, so the topical treatment should be for at least this much duration. Topical therapy is preferred for children and is less expensive; however, compliance for the duration of therapy is a problem. Oral treatment is recommended for those with extensive involvement, who did not respond to topical treatment and have frequent recurrences (Table 2). Ultraviolet B (UVB) as well as psoralen-UVA with 8-methoxypsoralen have both been tried for treatment of residual hypomelanosis after fungal elimination; results are unpredictable.

Chemoprophylaxis

Systemic prophylaxis is not routinely recommended and is reserved for highly recurrent cases that are severe enough to cause significant distress in patients with good liver function (Table 2).

Table 2: Antifungal Therapy for Pityriasis Versicolor

Nonspecific topical antifungal therapy	Specific antifungal therapy		Chemoprophylaxis
• (Acts by physically and/or chemically removing infected dead tissue and by preventing the invasion of newly formed or forming keratinized tissues)	• Topical	• Systemic therapy	
• Selenium sulfide 2.5% suspension applied from neck to waist and other affected area(s), rinsed thoroughly with water after 15 minutes; applied once daily for 7 days; and repeated weekly for 1 month, then monthly for maintenance • 50% propylene glycol in water applied twice daily for 2 weeks • Zinc pyrithione 1% shampoo applied daily for 2 weeks	• Ketoconazole 2% shampoo should be applied to the entire skin surface from the hairy scalp area down to the thighs and should be left in place for 5 minutes and then rinsed thoroughly for 4 weeks • Topical imidazole antifungals (e.g., clotrimazole, econazole, miconazole) up to 4 weeks • Terbinafine 1% cream twice daily for 15 days	• Ketoconazole 200 mg once daily for 5 days, or 400 mg/week for 2 weeks • Fluconazole 400 mg stat dose • Itraconazole 200 mg/day for 5 days or 400 mg stat dose • Systemic terbinafine and griseofulvin is ineffective in pityriasis versicolor	• Ketoconazole (400 mg orally, every 14 day or 200 mg orally, for 3 consecutive days per month) • Itraconazole (200 mg orally, twice daily, 1 day per month) • Fluconazole (400 mg, 1 day per month)

Course and Prognosis

The prognosis is good, with complete mycological cure after 3–4 weeks of treatment. Without therapy, pityriasis versicolor is a chronic disease and recurrence after treatment is 60% after 1 year and 80% after 2 years. Patients should be informed that the hypopigmented areas will not disappear immediately after treatment and that it may take them several months to regain their pigmentation.[6,40-54]

CONCLUSION

Each of the superficial cutaneous fungal infections has a characteristic clinical picture. All generally favor the tropical climate. These can be easily diagnosed with a firm clinical suspicion augmented with the KOH mount and microscopy, Wood's lamp, and dermoscopy. Histopathological examination and culture is rarely required in doubtful cases. While these infections are easily treatable, an early diagnosis and treatment is imperative. Both topical and systemic antifungals work quite well with little known resistance so far.

Editor's Comment

The article is a precise overview of important superficial fungal infections other than dermatophytosis, in clinical practice. It describes the entities in a concise and accurate manner with their management. These superficial infections although not so common as their dermatophytic counterparts, are important for the treating dermatologist. Drs Sumit Sethi and Tanvi Gupta have made sure the text is supplemented by useful tables and clinical pictures which makes an interesting read. The article will benefit everyone practising in areas where these fungal infections are commonly seen and help them to differentiate these from other entities. Knowledge about these conditions will help the clinician to clinch the diagnosis when in doubt.

Rashmi Sarkar, Seemal R Desai

REFERENCES

1. Gupta AK, Chaudhry M, Elewski B. Tinea corporis, tinea cruris, tinea nigra, and piedra. *Dermatol Clin.* 2003;21(3):395-400.
2. Hay RJ, Ashbee HR. Mycology. In: Burns T, Breathnach S, Cox N, Griffiths C, editors. Rook's Textbook of Dermatology. 8th ed. West Sussex: Wiley-Blackwell; 2010. pp. 36.1-36.93.
3. Elewski BE, Hughey LC, Sobera JO, Hay R. Fungal diseases. In: Bolognia JL, Jorizzo JL, Schaffer JV, editors. Dermatology. 3rd ed. Philadelphia, PA: Mosby Elsevier; 2012. pp. 1251-84.
4. Kalter DC, Tschen JA, Cernoch PL, McBride ME, Sperber J, Bruce S, et al. Genital white piedra: epidemiology, microbiology and therapy. *J Am Acad Dermatol.* 1986;14(6):982-93.

5. Verma S, Heffernan MP. Superficial fungal infection: dermatophytosis, onychomycosis, tinea nigra, piedra. In: Wolff K, Goldsmith LA, Katz SI, Gilchrest BA, Paller AS, Leffell DJ, editors. Fitzpatrick's Dermatology in General Medicine. 7th ed. New York: McGraw-Hill; 2008. pp. 1807-21.
6. James WD, Berger TG, Elston DM. Diseases resulting from fungi and yeasts. In: Andrews' Diseases of the Skin: Clinical Dermatology. 11th ed. Philadelphia, PA: Saunders Elsevier; 2011. pp. 287-321.
7. Schwartz RA. Superficial fungal infections. *Lancet.* 2004;364(9440):1173-82.
8. Bonifaz A, Gómez-Daza F, Paredes V, Ponce RM. Tinea versicolor, tinea nigra, white piedra, and black piedra. *Clin Dermatol.* 2010;28(2):140-5.
9. Drake LA, Dinehart SM, Farmer ER, Goltz RW, Graham GF, Hordinsky MK, et al. Guidelines of care for superficial mycotic infections of the skin: piedra. Guidelines/Outcomes Committee. American Academy of Dermatology. *J Am Acad Dermatol.* 1996;34(1):122-4.
10. Chagas-Neto TC, Chaves GM, Colombo AL. Update on the genus Trichosporon. *Mycopathologia.* 2008;166(3):121-32.
11. Guého E, Improvisi L, de Hoog GS, Dupont B. Trichosporon on humans: a practical account. *Mycoses.* 1994;37(1-2):3-10.
12. Pegas JR, Criado PR, Lucena SK, de Oliveira MA. Tinea nigra: report of two cases in infants. *Pediatr Dermatol.* 2003;20(4):315-7.
13. Van Velsor H, Singletary H. Tinea nigra palmaris: a report of 15 cases from coastal North Carolina. *Arch Dermatol.* 1964;90:59-61.
14. Bonifaz A, Badali H, de Hoog GS, Cruz M, Araiza J, Cruz MA, et al. Tinea nigra by *Hortaea werneckii*, a report of 22 cases from Mexico. *Stud Mycol.* 2008;61:77-82.
15. Perez C, Colella MT, Olaizola C, Hartung de Capriles C, Magaldi S, Mata-Essayag S. Tinea nigra: report of twelve cases in Venezuela. *Mycopathologia.* 2005;160(3):235-8.
16. Blank H. Tinea nigra: a twenty-year incubation period? *J Am Acad Dermatol.* 1979;1(1):49-51.
17. Petavy AF, Guillot J, Grosshans E, Coulet M, Rey M. A case of bilateral tinea nigra palmaris contracted in the Ivory Coast; treatment with clotrimazole and miconazole nitride. *Ann Dermatol Venereol.* 1977;104(5):400-2.
18. Julián-González R, Vargas-de Julián V. Tinea nigra in an unusual anatomic location. *An Pediatr (Barc).* 2013;79(5):340-1.
19. Piliouras P, Allison S, Rosendahl C, Buettner PG, Weedon D. Dermoscopy improves diagnosis of tinea nigra: a study of 50 cases. *Australas J Dermatol.* 2011;52(3):191-4.
20. Gupta G, Burden AD, Shankland GS, Fallowfield ME, Richardson MD. Tinea nigra secondary to Exophiala werneckii responding to itraconazole. *Br J Dermatol.* 1997;137(3):483-4.
21. Rossetto AL, Cruz RC. Spontaneous cure in a case of Tinea nigra. *An Bras Dermatol.* 2012;87(1):160-2.
22. Sayegh-Carreño R, Abramovits-Ackerman W, Girón GP. Therapy of tinea nigra plantaris. *Int J Dermatol.* 1989;28(1):46-8.
23. Rossetto AL, Cruz RC, Haddad Junior V. Double-blind study with topical isoconazole and terbinafine for the treatment of one patient with bilateral Tinea nigra plantaris and suggestions for new differential diagnosis. *Rev Inst Med Trop Sao Paulo.* 2013;55(2):125-8.
24. Gökalp AS, Aldirmaz C, Oğuz A, Gültekin A, Bakici MZ. Relation between the intestinal flora and diaper dermatitis in infancy. *Trop Geogr Med.* 1990;42(3):238-40.
25. Tan HH. Superficial fungal infections seen at the National Skin Centre, Singapore. *Nihon Ishinkin Gakkai Zasshi.* 2005;46(2):77-80.
26. Naglik JR, Moyes DL, Wächtler B, Hube B. *Candida albicans* interactions with epithelial cells and mucosal immunity. *Microbes Infect.* 2011;13(12-13):963-76.
27. Tsui C, Kong EF, Jabra-Rizk MA. Pathogenesis of Candida albicans biofilm. *Pathog Dis.* 2016;74(4):ftw018.
28. Morales DK, Hogan DA. Candida albicans interactions with bacteria in the context of human health and disease. *PLoS Pathog.* 2010;6(4):e1000886.
29. Bianchi CMP de C, Bianchi HA, Tadano T, de Paula CR, Hoffmann-Santos HD, Leite DP Jr, et al. Factors related to oral candidiasis in elderly users and non-users of removable dental prostheses. *Rev Inst Med Trop São Paulo.* 2016;58:17.

30. Leibovici V, Alkalay R, Hershko K, Ingber A, Westerman M, Leviatan-Strauss N, et al. Prevalence of Candida on the tongue and intertriginous areas of psoriatic and atopic dermatitis patients. *Mycoses.* 2008;51(1):63-6.
31. Rajendran R, Sherry L, Deshpande A, Johnson EM, Hanson MF, Williams C, et al. A Prospective Surveillance Study of Candidaemia: epidemiology, risk factors, antifungal treatment and outcome in hospitalized patients. *Front Microbiol.* 2016;7:915.
32. Mushi MF, Mtemisika CI, Bader O, Bii C, Mirambo MM, Groß U et al. High oral carriage of non-albicans Candida spp. among HIV-infected individuals. *Int J Infect Dis.* 2016;49:185-8.
33. Shivaswamy U, Neelambike SM. A study of candidiasis in HIV reactive patients in a tertiary care hospital, Mysore—South India. *Indian J Dermatol Venereol Leprol.* 2014;80(3):278.
34. Heidrich D, Stopiglia CD, Magagnin CM, Daboit TC, Vettorato G, Amaro TG, et al. Sixteen years of dermatomycosis caused by spp. in the metropolitan area of Porto Alegre, southern Brazil. *Rev Inst Med Trop Sao Paulo.* 2016;58:14.
35. Bluestein J, Furner BB, Phillips D. Granuloma gluteale infantum: case report and review of the literature. *Pediatr Dermatol.* 1990;7(3):196-8.
36. Costa-Orlandi CB, Magalhães GM, Oliveira MB, Taylor EL, Marques CR, de Resende-Stoianoff MA. Prevalence of dermatomycosis in a Brazilian tertiary care hospital. *Mycopathologia.* 2012;174(5-6):489-97.
37. Darmstadt GL, Dinulos JG, Miller Z. Congenital cutaneous candidiasis: clinical presentation, pathogenesis, and management guidelines. *Pediatrics.* 2000;105(2):438-44.
38. Del Rosso JQ, Kircik LH. Optimizing topical antifungal therapy for superficial cutaneous fungal infections: focus on topical naftifine for cutaneous dermatophytosis. *J Drugs Dermatol.* 2013;12(11 Suppl):s165-71.
39. Tosti A, Piraccini BM, Lorenzi S, Iorizzo M. Treatment of nondermatophyte mold and onychomycosis. *Dermatol Clin.* 2003;21:491-7.
40. Faergemann J, Fredriksson T. Tinea versicolor: some new aspects on etiology, pathogenesis, and treatment. *Int J Dermatol.* 1982;21(1):8-11.
41. Kallini JR, Riaz F, Khachemoune A. Tinea versicolor in dark-skinned individuals. *Int J Dermatol.* 2014;53(2):137-41.
42. Karaoui R, Bou-Resli M, Al-Zaid NS, Mousa A. Tinea versicolor: ultrastructural studies on hypopigmented and hyperpigmented skin. *Dermatologica.* 1981;162(2):69-85.
43. Gupta AK, Bluhm R, Summerbell R. Pityriasis versicolor. *J Eur Acad Dermatol Venereol.* 2002;16(1):19-33.
44. Gupta AK, Batra R, Bluhm R, Faergemann J. Pityriasis versicolor. *Dermatol Clin.* 2003;21(3):413-29, v-vi.
45. Faergemann J. Management of seborrheic dermatitis and pityriasis versicolor. *Am J Clin Dermatol.* 2000;1(2):75-80.
46. Faergemann J. Pityrosporum infections. *J Am Acad Dermatol.* 1994;31(3 Pt 2):S18-20.
47. Gupta AK, Batra R, Bluhm R, Boekhout T, Dawson TL Jr. Skin diseases associated with Malassezia species. *J Am Acad Dermatol.* 2004;51(5):785-98.
48. Geis PA. Epidemiology, etiology, clinical aspects, and diagnosis of tinea versicolor. *Int J Dermatol.* 1999;38(7):558.
49. Mendez-Tovar LJ. Pathogenesis of dermatophytosis and tinea versicolor. *Clin Dermatol.* 2010;28(2):185-9.
50. Vander Straten MR, Hossain MA, Ghannoum MA. Cutaneous infections dermatophytosis, onychomycosis, and tinea versicolor. *Infect Dis Clin North Am.* 2003;17(1):87-112.
51. Ljubojević S, Skerlev M, Lipozencić J, Basta-Juzbasić A. The role of Malassezia furfur in dermatology. *Clin Dermatol.* 2002;20(2):179-82.
52. Hu SW, Bigby M. Pityriasis versicolor: a systematic review of interventions. *Arch Dermatol.* 2010;146:1132-40.
53. Silva-Lizama E. Tinea versicolor. *Int J Dermatol.* 1995;34(9):611-7.
54. Borelli D, Jacobs PH, Nall L. Tinea versicolor: epidemiologic, clinical, and therapeutic aspects. *J Am Acad Dermatol.* 1991;25(2 Pt 1):300-5.

World Clin Dermatol. 2016;3(1):60-79.

Onychomycoses

Vishalakshi Viswanath MD DNB DDV, *Pradnya R Joshi MD DVL

Department of Dermatology, Rajiv Gandhi Medical College and Chatrapati Shivaji Maharaj Hospital
Thane, Maharashtra, India

ABSTRACT

Onychomycoses, one of the most common infective nail disorders, are caused by dermatophytes, nondermatophyte molds (NDMs), and *Candida* species.

Dermatophytes onychomycosis is most common followed by NDMs and *Candida* spp. Characteristic clinical patterns have been noted with different organisms. Based on the pattern of nail invasion and characteristic clinical features, onychomycoses can be classified into various clinical types, DLSO being the most common type. A clinical suspicion of onychomycosis should be confirmed by laboratory diagnosis. Dermoscopy of nails (onychoscopy) is a new method that can aid the dermatologists in diagnosis; a typical fringed proximal margin is a characteristic feature in onychomycosis.

Treatment is chosen depending on the clinical type, the number of involved nails, and the severity of the infection. The current recommendation is use of oral antifungals but these are often limited by drug interactions, and the topical antifungal lacquers show less efficacy. Hence a combination of both topical and systemic treatment is often the best choice. Newer treatment modalities such as lasers, light therapy, penetration enhancers etc. are still being investigated and may prove useful adjuncts in treatment of onychomycoses.

INTRODUCTION

Onychomycoses (infection of the nail plate by fungi) are one of the most common infective nail disorders presenting to the dermatologist and caused by dermatophytes, nondermatophyte molds (NDMs), and *Candida* species. Characteristic clinical patterns have been noted with different organisms. Though mycological diagnosis is the gold standard, use of newer techniques

*Corresponding author
Email: drpradnyalondhe@gmail.com

© 2016 Jaypee Brothers Medical Publishers. All rights reserved.

such as onychoscopy has simplified the approach towards diagnosis. Treatment of onychomycoses is a challenge and has improved with the advent of newer drug delivery systems.

EPIDEMIOLOGICAL FACTORS

The prevalence of onychomycoses due to dermatophytes varies between 6 and 25%, those due to NDM is between 10 and 15%, whereas *Candida* onychomycoses occur in presence of predisposing factors such as diabetes, immunosuppression, or prolonged water contact.[1,2] Onychomycoses is uncommon in children and is more prevalent in males and in elderly population.

Predisposing factors for developing onychomycosis include elderly population, diabetes, immunosuppression, and trauma. Elderly population is prone due to poor peripheral circulation, repeated trauma, and slow linear nail growth. High prevalence in diabetics is due to a combination of host factors including impaired glycemic index, ischemia, neuropathy, and local immunosuppression. Avid sports participation is another contributory factor and seen with increasing use of health clubs, swimming pools, and occlusive footwear for exercise.[3] Toenails are more frequently affected than fingernails, especially in infections due to dermatophytes and NDM. *Trichophyton rubrum* is responsible for approximately 90% of cases of toenail onychomycosis.[4] Infections due to *Candida* is common in fingernails. Candidal paronychia develops and worsens on prolonged contact with moisture, and additionally bacterial infection or contact dermatitis can aggravate an existing paronychia. For *Candida* onychomycoses, other predisposing conditions include Raynaud's phenomenon or disease and Cushing syndrome.

ETIOPATHOGENESIS[1]

Various fungal organisms and species causing onychomycoses have been outlined in table 1.

Table 1: Causative Organisms in Onychomycoses

Fungi	Species
Dermatophytes	*Trichophyton rubrum, T. mentagrophytes, T. soudanense, T. violaceum, T. interdigitale, Epidermophyton floccosum*
Non-dermatophyte molds	*Fusarium* spp., *Neoscytalidium* spp., *Scopulariopsis brevicaulis, Alternaria* spp., *Aspergillus* spp., *Sarocladium (previously Acremonium) strictum* Uncommon: *Onychocola canadensis, Pseudeurotium ovalis, Pyrenochaeta unguis-hominis, Lasiodiplodia theobromae, Cochliobolus (previously Curvularia) lunata*
Candida species	*Candida albicans, Candida parapsilosis*

Nail infection may be the only manifestation of infection with dermatophytes or it may be accompanied by cutaneous lesions. Skin involvement in the form of tinea manuum or tinea pedis is frequently seen with onychomycosis due to dermatophytes with *T. rubrum*, *T. interdigitale*, and rarely, *Epidermophyton floccosum*. Scalp infections are seen in onychomycoses due to *T. tonsurans, T. violaceum, and T. soudanense*. Amongst the dermatophytes, *T. rubrum* invades the nail plate easily. Invasion commonly occurs from the lateral nail fold or free edge and causes opacity and destruction of the nail plate. In cases of NDM, skin involvement is infrequent. Onychomycoses due to *Candida* or *Neoscytalidium* spp. may be accompanied by paronychia or inflammation of the nail folds.

CLINICAL TYPES AND DIFFERENTIAL DIAGNOSIS

Based on the pattern of nail invasion and characteristic clinical features, onychomycoses can be classified into various clinical types. The causative organisms, clinical features, and differential diagnosis of various clinical types have been described in table 2[1,5] (Figures 1 to 5).

Classification

- Distal and lateral subungual onychomycoses (DLSO)
- Proximal subungual onychomycoses (PSO)
- Superficial white onychomycoses (SWO)
- Total dystrophic onychomycoses (TDO)
- Endonyx
- Mixed onychomycoses
- Paronychia with onychomycoses.

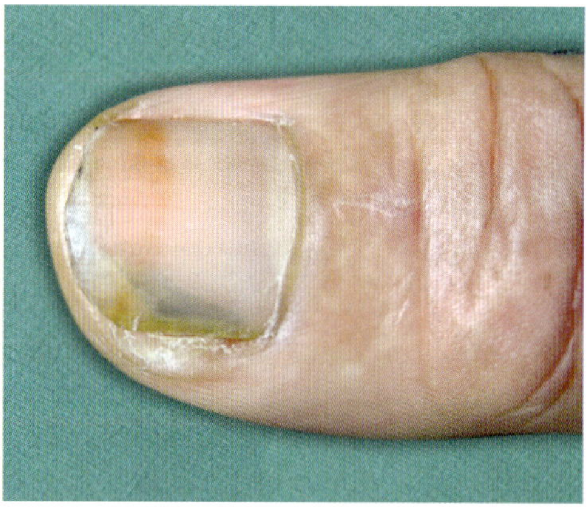

Figure 1: Distal and lateral subungual onychomycoses.

Table 2: Onychomycoses: Types, Causative Organism, Clinical Features, and Differential Diagnosis

Types/causative organism	Clinical features	Differential diagnosis
Distal and lateral subungual onychomycoses (DLSO): *Trichophyton rubrum, T. mentagrophytes, Candida albicans, Fusarium* spp., *Neoscytalidium* spp., *Scopulariopsis brevicaulis*	• Most common pattern of infection • Fungi invade undersurface of the nail unit from distal and lateral edge of the nail • Nail plate appears yellow-white, is detached due to onycholysis, becomes thickened with subungual hyperkeratosis • Often affects toenails and may be seen with tinea pedis	• Traumatic onycholysis • Psoriasis
Proximal subungual onychomycoses (PSO): *T. rubrum*, *Fusarium* spp.	• White area under the proximal nail plate, in the lunula area • Common in human immuno-deficiency virus patients • Periungual inflammation may be seen	• Acute bacterial paronychia • Pustular psoriasis of the nail
Superficial white onychomycoses (SWO): *T. mentagrophytes*, *T. rubrum*, *T. interdigitale*, *Fusarium* spp., *Acremonium*, *Neoscytalidium*	• Less common • Fungi invade the dorsal nail plate and form colonies • White opaque formations which can be easily scraped	• Superficial nail fragility due to prolonged wearing of nail polish • Transverse toenail leukonychia due to trauma
Total dystrophic onychomycoses: *T. mentagrophytes, T. rubrum, C. albicans, Neoscytalidium* spp.	• Most severe stage, can result from a long-standing DLSO or PSO • The nail plate is diffusely thickened, friable, and yellowish	• Psoriasis • Twenty nail dystrophy
Endonyx *T. soudanense, T. violaceum*	• Rare infection, invasion of nail plate without nail bed involvement • Nail plate shows pitting and lamellar splits	• Psoriasis • Leukonychia
Mixed onychomycoses *T. rubrum, Fusarium* spp.	• More than one pattern of nail invasion (DLSO + SWO, DLSO + PSO, PSO + SWO)	• Psoriasis • Traumatic
Paronychia with onychomycoses *Candida* spp., *Fusarium* spp., *Neoscytalidium*	• DLSO or PSO type with proximal nail fold inflammation	• Acute bacterial paronychia • Pustular psoriasis

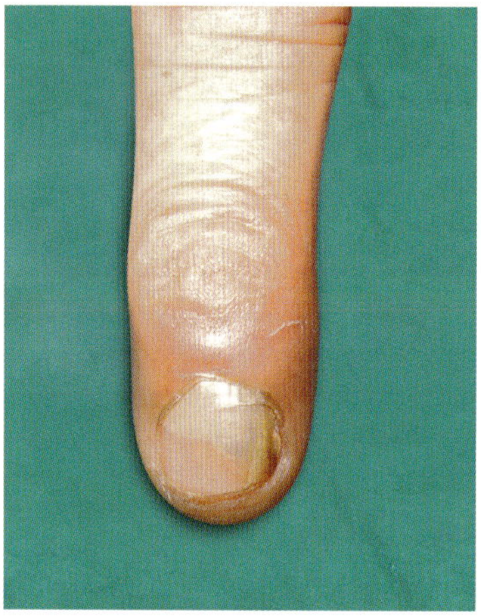

Figure 2: Proximal subungual onychomycoses.

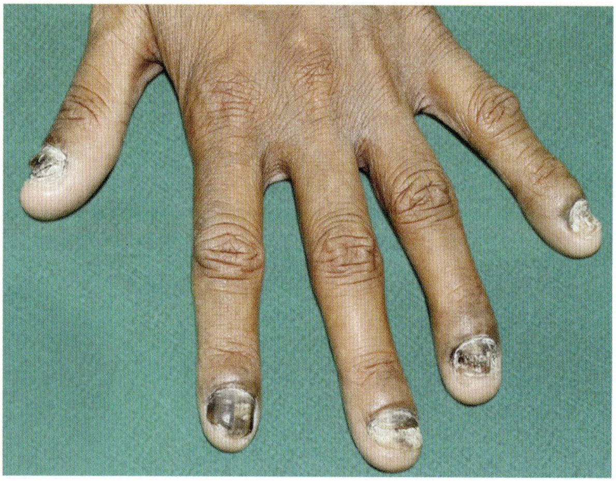

Figure 3: Total dystrophic onychomycoses.

Amongst the various clinical types, dermatophytes frequently cause DLSO, and TDO. Proximal subungual onychomycoses is common in human immunodeficiency virus patients whereas SWO and endonyx are less common infections. Dermatophytoma, a variant of DLSO, responds poorly to treatment. It is characterized by subungual accumulation of hyphae and scales and requires excision of the area and systemic treatment. Fungal melanonychia is a rare variant characterized by black pigmentation of the nail and may be associated with the melanoides variant of *T. rubrum* or other fungi that produce melanin, such as *Neoscytalidium dimidiatum*, *Aspergillus niger*, *Alternaria*, and *Exophiala*.[6]

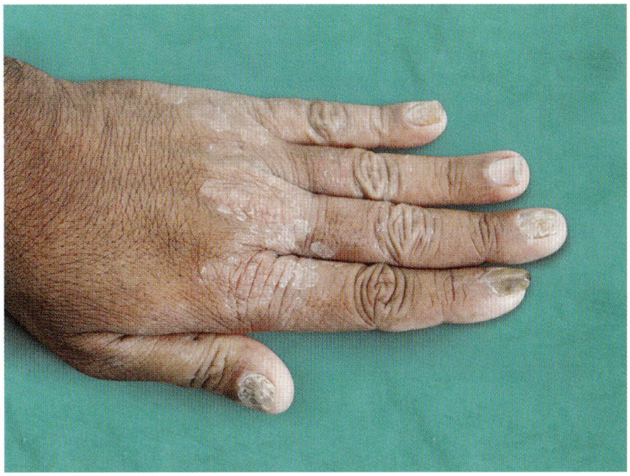

Figure 4: Total dystrophic onychomycoses with tinea manuum.

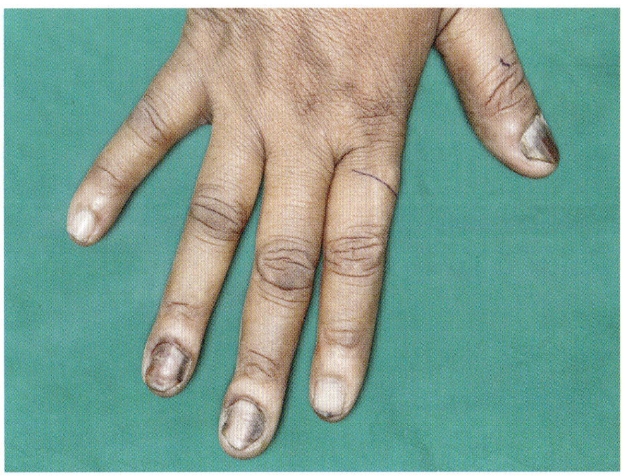

Figure 5: Paronychia with onychomycoses.

Nondermatophyte molds frequently cause toenail infections without skin involvement with *Fusarium* spp. being commonly implicated. *Scopulariopsis brevicaulis* infections usually infects the great toenail and can coexist with or may be indistinguishable from those of a dermatophyte infection; but in heavy invasions, a cinnamon color of the nail plate may be seen. Other NDMs usually cause SWO, in contrast to *Scopulariopsis* infections; secondary mold invasion often affects several nails. Mold infections are difficult to treat; a dystrophic nail caused by ischemia and secondarily colonized by *Aspergillus* may regrow abnormally even after nail avulsion.

Onychomycoses due to *Candida* commonly manifests as DLSO associated with paronychia. It may manifest as erosion of the distal and lateral nail plate of the fingernails, especially in women and it does not progress to total nail dystrophy. In chronic mucocutaneous candidosis, complete destruction of the nail plate can occur. *Candida* granuloma is an uncommon variant seen in immunocompromised patients due to direct invasion by the organisms. Thickening of the nail plate and associated paronychia may be seen initially and in severe cases swelling of the digit may give rise to pseudo clubbing or "chicken drumstick" appearance.[7]

Differential Diagnosis

The clinical conditions which can mimic onychomycoses is outlined in table 3.[8] The mimickers based on the clinical types of onychomycoses have been outlined in table 2. Psoriasis, lichen planus, and traumatic conditions are common clinical mimickers, and mycological diagnosis is the gold standard for confirmation of diagnosis and initiation of treatment.

INVESTIGATIONS

The investigations in onychomycoses are outlined in table 4.

Table 3: Differential Diagnosis
Infections: Acute/chronic paronychia, viral warts
Inflammatory conditions: Psoriasis, lichen planus, eczemas, twenty nail dystrophy
Traumatic: Occlusive footwear, nail procedures/cosmetic use
Tumors: Bowen's disease, fibroma, melanoma
Others: Systemic diseases (hyperthyroidism, diabetes), drugs causing onycholysis or pigmentation (tetracyclines, cytostatics, retinoids), nutritional deficiencies

Table 4: Investigations in Onychomycoses

Laboratory diagnostic methods	Newer techniques
• Direct microscopy (KOH test)	• Dermoscopy
• Nail plate biopsy for PAS stain	• Polymerase chain reaction (molecular diagnostics)
• Fungal culture	• Confocal laser-scanning microscopy
	• Dermatophyte test strip
	• Fluorescence microscopy
	• Raman spectroscopy

KOH, potassium hydroxide; PAS, periodic acid-Schiff.

Laboratory Diagnostic Methods

Samples for microscopy, culture, or histopathology can be collected from the nail plate or subungual debris. Standard mycological tests, potassium hydroxide (KOH) (for detection of hyphae), and fungal culture (for species identification) are usually done simultaneously; these may yield false-negative or false-positive results. Fungi grow readily on simple media containing glucose and preferably an organic nitrogen source. Many laboratories select a simple glucose/peptone agar, either with 4% sugar, 1% peptone, and an acid, pH (Sabouraud's dextrose agar) or with 2% sugar, 1% peptone, and a neutral pH (Emmons' modification). Antibacterial such as gentamicin (0.0025%) and/or chloramphenicol (0.005%) may be added to reduce contamination and, with (for isolating dermatophytes alone) or without (if NDM or candidosis is suspected) addition of cycloheximide (0.04%).[1]

Culture is advisable in following instances:

- In patients on long-term treatment without improvement
- Negative direct microscopical results
- Suspected infection by NDM
- Mixed infections (dermatophytes and NDM).

Fungal cultivation is a slow process (4 weeks) and may generate false-negative results in 40% of cases that are microscopically positive.[9] As an alternative, periodic acid-Schiff (PAS) stain of nail plate can detect presence of dermatophytes, provides quicker results, and is more sensitive.[10]

Newer Techniques

Newer diagnostic techniques can overcome the drawbacks of lack of specific and rapid methods of pathogen identification.

Dermoscopy

Dermoscopy shows two characteristic findings described as nail plate and free edge dermoscopy. Nail plate dermoscopy reveals a jagged-edge appearance of the proximal margin of onycholytic area with spikes directed to the proximal nail fold, and overall irregular pigmentation in longitudinal striae of different colors, giving an appearance similar to the aurora borealis.[11] Dermoscopy of the frontal margin of the affected nail plate shows a "ruin appearance" of the subungual hyperkeratosis.[12] Longitudinal, parallel white lines, splinter hemorrhages, and woodworm-like cavities at the distal free edge, corresponding to nail plate channels produced by tumor extension are findings present in onychomatricoma.[13]

Polymerase Chain Reaction

When the mycological analyses are negative and the clinical picture is highly suggestive of onychomycosis, polymerase chain reaction (PCR) demonstrating a sensitivity rate of 84% method is a good option.[14] Polymerase chain reaction detects specific deoxyribonucleic acid (DNA) sequence and fungi species-specific PCR methods are available. Deoxyribonucleic acid is extremely resistant and can persist even in the absence of viable hyphae; hence, DNA amplification techniques such as PCR are useful.

Confocal Laser-scanning Microscopy

Dermatophytes appear as a network of lengthy structures with high reflection and typical shape of hyphae, with demonstration of location and density of the fungi and quantifying fungal load.[15] Drawback is its inability to differentiate between dermatophytes and molds and yeasts.

Optical Coherence Tomography

Optical coherence tomography is a quick and noninvasive optical method but has low specificity (43%). White, lengthy or thready, structures with high reflection or round aggregated white structures are suggestive of onychomycosis.[16]

Dermatophyte Test Strip

This is an immunochromatography test that uses a monoclonal antibody and reacts with *Trichophyton* spp. by giving a positive signal on contact with one of these dermatophytes within 15 minutes.[17]

Fluorescence Microscopy

On fluorescent microscopy, nail clippings from suspected onychomycosis stained with PAS gives superior results than the classic KOH method.[18]

Raman Spectroscopy

Vibrational spectroscopic technique detects the molecular composition of samples based on the molecular specificity of spectral bands.[19]

TREATMENT MODALITIES

Pharmacological Therapy

Treatment of onychomycosis depends on the clinical type, the number of involved nails, and the severity of the infection.

The current recommendation is the use of an oral antifungal (terbinafine or itraconazole) because they are more effective than topical agents. However, oral treatments are limited by drug interactions and potential hepatotoxicity, especially in the elderly where the disease is most prevalent. A combination of both oral and systemic treatment is often the best choice. Monotherapy with topical antifungals is limited in following cases:[20]

- Superficial white, except in transverse or striate infections
- Distal lateral subungual onychomycosis, except in the presence of longitudinal streaks, when less than 80% of the nail plate is affected with lack of involvement of the lunula
- Contraindication to systemic antifungal.

Topical and systemic therapies of onychomycoses are outlined in tables 5 and 6.

The poor nail unit penetration limits the use of topical antifungals, and results in relapses and reinfections in 20–25% of patients.[21] Hence, penetration of a topical antifungal through the nail plate requires a vehicle that is specifically formulated for transungual delivery. Chemical penetration enhancers, such as dimethyl sulfoxide, urea, and bioadhesive polymers, are often used to improve delivery. A combination with systemic antifungals, debridement, or nail avulsion in severe onychomycosis reduces the treatment duration and increases the cure rate.[22]

Cure rates with efinaconazole 10% solution are comparable with oral itraconazole.[23] Efinaconazole and tavaborole were approved by FDA in 2014 as topical treatment of toenail onychomycosis. A phase 2b/3 study with topical luliconazole (10%) is ongoing.[24]

A large clinical trial has shown better efficacy with terbinafine than itraconazole.[25] A meta-analysis has concluded that although continuous terbinafine is generally more effective than a pulse regimen for mycological cure, both are equally effective for complete clinical cure of toenail onychomycosis.[26]

In *Candida* onychomycosis, itraconazole and fluconazole produce the best responses and terbinafine is not used as the yeast is not sensitive.[1] A careful evaluation of the patient is a must, as *Candida* onychomycosis is frequently associated with diabetes or immunodepression. In cases of lateral nail plate involvement, dermatophytomas or dystrophic onychomycosis, surgical or chemical avulsion of the nail plate combined with topical or systemic treatment may be needed.[27]

The second-generation triazoles (voriconazole, posaconazole, ravuconazole, albaconazole, pramiconazole) have broad spectrum antifungal activity, particularly to yeasts and NDMs. They have an improved safety profile and fewer drug interactions than the first-generation triazoles. However, their utility is restricted by their high cost, and these have been reserved primarily for therapy of invasive opportunistic fungal infections in immunocompromised.[20]

Table 5: Topical Therapy

Drug	Formulation	Application	Treatment duration	Organisms	Properties
Amorolfine 5%	Non-water-soluble lacquer	Once a week	6–12 months	Dermatophytes, non-dermatophyte molds and yeast	Fungistatic and fungicidal
Ciclopirox 8%	Non-water-soluble lacquer, water-soluble lacquer (improved the nail permeability)	Once daily	Fingernails: 24 weeks Toenails: 48 weeks	*Trichophyton rubrum, Scopulariopsis brevicaulis, Candida*	Fungicidal, anti-inflammatory, and anti-allergic
Efinaconazole 10%	Solution	Once daily	48 weeks	Dermatophytes, *Acremonium, Fusarium, Paecilomyces, Pseudallescheria, Scopulariopsis, Aspergillus, Cryptococcus, Trichosporon, Candida*	Fungicidal
Tavaborole 5%	Water-soluble nail solution	Once daily	48 weeks	*Candida albicans, T. rubrum, T. mentagrophytes*	Fungicidal
Tioconazole 28%	solution	Twice daily	6–12 months	Dermatophytes, *Candida, Aspergillus, Cryptococcus neoformans*	Fungistatic
Terbinafine 1%	nail solution, spray	Twice daily	Not yet established	Broad spectrum	Fungistatic and fungicidal
Tavaborole 5%	alcohol-based solution	Once daily	48 weeks	Broad spectrum	Fungicidal
Luliconazole 10%	cream	Once daily	Not yet established	*T. rubrum, Epidermophyton floccosum, C. albicans, Malassezia* subspecies, and *Aspergillus fumigatus*	fungicidal and fungistatic

Table 6: Systemic Therapy

Drugs/pregnancy category	Organisms	Dosage	Length of treatment	Common side effects	Monitoring/other
Itraconazole category C	• Dermatophytes, some • NDM, *Candida* spp.	• 200 mg per day • Pulse: 200 mg twice daily for 1 week each month	• 12 weeks continuously • Pulse • Fingernails: 6 weeks • Toenails: 12 weeks	• Headache • Diarrhea • Dyspepsia • Flatulence • Abdominal pain • Dizziness • Rash	• Pretreatment liver function test in patients with known hepatic abnormality
Terbinafine category B	• Dermatophytes, some • NDM, not *Candida* spp.	• 250 mg daily • Pulse: 500 mg daily for 1 week each month (1 pulse)	• Fingernails: 6 weeks • Toenails: 12 weeks • 2 pulses for fingernails • 4 pulses for toenails	• Gastrointestinal disturbance • Rash • Nausea • Diarrhea • Taste disturbances	• Pretreatment liver function test • Complete blood count in immune-suppressed patients
Fluconazole category D*	• Dermatophytes, • some • NDM, *Candida* spp.	• 150–450 mg • weekly	• Fingernails: 6–9 months • Toenails: 12–18 months	• Nausea • Headache • Rash • Vomiting • Diarrhea	• Pretreatment liver function test in patients with known hepatic abnormality • Not FDA-approved for onychomycosis
Griseofulvin category X	• Dermatophyte	• 500–1,000 mg daily	• Until infection clears	• Rash • Urticaria • Nausea • Vomiting • Diarrhea • Headache	• Liver function tests • Renal function tests • Complete blood count every 6–8 weeks

*For dose more than 150 mg throughout pregnancy.
NDM, non-dermatophyte mold; FDA, Food and Drug Administration.

Topical medications are recommended during pregnancy and lactation. Azoles are usually avoided during first trimester in nonmeningeal infections. Fluconazole should ideally be started after delivery, and, if not possible, after the first trimester. Itraconazole should be avoided during pregnancy and in particular, during the first trimester, and effective contraception should be continued throughout treatment and for 2 months thereafter in females of childbearing age.[28] Several modalities can be used in diabetic patients. Azole antifungals, including itraconazole and fluconazole, can elevate levels of oral hypoglycemic drugs. Terbinafine does not have significant interactions with oral hypoglycemic drugs. As there is increased prevalence of cardiac disease in diabetics, terbinafine is preferred over itraconazole.[29] Topical antifungals are safe in hepatic and renal impairment. In elderly patient with comorbidities, the following factors should be considered during systemic therapies:[20]

- Terbinafine and fluconazole: Contraindicated in hepatic and renal impairment
- Itraconazole: Contraindicated in hepatotoxicity and cardiac failure
- Griseofulvin: Contraindicated in hepatic impairment.

The current therapeutic guidelines with levels of recommendation are outlined in table 7:[20]

Table 7: British Association of Dermatologists Guidelines (2014)

Strength of recommendation	Treatment in adults
	Systemic
A	Itraconazole: First line of treatment for dermatophyte onychomycosis
B	Terbinafine: First line of treatment for dermatophyte onychomycosis, and generally preferred over itraconazole
C	Fluconazole: May be a useful alternative in patients unable to tolerate terbinafine or itraconazole
D	Griseofulvin: Lower efficacy and higher relapse rates compared with terbinafine and itraconazole
D	Combination treatment: Recommended if response to topical monotherapy is likely to be poor
	Topicals*
	Amorolfine: Useful for superficial and distal onychomycosis
	Ciclopirox: Useful for superficial and distal onychomycosis and for patients in whom systemic therapy is contraindicated
	Tioconazole: Useful for superficial and distal onychomycosis

Continued

Continued

Table 7: British Association of Dermatologists Guidelines (2014)	
	Treatment in children
	Systemic
A	Itraconazole: First line of treatment for dermatophyte onychomycosis
A	Terbinafine: First line of treatment for dermatophyte onychomycosis, and generally preferred over itraconazole
B	Fluconazole: Considered as second line if itraconazole and terbinafine is contraindicated or not tolerated
C	Griseofulvin: Considered as second line if itraconazole and terbinafine is contraindicated or not tolerated

*Tavaborole was not available at the time of the guidelines' publication, and luliconazole was undergoing a phase 3 clinical trial for onychomycosis.

Procedural Therapies

Debridement and the mechanical reduction of toenail length and thickness using nail nipper or rotating burr in combination with topical ciclopirox helps in mycological cure.[30] Benefits are due to reduced fungal load, and enhanced penetration of topical drugs into the nail unit. For patients who opt against pharmacologic treatment, debridement allows more comfort in shoe gear and reduces potential pressure on the nail bed, especially if diabetic neuropathy is present.

Nail avulsion, the separation of the nail plate from the nail bed, can be achieved nonsurgically with daily application of topical 40% urea for 1–2 weeks.[31] It is followed by application of topical antifungal once the toenail has been removed. This procedure can be useful in patients who have a needle/procedure phobia, which have peripheral vascular disease or another comorbidity precluding pharmacologic intervention, or have a single nail infected. However, removal of the nail itself will not result in clearance of the infection, even when followed by topical antifungal therapy.

Newer Treatment Modalities

Lasers

Laser systems produce cellular photodamage in the absence of exogenous dyes or other photosensitizing drugs. The laser causes photoinactivation of the fungal pathogens at a depth below the nail tissue surface leaving the surrounding tissue intact. Lasers used include:

- Carbon dioxide laser

- Neodymium-doped yttrium aluminum garnet laser
- Diode 870-nm, 930-nm laser
- Femtosecond infrared titanium sapphire laser (deeper level of penetration).

Advantages

- Food and Drug Administration approved, for improvement of the cosmetic appearance of the nail and not for mycological cure
- Minimally-invasive nature
- Few number of requested treatment sessions required.

A systematic review on the use of lasers on onychomycosis has been published, majority of cases using the 1,064 nm neodymium laser.[32] There are no studies published comparing lasers with more traditional therapies. Lasers are showing promising results in the treatment of onychomycosis, but recommendations cannot be made at this stage as the evidence is poor.

Light Therapy[33]

Light therapy includes:

- Photodynamic therapy
- Ultraviolet light therapy (UVC radiation)
- Near infrared photoinactivation therapy.

Penetration Enhancers[33]

These are novel drug delivery systems and include:

- Iontophoresis
- Low frequency ultrasound
- Microporation.

Combination Therapy[33]

It produces better treatment outcomes due to different mechanisms of action and drug synergy.

- Combination of topical and systemic antifungals: The following combinations have proved better than standalone therapies:
  - Itraconazole 200 mg daily for 3 months plus weekly applications of amorolfine 5% nail lacquer for 6 months
  - Terbinafine 250 mg daily for 3 months plus weekly applications of amorolfine 5% nail lacquer for 15 months

- Combination of surgical and medical treatment: Surgical or chemical nail avulsion (using 40% urea) in combination with oral antifungal is suitable for thick painful nails. However, the procedure itself may cause pain and disfigurement of the nail. The overall clinical results using this mode of therapy may not be satisfactory. Other combinations are chemical avulsion, with 40% urea paste combined with 1% bifonazole and combined surgical and topical therapy (ketoconazole or oxiconazole)
- Boosted antifungal therapies: Due to their inactive state, the resting fungal spores are resistant to drugs, hence, are widely considered to be responsible for low cure rates and higher rates of relapse. Boosted antifungal therapy targets the resting fungal spores by converting them into drug responsive hyphae. For this, a piece of Sabouraud's agar is applied to the nail followed by topical (boosted antifungal topical treatment–BATT) or systemic antifungal therapy (boosted oral antifungal treatment–BOAT). Pilot studies on these modalities have shown promising results.[34,35]

Treatment Endpoint

Treatment success is difficult to measure as the definition of cure for onychomycosis is variable.

- Mycological cure: Absence of fungi posttreatment, detected on negative KOH microscopy and negative mycological culture
- Clinical cure: Minimal or no residual signs and symptoms, or as 90–100% clinical improvement
- Complete cure: Combination of clinical cure and mycological cure.

After treatment initiation, clinically normal nail plate can be seen growing at the proximal end of the nail. The duration for the entire nail to grow and appear normal may take anytime between 6 months for the fingernails and up to a year or more for toenails. This is the average nail plate growth turnover rate, which is the time taken to replace the damaged nail. Ageing, consumption of chemotherapeutic drugs such as methotrexate or azathioprine, and preexisting nail diseases such as yellow nail syndrome, lichen planus, and onychomycosis itself can slow down the linear growth of nails, and hence, delay the much-anticipated treatment response.[36]

Prognosis

Prognostic indicators are enlisted in table 8.[33]

Table 8: Prognostic Indicators		
Factors	**Poor prognosis**	**Good prognosis**
Morphological	Total dystrophic variety, lateral edge involvement, thick nail plate, dermatophytoma	Superficial white onychomycosis
Host factors	Old age, immunosuppression, poor peripheral circulation, other dermatoses, e.g., nail psoriasis, genetic predisposition	Younger population
Agent factors	Nonresponsive organisms (nondermatophyte mold), drug resistance, environmental and occupational factors, occlusive footwear, prolonged contact with moisture	Dermatophytes

Recurrence, Relapse, Prophylaxis, and Prevention

Recurrence in onychomycosis is high (10–53%).[37] It could be due to relapse, which is due to inadequate or inappropriate treatment or reinfection (new infection after completing treatment). Recurrence secondary to NDM is common because of the lack of definitive treatment for these fungi.[38] A meta-analysis found that relapses are more common after treatment with itraconazole compared to terbinafine.[39] Drug resistance to antifungal agents and occurrence of biofilms is another possibility.[40,41]

Prevention of onychomycosis includes adequate treatment of concurrent tinea, screening and treating family members for coexisting tinea.[38] Recurrences can be prevented by improving feet hygiene, that is, keeping it dry, trimming nails short, using regular topical antifungals, and avoiding walking barefoot. Post-treatment prophylaxis with topical lacquer amorolfine is helpful.[37]

Treatment of Nondermatophyte Mold Onychomycoses

Nondermatophyte mold is a common pathogen isolated in cases of onychomycosis in tropical climates.[42] Also, the presence of NDM detected on culture poses a diagnostic dilemma as these pathogens are sometimes considered as contaminants. Hence, isolation of NDMs may require repeat cultures and a clinical correlation is required to determine its significance.[43] Six major criteria are generally used for the identification of NDMs. These are microscopic identification of the NDM using KOH preparation, isolation by culture, repeat isolation by culture, inoculum counting, failure to isolate a dermatophyte in culture, and histology.[2] Gupta et al. have recommended using three out of these six criteria for a definitive diagnosis of NDM, two of which should include positive microscopy and culture.[2] In general, NDM do not respond to systemic antifungals, the best choice is topical therapy associated with periodic removal of the affected nail plate. Recent studies suggest that terbinafine and itraconazole are efficacious agents for NDMs, especially for *S. brevicaulis* and *Aspergillus* species.[1]

CONCLUSION

Onychomycosis has various causative agents, presentations, and risk factors. Consequently, there is no single gold standard for the treatment of this condition. The choice of the best treatment should be made on a case-by-case basis, with consideration given to the causative agent, the number of nails involved, and the risks and benefits associated with the different treatments. An accurate diagnosis of onychomycosis that fulfils both the clinical and laboratory criteria is mandatory before initiating treatment in view of long treatment duration and the potential side effects of the antifungal agents. Consideration should also be given to the prevention of reinfection and recurrence of this chronic, difficult to eradicate condition.

Editor's Comment

Of all the types of superficial fungal infections,onychomycosis takes the longest to treat and affects the quality of life of the afflicted patient because of cosmetic disfigurement. Dr Vishalakshi Vishwanath rightly points out that both topical and medical management as well as a medical as well as surgical management leads to improvement of the condition.The different types of onychomycosis as well as their laboratory diagnosis and problem of recurrence is addressed.

Rashmi Sarkar, Seemal R Desai

REFERENCES

1. Hay RJ, Ashbee HR. Fungal infections. In: Griffiths C, Barker J, Bleiker T, Chalmers R, Creamer D, editors. Rook's Textbook of Dermatology. 9th ed. London: Wiley Blackwell; 2016. pp. 32.6-32.66.
2. Gupta AK, Drummond-Main C, Cooper EA, Brintnell W, Piraccini BM, Tosti A. Systematic review of nondermatophyte mold onychomycosis: diagnosis, clinical types, epidemiology, and treatment. *J Am Acad Dermatol.* 2012;66:494-502.
3. Proceedings of the international summit on cutaneous antifungal therapy and mycology workshop. San Francisco, California, October 21-24, 1993. *J Am Acad Dermatol.* 1994;31:S1-116.
4. Scher RK, Rich P, Pariser D, Elewski B. The epidemiology, etiology, and pathophysiology of onychomycosis. *Semin Cutan Med Surg.* 2013;32:S2-4.
5. Piraccini B, Alessandrini A. Onychomycosis: A review. *J Fungi.* 2015;1:30-43.

6. Finch J, Arenas R, Baran R. Fungal melanonychia. *J Am Acad Dermatol.* 2012;66:830-41.
7. Kaur R, Kashyap B, Bhalla P. Onychomycosis--epidemiology, diagnosis and management. *Indian J Med Microbiol.* 2008;26:108-16.
8. Allevato MA. Diseases mimicking onychomycosis. *Clin Dermatol.* 2010;28:164-77.
9. Fletcher CL, Hay RJ, Smeeton NC. Onychomycosis: the development of a clinical diagnostic aid for toenail disease. Part I. Establishing discriminating historical and clinical features. *Br J Dermatol.* 2004;150:701-5.
10. Reisberger EM, Abels C, Landthaler M, Szeimies RM. Histopathological diagnosis of onychomycosis by periodic acid-Schiff-stained nail clippings. *Br J Dermatol.* 2003;148:749-54.
11. Piraccini BM, Balestri R, Starace M, Rech G. Nail digital dermoscopy (onychoscopy) in the diagnosis of onychomycosis. *J Eur Acad Dermatol Venereol.* 2013;27:509-13.
12. De Crignis G, Valgas N, Rezende P, Leverone A, Nakamura R. Dermatoscopy of onychomycosis. *Int J Dermatol.* 2014;53:e97-9.
13. Lesort C, Debarbieux S, Duru G, Dalle S, Poulhalon N, Thomas L. Dermoscopic features of onychomatricoma: a study of 34 cases. *Dermatology.* 2015;231:177-83.
14. Arca E, Saracli MA, Akar A, Yildiran ST, Kurumlu Z, Gur AR. Polymerase chain reaction in the diagnosis of onychomycosis. *Eur J Dermatol.* 2004;14:52-5.
15. Arrese JE1, Quatresooz P, Piérard-Franchimont C, Piérard GE. Nail histomycology. Protean aspects of a human fungal bed. *Ann Dermatol Venereol.* 2003;130:1254-9.
16. Confocal laser scanning microscopy as a new valuable tool in the diagnosis of onychomycosis - comparison of six diagnostic methods. *Mycoses.* 2013;56:47-55.
17. Tsunemi Y, Takehara K, Miura Y, Nakagami G, Sanada H, Kawashima M. Screening for tineaunguium by Dermatophyte Test Strip. *Br J Dermatol.* 2014;170:328-31.
18. Idriss MH, Khalil A, Elston D. The diagnostic value of fungal fluorescence in onychomycosis. *J Cutan Pathol.* 2013;40:385-90.
19. Smijs TG, Jachtenberg JW, Pavel S, Bakker-Schut TC, Willemse-Erix D, de Haas ER, et al. Detection and differentiation of causative organisms of onychomycosis in an ex vivo nail model by means of Raman spectroscopy. *J Eur Acad Dermatol Venereol.* 2013;28:1492-9.
20. Ameen M, Lear JT, Madan V, Mohd Mustapa MF, Richardson M. British Association of Dermatologists' guidelines for the management of onychomycosis 2014. *Br J Dermatol.* 2014;171:937-58.
21. Del Rosso JQ. The role of topical antifungal therapy for onychomycosis and the emergence of newer agents. *J Clin Aesthet Dermatol.* 2014;7:10-8.
22. Tietz HJ, Hay R, Querner S, Delcker A, Kurka P, Merk HF. Efficacy of 4 weeks topical bifonazole treatment for onychomycosis after nail ablation with 40% urea: A double-blind, randomized, placebo-controlled multicenter study. *Mycoses.* 2013;56:414-21.
23. Tosti A. Efinaconazole solution 10%: topical antifungal therapy for toenail onychomycosis. *Cutis.* 2013;92:203-8.
24. Scher RK, Nakamura N, Tavakkol A. A review of a new antifungal agent for the topical treatment of onychomycosis. *Mycoses.* 2014;57:389-93.
25. Evans EG, Sigurgeirsson B. Double blind, randomised study of continuous terbinafine compared with intermittent itraconazole in treatment of toenail onychomycosis. The LION Study Group. *BMJ.* 1999;318:1031-5.
26. Gupta AK, Paquet M, Simpson F, Tavakkol A. Terbinafine in the treatment of dermatophyte toenail onychomycosis: a meta-analysis of efficacy for continuous and intermittent regimens. *J Eur Acad Dermatol Venereol.* 2013;27:267-72.
27. Lecha M, Effendy I, Feuilhade de Chauvin M, Di Chiacchio N, Baran R; Taskforce on Onychomycosis Education. Treatment options—development of consensus guidelines. *J Eur Acad Dermatol Venereol.* 2005 Sep;19:25-33.
28. Cottreau JM, Barr VO. A Review of Antiviral and Antifungal Use and Safety during Pregnancy. *Pharmacotherapy.* 2016;36:668-78.
29. Winston JA, Miller JL. Treatment on onychomycosis in diabetic patients. *J Clinical Diabetes.* 2006;24:160-6.

30. Malay DS, Yi S, Borowsky P, Downey MS, Mlodzienski AJ. Efficacy of debridement alone versus debridement combined with topical antifungal nail lacquer for the treatment of pedal onychomycosis: a randomized, controlled trial. *J Foot Ankle Surg.* 2009;48:294-308.
31. Gupta AK, Paquet M, Simpson FC. Therapies for the treatment of onychomycosis. *Clin Dermatol.* 2013;31:544-54.
32. Bristow IR. The effectiveness of lasers in the treatment of onychomycosis: a systematic review. *J Foot Ankle Res.* 2014;7:34.
33. Grover C, Khurana A. An update on treatment of onychomycosis. *Mycoses.* 2012;55:541-51.
34. Pierard GE, Pierard-Franchimont C, Arrese JE. The boosted antifungal topical treatment (BATT) for onychomycosis. *Med Mycol.* 2000;38:391-2.
35. Pierard GE, Pierard-Franchimont C, Arrese JE. The boosted oral antifungal treatment for onychomycosis beyond the regular itraconazole pulse dosing regimen. *Dermatology.* 2000;200:185-7.
36. Geyer AS, Onumah N, Uyttendaele H, Scher RK. Modulation of linear nail growth to treat diseases of the nail. *J Am Acad Dermatol.* 2004;50:229-34.
37. Sigurgeirsson B, Olafsson JH, Steinsson JB, Paul C, Billstein S, Evans EG. Long-term effectiveness of treatment with terbinafine vs itraconazole in onychomycosis: a 5-year blinded prospective follow-up study. *Arch Dermatol.* 2002;138:353-7.
38. Tosti A, Hay R, Arenas-Guzman R. Patients at risk of onychomycosis–risk factor identification and active prevention. *J Eur Acad Dermatol Venereol.* 2005;19:13-6.
39. Yin Z, Xu J, Luo D. A meta-analysis comparing long-term recurrences of toenail onychomycosis after successful treatment with terbinafine versus itraconazole. *J Dermatolog Treat.* 2012;23:449-52.
40. Mendez-Tovar LJ, Manzano-Gayosso P, Velasquez-Hernandez V, Millan-Chiu B, Hernández-Hernández F, Mondragón-González R, et al. Resistance to azolic compounds in clinical Trichophyton spp. strains. *Rev Iberoam Micol.* 2007;24:320-2.
41. Gupta AK, Daigle D, Carviel JL. The role of biofilms in onychomycosis. *J Am Acad Dermatol.* 2016;74:1241-6.
42. Leelavathi M, Tzar MN, Adawiyah J. Common organisms causing onychomycosis in tropical climate. *Sains Malaysiana.* 2012;41:697-700.
43. de Berker D. Clinical practice. Fungal nail disease. *N Engl J Med.* 2009;360:2108-1.

World Clin Dermatol. 2016;3(1):80-109.

Systemic Mycoses

Vikram K Mahajan MD

Department of Dermatology, Venereology, and Leprosy,
Dr R.P. Government Medical College, Kangra, Himachal Pradesh, India

ABSTRACT

The systemic mycoses in humans represent a diverse group of infections from fungi that are mainly saprophyte to soil and decaying vegetable material. Thus, predisposing individuals in rural areas, those involved in agricultural work and personnel handling plant material. Most reports have adult males infected frequently owing to their higher exposure risk than gender susceptibility. Although many of these infections present with cutaneous manifestations, systemic manifestations occur and may be protean.

They are broadly classified as "superficial" and "deep" mycoses depending on the tissues/sites involved. Superficial mycoses (mostly dermatophytic) involve mainly the superficial layers of skin and appendages (hair and nails) and account for more than 99% of all mycoses cases in practice. The deep mycoses are not uncommon and account for about 1% of the total mycoses cases. They can present as subcutaneous mycoses involving skin and subcutaneous tissues that may be locally invasive affecting fascial planes and bones or systemic mycoses that involve various organ systems and may also have cutaneous lesions.

Etiologically, systemic fungal infections are broadly classified as endemic mycoses due to true pathogenic fungi or opportunistic fungal infections due to several saprophytic fungi.

Opportunistic pathogens are less virulent as compared to true pathogens and infect individuals with primary or secondary immune deficiencies. Clinically, aspergillosis, zygomycosis, systemic candidiasis, penicilliosis, and pneumocystosis are common opportunistic systemic fungal infection, whereas cryptococcosis occurs both as endemic mycoses and the opportunistic infection.

Email: vkm1@rediffmail.com

© 2016 Jaypee Brothers Medical Publishers. All rights reserved.

These infections are not uncommon, have protracted clinical course, significant morbidity and poor quality of life. The prevalence of deep mycoses has increased in the present era of immune suppression. As they do not have a very characteristic clinical picture, the diagnosis depends upon high clinical suspicion, demonstration of the fungus by direct microscopy, culture or histopathology.

INTRODUCTION

Fungi with typical eukaryotic features represent a separate kingdom distinct from plants and animals and are ubiquitous. They generally help in decomposition and recycling of organic matter. Only fewer than 100 of estimated thousands of species of fungi are pathogenic to humans. Depending on the type of pathogen, conditions conducive for their growth, opportunity to infect humans, and host immune status, they will present as superficial or deep mycosis depending on the tissues/sites involved. Superficial mycoses account for more than 99% cases, involvement of superficial layers of skin, hair, and nails occurs from mostly dermatophytes. The remaining 1% are the deep mycoses, which are a group of infections involving the skin, subcutaneous tissue, fascial planes following traumatic inoculation of pathogen and present as subcutaneous mycoses, or deep/systemic mycoses representing hematogenous spread of organisms including opportunistic pathogens to osteoarticular or other organ systems, especially in immunocompromised hosts. Etiologically, systemic fungal infections are broadly classified as endemic mycoses due to true pathogenic fungi or opportunistic fungal infections due to several saprophytic fungi.

The systemic mycoses such as histoplasmosis, blastomycosis, coccidioidomycosis, and paracoccidioidomycosis are due to true pathogens with geographically defined endemic areas (Figure 1). The systemic disease primarily occurs from inhalation of the causative fungi in form of pulmonary symptoms and pneumonitis. A vast majority of infections resolve spontaneously in immune competent individuals but disseminated histoplasmosis and coccidioidomycosis may occur in immune compromised. These fungi exhibit temperature dimorphism. They exist as molds having septate hyphae with conidia at 25–30°C and in natural environment or as yeast form at 37°C and in living tissues. They are mainly saprophyte to soil and plant detritus, predisposing individuals in rural areas, those involved in agricultural work and personnel handling plant material to contracting these infections. Although both genders are exposed equally to the infection, most reports have adult males infected frequently owing to their higher exposure risk than gender susceptibility.

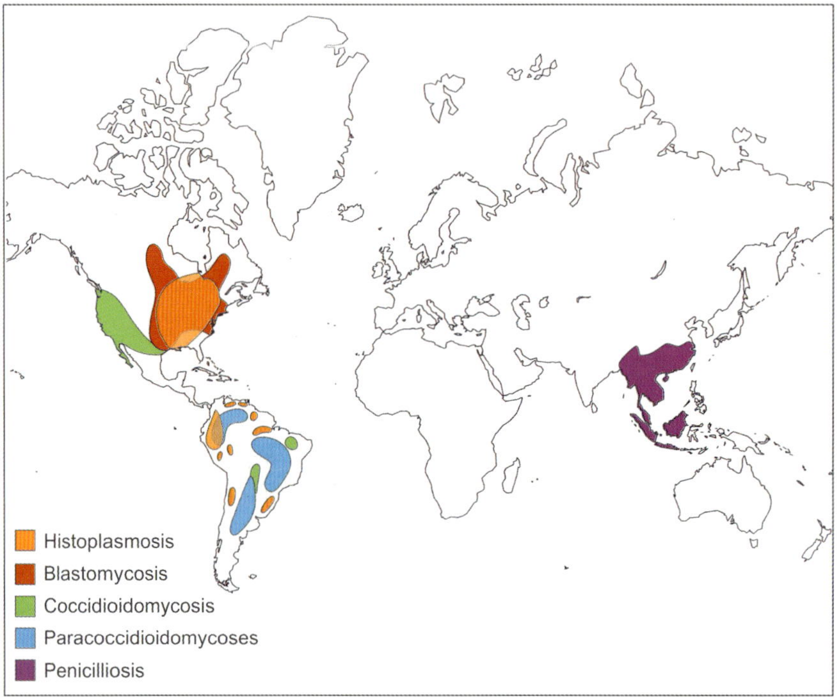

Figure 1: Geographically defined endemic areas for systemic mycoses. Source: Gupta D, Thappa DM. Deep fungal infections. Singal A, Grover C (Eds). Comprehensive Approach to Infections in Dermatology, 1st edition. New Delhi: Jaypee Brothers Medical Publishers (P) Ltd.; 2015. pp. 158-84, *with permission.*

Opportunistic pathogens are less virulent as compared to true pathogens and infect individuals with primary or secondary immune deficiencies. They impart no specific protective immunity to the infected. Clinically, systemic candidiasis, aspergillosis, zygomycosis, penicilliosis, and pneumocystosis are common opportunistic fungal infections. Cryptococcosis occurs both as endemic mycoses and the opportunistic infection.

Treatment in most cases remains unsatisfactory despite availability of several antifungal agents (Table 1). The infecting pathogen, system affected, disease severity, cost and ease of drug administration, and drug toxicity often dictate selection of a therapeutic agent. However, severe life-threatening infections will require intensive treatment. Nevertheless, recurrences are common as there are no well-defined treatment protocols and criteria for cure or treatment completion leading to protracted clinical course.

Table 1: Systemic Antifungal Agents for Treatment of Deep Mycoses

Class of drugs	Drug name	Dose (route of administration)	Adverse effects	Important drug interactions needing caution	Contraindications	Use in pregnancy and lactation
Chemical compound having iodine (76%) and potassium (23%) w/w	SSKI	30–40 drops TID daily, starting and increasing doses by 5 drops TID daily (oral)	Metallic taste, flu-like symptoms, lacrimation, gastrointestinal upsets, parotid swelling, acneiform, iododerma, hypothyroidism, pulmonary edema, and heart failure	ACE inhibitors, potassium-sparing diuretics	Known hypersensitivity, intolerance for SSKI, dermatitis herpetiformis, renal and cardiopulmonary disorders	• Pregnancy category D drug
Azoles	Itraconazole	200–400 mg/day (oral)	Abdominal discomfort, epigastric pain, vomiting, constipation, headache, liver toxicity, hypersensitivity rash, Stevens-Johnson syndrome (SJS)	Rifampicin, isoniazid, phenytoin, carbamazepine, phenobarbitone, terfenadine, astemizole, H2 blockers, proton pump inhibitors, cisapride, quinidine, pimozide, midazolam, alprazolam, triazolam, oral anticoagulants (warfarin), protease inhibitors (ritonavir, indinavir, saquinavir), zidovudine, verapamil, statins, oral antidiabetic drugs (sulfonylurea, thiazolidinediones) clarithromycin, cyclosporin, digoxin, buspirone, methylprednisolone, sirolimus, tacrolimus	Known hypersensitivity to azoles, hepatic/renal impairment	• Voriconazole is pregnancy category D drug • All other azoles are pregnancy category C drugs. They are contra-indicated in pregnancy • Itraconazole is less teratogenic than fluconazole and ketoconazole • Itraconazole is contra-indicated in lactating women but fluconazole and ketoconazole can be used • For voriconazole and posaconazole data is limited

Continued

Continued

Table 1: Systemic Antifungal Agents for Treatment of Deep Mycoses

Class of drugs	Drug name	Dose (route of administration)	Adverse effects	Important drug interactions needing caution	Contraindications	Use in pregnancy and lactation
	Fluconazole	200–600 mg/day (oral)				
	Voriconazole	4–6 mg/kg 12 hourly (IV) for severe infections followed by 100–200 mg every 12 hour orally Maintenance dose-3 mg/kg every 12 hourly IV or 50–100 mg every 12 hour (oral)	Similar to other azoles and may cause visual disturbances additionally			
	Posaconazole	Initially 200 mg 4 times/day, then 400 mg twice/day (oral)	Flu-like symptoms, gastrointestinal upset, hepatorenal toxicity, headache, confusion, uneven heart rate, easy bruising	As above and ergotamine, bromocriptine, efavirenz		
	Ravuconazole	200 mg/day (oral)	Have a similar spectrum of activity to voriconazole but limited activity against Fusarium, Scedosporium and Zygomycetes spp. in in vitro studies		Not yet approved for human use	
	Ketoconazole	It is ineffective in most of subcutaneous mycoses and not used/recommended (oral)				

Continued

Continued

Table 1: Systemic Antifungal Agents for Treatment of Deep Mycoses

Class of drugs	Drug name	Dose (route of administration)	Adverse effects	Important drug interactions needing caution	Contraindications	Use in pregnancy and lactation
Allylamines	Terbinafine	500–1,000 mg/day (oral)	Nausea, diarrhea, dyspepsia, SJS, hepatitis, headache, pruritus, hypersensitivity rash, urticaria, visual disturbances, SLE flare-up	Rifampicin, ondansetron, cimetidine, cyclosporine, antiarrhythmic (propafenone, mexiletine, flecainide, debrisoquine), tricyclic antidepressants (imipramine, clomipramine, nortriptyline, doxepin), β-blockers, narcotics (dextromethorphan, codeine, methadone, tramadol)	• Known drug hypersensitivity • Chronic or active hepatorenal disease	• Pregnancy category D drug and is contraindicated • Contraindicated in lactation
Polyenes	Liposomal Amphotericin B	Initially, 1.0 mg/kg/day (use up to 1.5 mg/kg/day for systemic infections); increased to 3–5 mg/kg/day (IV)	Chills, fever, vomiting, flushing, anaphylaxis, muscle, joint pains, renal toxicity, hypokalemia, bone marrow depression, and phlebitis at infusion site	Other nephrotoxic drugs, corticosteroids, flucytosis	Known hypersensitivity to the drug	• Safe in pregnancy and lactation • Pregnancy category C drug. Its secretion in human breast milk is not known. Use with caution
Fluorinated pyrimidine antimetabolite	5-fluorocytosine or flucytosine	50–150 mg/kg/day given four times daily (mostly combined with amphotericin B or rarely with itraconazole/fluconazole), (oral)	Gastrointestinal intolerance, bone marrow toxicity (especially in the presence of compromised renal function), photosensitivity, hypersensitivity, urticaria and angioedema, confusion or hallucinations, sedation, hearing loss	Nephrotoxic drugs, cytosine inactivates it, amphotericin B	Known hypersensitivity to the drug, renal dysfunction	

Continued

Continued

Table 1: Systemic Antifungal Agents for Treatment of Deep Mycoses

Class of drugs	Drug name	Dose (route of administration)	Adverse effects	Important drug interactions needing caution	Contraindications	Use in pregnancy and lactation
Echinocandin	Caspofungin	70 mg/m^2 on day 1 followed by 50 mg/m^2/day, (IV infusion)	• Fever, rash, nausea, vomiting, diarrhea, transient hepatorenal function derangement, hypokalemia, anemia, tachycardia, edema, cough, pleural effusion, and dyspnea • Phlebitis at infusion site • Histamine releasing drug	• Cyclosporine increases its effect/liver toxicity • Synergistic effect with amphotericin B, fluconazole, itraconazole, posaconazole, and voriconazole	• Known hypersensitivity to the drug • Safety and efficacy not established in neonates and infants more than 3 months of age	• Pregnancy category C drug. Its secretion in human breast milk is not known. Use with caution

SSKI, saturated solution of potassium iodide; TID, three times a day; IV, intravenous; ACE, angiotensin converting enzyme; SLE, systemic lupus erythematosus..
Source: Mahajan VK. Subcutaneous mycoses. Singal A, Grover C (Eds). Comprehensive Approach to Infections in Dermatology, 1st edition. New Delhi: Jaypee Brothers Medical Publishers (P) Ltd.; 2015. pp. 116-57, *with permission*.

HISTOPLASMOSIS

Histoplasmosis (synonyms: Darling's disease, Cave disease, Ohio valley disease, reticuloendotheliosis) is caused by dimorphic fungus *Histoplasma capsulatum* var. *capsulatum*.

Epidemiology

Histoplasma capsulatum infection is contracted through exposure to fungal spores in soil contaminated with bird and bat droppings in warm and moist climates. Birds, fowl, and bats are the significant reservoirs for histoplasmosis and endemic areas can harbor infectious fungal spores. The disease is endemic in the East central part of the United States (Mississippi, Missouri, and Ohio valleys) and *H. capsulatum* var. *capulatum* coexists with another variety, *H. capsulatum* var. *duboisii*, in the western and central regions of sub-Saharan Africa. *Histoplasma capsulatum* is endemic in East Indian states like West Bengal but new endemic foci are being identified among human immunodeficiency virus (HIV)/acquired immunodeficiency syndrome (AIDS) affected.

Clinical Features

Although immune competent hosts can contract the disease, there is increased risk for the disseminated form in immune compromised hosts. Clinically, the infection follows inhalation of fungal spores presenting as acute, chronic cavitary and disseminated pulmonary histoplasmosis. The infection spreads further to lymph nodes, spleen, and other systems via hematogenous spread. Rarely, primary cutaneous histoplasmosis occurs from direct cutaneous inoculation of the pathogen.

The acute pulmonary histoplasmosis has usual symptoms of acute lung infection and shows diffuse mottling or localized infiltration in chest roentgenogram. It may be associated with erythema multiforme or erythema nodosum. However, acute pulmonary form is usually considered uncommon as a majority of infected persons in endemic areas are asymptomatic despite positive reactions to histoplasmin testing. Chronic pulmonary histoplasmosis usually affects adults presenting with pulmonary consolidation and cavitation mimicking tuberculosis.

The disseminated histoplasmosis is uncommon but frequently a fatal form of disease. Its acute form mostly occurs in infants or immunosuppressed patients especially HIV/AIDS affected persons with low (<200 cells/mm^3) CD4 counts. The lungs show features of consolidation and have associated fever, anemia, loss of appetite, generalized lymphadenopathy, and enlarged liver and spleen. Polymorphic skin lesions in the form of papules, small nodules or small molluscum-like lesions often develop as a manifestation of disseminated infection (Figure 2) and may

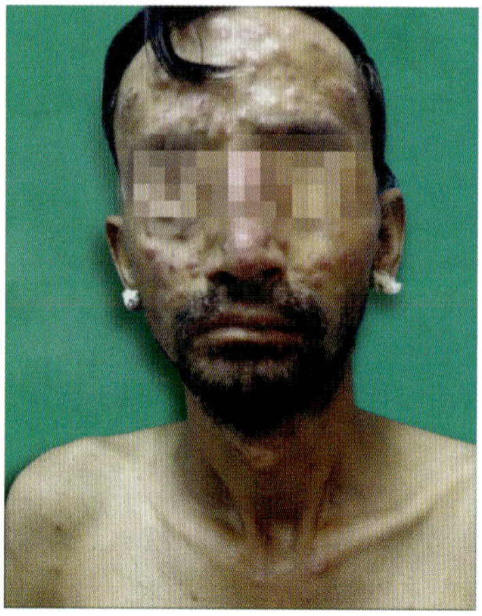

Figure 2: Disseminated polymorphic skin lesions as papules, small nodules, few crusted lesions in a human immunodeficiency virus/acquired immune deficiency syndrome patient. He also had similar lesions over trunk and extremities.

subsequently form shallow ulcers. The chronic disseminated form may appear months or years after a patient has left an endemic area. The most common presenting features are oral or pharyngeal ulceration, hepatosplenomegaly, and adrenal insufficiency.

Primary cutaneous histoplasmosis is uncommon and a nodule or indurated ulcer develops at the site of traumatic inoculation of the organism, often accompanied by local lymphadenopathy.

Diagnosis

The diagnosis of pulmonary histoplasmosis is based on clinical suspicion in the setting of failed antitubercular therapy and immune suppression. The primary pulmonary histoplasmosis resembles tuberculosis at all stages and pneumonias of viral/bacterial origin, while the disseminated form may mimic visceral leishmaniasis, brucellosis, and malaria. The cutaneous and mucocutaneous lesions need differentiation from sporotrichosis and other mycoses, syphilis, toxoplasmosis, and neoplasias.

Pathology

Microscopic examination of biopsy specimens will show a diffuse infiltrate comprising predominantly of histiocytes admixed with plasma cells, few lymphocytes, and eosinophils with characteristic intracellular small (2–4 μm)

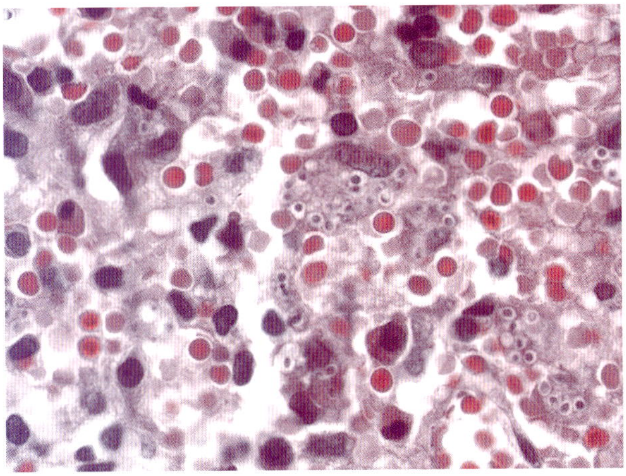

Figure 3: Numerous yeast cells of *Histoplasma capsulatum* are visualized in histology sections from skin biopsy (H&E, x400).

sized eosinophilic round/ovoid yeast forms with a rim of clearing often within the macrophages (Figure 3). Demonstration of fungus in cytology smears from skin lesions/lymph node appears useful for rapid diagnosis. These are easily identified in tissue sections stained with periodic acid-Schiff (PAS) or Gomori methenamine silver or sputum direct smears/potassium hydroxide (KOH) mounts from clinical samples (pus, skin scrapings, lymph node aspirates). Mycelial forms are seen rarely in tissue.

Culture of Causative Fungus

The confirmation of diagnosis of histoplasmosis depends upon the isolation by culture in laboratory and identification of the small intracellular yeast-like cells of *Histoplasma* from clinical samples such as sputum, peripheral blood, bone marrow, or biopsy specimens (Figure 4). The fungus grows in mold form at room temperature as white, cottony colonies on Sabouraud's dextrose agar (SDA) and produces two types of spores: (i) the typical large (8–15 µm), rounded, tuberculate macroconidia and (ii) small microconidia that are infectious, can be visualized in lactophenol cotton blue (LCB) mounts (Figure 5). It also demonstrates temperature dimorphism.

Other Diagnostic Methods

Serology is often useful in diagnosis and a rising complement-fixation titer indicates dissemination. As the presence of antibodies to specific H and M antigens correlates well with active or recent infection, detection of precipitins

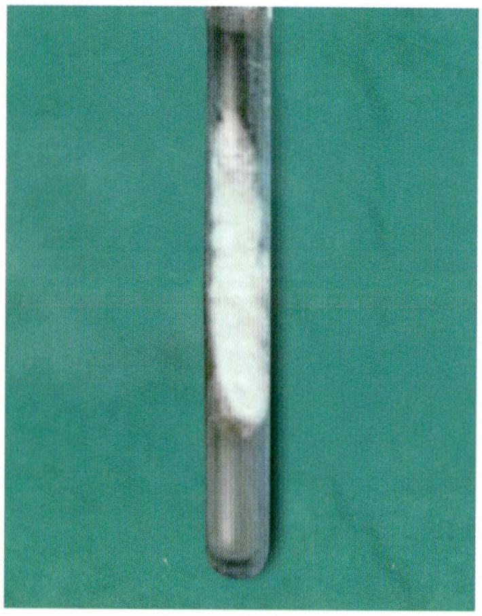

Figure 4: Cottony white colonies of *Histoplasma capsulatum* on Sabouraud's dextrose agar at 30°C.

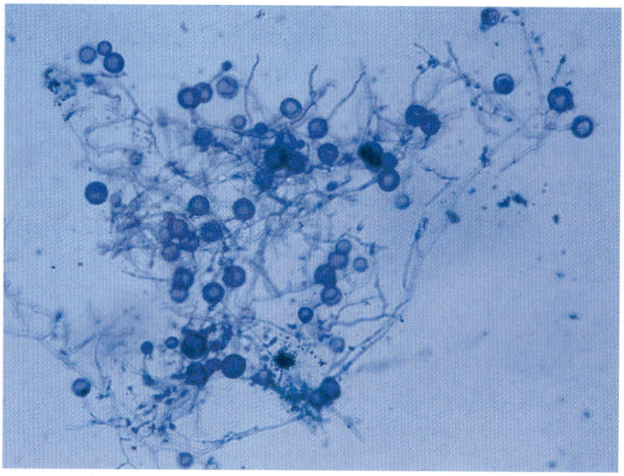

Figure 5: Large, rounded, unicellular, tuberculate macroconidia spores of *Histoplasma capsulatum* in lactophenol cotton blue mount (x400).

by immunodiffusion is valuable diagnostic tool. Similarly, detection of circulating *Histoplasma* antigen by serologic or urine tests is particularly helpful in patients with AIDS.

The intradermal histoplasmin skin test is often negative and of no help in diagnosis in patients from endemic regions and with disseminated histoplasmosis.

Histoplasma antigen detected in the bronchoalveolar lavage (BAL) by polymerase chain reaction (PCR) provides a rapid diagnosis in chronic pulmonary histoplasmosis and in patients with progressive disseminated histoplasmosis.

Treatment

Treatment with amphotericin B is highly effective and recommended along with itraconazole for all forms of histoplasmosis for long-term survival. Surgical excision of primary cutaneous histoplasmosis lesion under amphotericin/ itraconazole coverage appears curative. However, immune compromised patients will need itraconazole prophylaxis for life. The use of highly active antiretroviral therapy (HAART) reduces the requirement for maintenance therapy in some cases. Posaconazole and fluconazole are useful alternatives. The acute pulmonary forms of histoplasmosis rarely require treatment with specific antifungals.

BLASTOMYCOSIS

Blastomycosis (synonyms: North American blastomycosis, Gilchrist's disease) is a chronic systemic mycosis caused by the dimorphic pathogen *Blastomyces dermatitidis*.

Epidemiology

The disease is particularly endemic in the Mississippi and Ohio River valleys of North America, Great Lakes region, and the Southeastern states. Sporadically, cases occur in Africa, Middle East, and India. Although *B. dermatitidis* has been isolated from bats in India, the soil is probably the most important source of infection.

Clinical Features

Three forms of blastomycosis: (i) primary cutaneous, (ii) pulmonary and (iii) disseminated occur clinically. The infection is via inhalation of the organism and lungs are typically the first site of infection. Nevertheless, secondary cutaneous dissemination is common and may be the first sign of disease, seen sometimes even in the absence of overt pulmonary disease.

Primary cutaneous blastomycosis is uncommon and results from direct traumatic inoculation of the pathogen as among workers or pathologists handling the material in a laboratory. An erythematous, indurated lesion with ulcer (chancre) develops at inoculation site in 1–2 weeks and is associated with lymphangitis and lymphadenopathy. Spontaneous healing may occur within a few weeks or months.

Pulmonary blastomycosis resembles tuberculosis and may show no symptoms or present with low-grade fever, chest pain, cough, and hemoptysis. Erythema nodosum occurs occasionally. It is not uncommon for pulmonary lesion to resolve spontaneously or there may be cavity formation with lung abscess. The untreated disease may disseminate often with fatal consequences.

The onset of disseminated blastomycosis commonly presents with skin lesions that are often multiple, distributed symmetrically usually over face and the extremities. The early lesion, a papule or nodule, evolving to pus discharging ulcer and enlarges to form a hyperkeratotic lesion over a period. The lesions tend to heal in the center with scarring and spread at the periphery. In addition to skin, dissemination may occur to involve bones, epididymis, and the adrenal glands. Though uncommon, widespread blastomycosis may occur in AIDS patients.

Diagnosis

The chronic granulomatous skin lesions need differentiation from tuberculosis, other deep mycoses, syphilis, leprosy, pyoderma gangrenosum, iododerma, and neoplasia. Pulmonary lesions necessitate differentiation from tuberculosis and other infections.

Pathology

Histology of skin lesion demonstrates pseudoepitheliomatous hyperplasia, suppurative and granulomatous inflammation and round yeast forms with characteristic broad-based budding and thick, double-contoured walls that help in differentiating blastomycosis from other fungal infections. The single budding yeasts can be better visualized in Gomori-Grocott and PAS-stained smears. The fungus can be visualized in KOH mounts from pus, skin scrapings, or sputum as refractile, rounded, thick-walled, budding spherical yeast cells.

Culture of Causative Organism

The fungus can be grown on SDA supplemented with antibiotics or potato dextrose agar at 25–30°C, and it exhibits temperature dimorphism. The colonies grow in 2 weeks and are waxy and cottony initially and become white to tan. Small (2–5 μm), rounded or pear-shaped conidia are visualized microscopically on short stalks arising at right angles from the hyphae.

Other Diagnostic Methods

A characteristic precipitin line, the E band, due to precipitating antibodies to *B. dermatitidis* in the sera of patients has been described in a significant number of proven cases. However, antibody testing has low sensitivity and specificity. Exoantigen testing and nucleic acid probes are safe and rapid methods to identify the organism most accurately especially in urine samples. A second-generation enzyme-linked immunosorbent assay (ELISA) for detection of antigen in BAL fluid is another useful test for diagnosing pulmonary blastomycosis.

Treatment

Oral itraconazole appears effective choice in most cases. Ketoconazole is an alternative therapy when tolerated. Amphotericin B is used for the treatment of widespread disseminated blastomycosis.

COCCIDIOIDOMYCOSIS

Coccidioidomycosis (synonyms: valley fever, desert rheumatism, San Joaquin valley fever, coccidioidal granuloma. Posadas' disease) is caused by fungal species *Coccidioides immitis* and *Coccidioides posadasii*.

Epidemiology

Coccidioidomycosis is endemic in deserts of the Southwestern states of America, and in parts of Central and South America climatic conditions of very high summer temperatures and low annual rainfall. The fungus *Coccidioides* is a soil saprophyte and the two species (i) *C. immitis* and (ii) *C. posadasii* are usually indistinguishable on clinical and microbiological characteristics alone. However, both are distinct in their endemic behavior; *C. immitis* occurs only in California and *C. posadasii* elsewhere. Exposure to infective organism may occur among visitors to an endemic area. In India, proven coccidioidomycosis was seen in patients returning from Arizona, an endemic area for coccidioidomycosis.

Clinical Features

The usual route of infection is inhalation of arthroconidia causing pulmonary infection. Cutaneous infection uncommonly occurs from direct implantation into skin from trauma.

Primary pulmonary coccidioidomycosis, the most common form may occur as asymptomatic infection, simulate influenza, or present as a lung infection associated with fever, cough, and pleuritic chest pain. While erythema nodosum and erythema multiforme are common cutaneous features, early, generalized, macular and erythematous rash occur in few. The symptom complex comprising skin lesions, fever and arthralgias is labeled as "valley fever" by locals in the San Joaquin valley of south central California. The chronic pulmonary disease resembles tuberculosis and presents with chronic cough and usually no skin lesions.

Disseminated coccidioidomycosis involving skin, subcutaneous tissues, bones, joints, and other organs develops in less than 0.5% of infected individuals and usually in immune suppressed patients. The skin lesions include papules, nodules, granulomas, abscesses, ulcers, or discharging sinuses with underlying bone or joint disease. Meningitis is another important complication of disseminated infection. Persistent pneumonia, skin lesions, and widespread dissemination can occur in AIDS patients.

Primary cutaneous coccidioidomycosis is rare infection and occurs following traumatic implantation of pathogen. After 1–3 weeks, an indurated nodule develops at the site of inoculation that is followed by regional lymphadenopathy.

Diagnosis

The chronic granulomatous skin lesions need differentiation from tuberculosis, other deep mycoses, syphilis, leprosy, pyoderma gangrenosum, iododerma, and neoplasia. Pulmonary infection requires differentiation from tuberculosis and other infections. The distinct feature is development of erythema nodosum early in the disease course. Coccidioidomycosis infection must be suspected in patients returning from endemic regions. The usual differentials to cutaneous involvement in disseminated disease the include other infective and noninfective granulomatous diseases and other mycotic infections.

Pathology

The biopsy findings of specific lesions are pathognomic and reveal characteristic endospore-containing double-walled spherules measuring 30–60 μm in diameter when mature and a suppurative granulomatous reaction with histiocytes, lymphocytes, and giant cells typically surrounds the spherules and released endospores. Immature spherules stain better with PAS and silver methenamine stains for easy identification. Mycelium is rarely seen in histopathologic sections.

The globular spherules can also be demonstrated in KOH mounts prepared from clinical samples such as sputum, cerebrospinal fluid or pus.

Culture of Causative Organism

The confirmation of diagnosis depends upon the isolation by culture on SDA, BHI agar, or potato dextrose agar 2–3 weeks after incubation at 28–30°C. The fast-growing colonies of *C. immitis* and *C. posadasii* are initially waxy then cottony and white to tan. Microscopically, chains of arthrospores at intervals on barrel-shaped mycelium are visualized.

Other Diagnostic Methods

Serologic tests for detection of immunoglobulin M (IgM) and IgG antibodies between 1 and 3 weeks and 2 and 28 weeks, respectively are of value in the diagnosis and prognosis of coccidioidomycosis. Precipitins develop in about 90% of infected individuals within 2–6 weeks but are short-lived. Other lab tests include enzyme immunoassays, immunodiffusion, and complement fixation. Complement-fixing antibodies are characteristic of more severe infections. Exoantigen testing and nucleic acid probes (AccuProbe assays), conventional nested PCR tests are used to identify the causative fungus.

Intradermal test with coccidioidin is of little diagnostic value but useful for epidemiological studies. Spherulin derived from the tissue form of *C. immitis* is superior to coccidioidin in detecting cutaneous hypersensitivity. Anergy suggests disseminated disease and is a poor prognostic sign.

Treatment

No specific therapy is necessary in the primary pulmonary infection and treatment with oral itraconazole or other azoles will not remit symptoms in patients with erythema nodosum. The outcome of systemic therapy with amphotericin B, itraconazole, or fluconazole for disseminated disease remains variable. Meningitis and progressive disseminated infection involving multiple sites are usually refractory to therapy. The usefulness of voriconazole and posaconazole in coccidioidomycosis is currently under evaluation.

PARACOCCIDIOIDOMYCOSIS

Paracoccidioidomycosis (synonyms: South American blastomycosis, Brazilian blastomycosis, Lutz-Splendore-Almeida disease) is caused by the dimorphic fungus *Paracoccidioides brasiliensis*.

Epidemiology

The disease is endemic in Central and South America (Argentina, Brazil, Colombia, Ecuador, and Venezuela). In most cases, infection occurs via inhalation of the conidia from the environment.

Clinical Features

It is acquired through the respiratory tract and is an insidious, chronic, and progressive systemic infection that primarily involves lungs manifesting as productive cough, fever, and weight loss while lymph nodes and mucocutaneous involvement is usually secondary as direct inoculation of the fungus into skin or mucous membranes is not common. Paracoccidioidomycosis is uncommon in AIDS patients and young adults or older children may develop widespread infection without recognizable predisposing factors.

The primary pulmonary disease (primary pulmonary complex) is subclinical or mild in most patients and acute form of pulmonary infection is rare. The pulmonary infection tends to be chronic and often slowly progressive. The pulmonary lesions may be bilateral and nodular on chest X-ray and there is often extensive fibrosis. The enlarged and tender cervical lymph nodes that are adherent to the overlying skin may eventually suppurate forming scrofuloderma-like chronic sinuses. Other systemic sites of involvement include the spleen, intestines, lungs, and liver.

Mucocutaneous involvement commonly occurs in progressive disseminated disease. Oral or circumoral lesions are common and may also occur in the nose, conjunctivae, or around the anus. These lesions may be small granulomatous papulonodules or ulcers that heal with scarring and considerable deformity.

Primary cutaneous paracoccidioidomycosis occurs from traumatic inoculation of causative fungus into the skin resulting in development of a verrucous papule, plaque or ulcer.

Diagnosis

The usual clinical differentials include tuberculosis, leishmaniasis, and other deep mycoses.

Pathology

Histologically, paracoccidioidomycosis needs differentiation from blastomycosis. Features include pseudoepitheliomatous hyperplasia accompanied by suppurative and granulomatous inflammation with yeast cells found within and outside of giant cells. Presence of large, thick-walled organisms (2–30 μm in size) with multiple narrow-based buds and budding pattern in tissue sections is diagnostic. The organisms can be visualized better in tissue sections stained with methenamine silver (Grocott modification).

Characteristic multiple round budding yeasts with parent cell surrounded by multiple small buds (captain's wheel appearance) can be visualized in KOH mounts from clinical samples such as sputum, exudates, and scrapings.

Culture of Causative Organism

The organism is dimorphic and produces a cottony mycelial-phase growth on SDA at room temperature, whereas the characteristic yeast phase can be induced on enriched media such as BHI agar at 37°C.

Other Diagnostic Methods

Serology using immunodiffusion assay and a complement-fixation test is helpful in confirming the diagnosis. Antigen-detection tests are useful in monitoring patients with disseminated disease. Immunoblot assay for detection of antibody to a 43 kDa antigen has high specificity.

Treatment

Itraconazole remains the treatment of choice in most cases leading to remissions in 3–6 months. Ketoconazole is an effective alternative when not contraindicated. However, relapses are common and requiring long-term follow-up. Intravenous amphotericin B is preferred for extensive disease, those with the progressive disseminated infection, and in severely ill patients. Residual severe pulmonary or intraoral fibrosis after treatment may occur.

CRYPTOCOCCOSIS

Cryptococcosis (synonyms: torulosis, European blastomycosis) is caused by an encapsulated yeast *Cryptococcus neoformans* comprising three variants: (i) *C. neoformans* var. *neoformans*, (ii) *C. neoformans* var. *gattii*, and (iii) *C. neoformans* var. *grubii*. The *C. neoformans* var. *neoformans* isolates have A, D, or AD capsular serotypes and *C. neoformans* var. *gattii* isolates are serotype B or C. It suggested that the *C. neoformans* var. *grubii* serotype A is a part of *C. neoformans* var. *neoformans*.

Epidemiology

The *C. neoformans* and *C. neoformans* var. *grubii* can be isolated from pigeon excreta and *C. neoformans* var. *gattii* is found in the debris of certain eucalyptus trees in the tropics and California. Cryptococcosis occurs worldwide including India and individuals with immune deficiency due to AIDS, malignant lymphomas, sarcoidosis, collagen disease, carcinoma, or on systemic immunosuppressive therapy are particularly susceptible. *C. neoformans* and *C. neoformans* var. *grubii* are isolated more commonly from patients with AIDS than *C. neoformans* var. *gattii*.

Clinical Features

The main portal of entry is through inhalation into the lungs and there is a marked predilection for the brain and meninges. The cutaneous lesions develop from dissemination or rarely due to direct inoculation.

The initial pulmonary disease is usually asymptomatic and limited. Pulmonary infection occurs in about 10% patients with meningitis. Chest signs include nodular shadows, cavitations, and pleural effusion in chest roentgenograms.

Involvement of CNS often predominates manifesting as chronic meningitis or as focal brain lesions simulating tumor. Meningitis is most common feature with signs of meningitis, altered consciousness, and cranial nerve palsies. These signs are usually expressed weakly in AIDS patients.

Mucocutaneous lesions occur in about 10% cases. They are polymorphic and are seldom pathognomonic. These are subcutaneous nodules, acneiform papules and pustules, molluscum contagiosum-like lesions, or abscesses that ulcerate. Punched out ulcers with distinct rolled edges may develop sometimes in primarily unaffected skin. Cutaneous lesions signify disseminated disease in patients with HIV/AIDS and require careful evaluation and long-term follow-up. Visceral cryptococcosis occurs from dissemination of fungus to any organ or tissue such as heart, testis, prostate, and eye. The prostate gland plays a significant role in persistence of genitourinary infection during treatment. Osseous cryptococcosis involving any bony site is seen in 5–10% of patients with disseminated disease. Involvement of vertebrae is the most common.

Primary cutaneous cryptococcosis is rare and occurs following direct inoculation of organisms into the skin. The lesions are usually solitary nodules that may ulcerate. Local lymphadenopathy also develops.

Diagnosis

The diagnosis is based on clinical suspicion especially in immune compromised individuals. Pulmonary and CNS cryptococcosis can be mistaken for pulmonary tuberculosis, other systemic mycoses, or other infective causes of meningitis. Cryptococcal skin lesions can mimic molluscum contagiosa or cutaneous neoplasia in AIDS patients. Imaging studies for pulmonary cryptococcosis will reveal parahilar infiltrate and dense spherical shadows (cryptococcomas).

Pathology

Two basic histologic patterns, gelatinous and granulomatous, occur depending upon age of the lesions. Early lesions are gelatinous and contain masses of encapsulated budding yeast cells with very little tissue reaction. The capsules of the cells can be stained using the mucicarmine or Alcian blue stains. Granulomatous pathology and a pronounced tissue reaction consisting of histiocytes with areas of necrosis usually suggests older lesion. The yeast cells are scanty and mainly intracellular within the giant cells and histiocytes.

Culture of Causative Fungus

It is imperative to culture suspicious clinical samples obtained from organ system involved in immune compromised patients for confirmation of clinical diagnosis. *Cryptococcus neoformans* grows well on SDA or BHI agar at 26 and 37°C. The colonies are soft, cream to pale brown and usually mucoid. Cryptococci are large (5–15 μm), budding yeast cells with distinct gelatinous capsules. The organism can also be visualized on direct microscopy in India ink or Nigrosin mounts from cerebrospinal fluid or pus. Its ability to produce urease or pigment on Guizotia seed medium (Staib medium) is characteristic biochemical feature.

Other Diagnostic Methods

Serological tests are rapid, specific, and particularly useful in disseminated or CNS infections. Serodiagnosis is dependent on the detection of cryptococcal capsular antigen by a latex agglutination test or an ELISA. While immune competent patients with single localized skin lesions are often antigen negative, high titers in serum and cerebrospinal fluid occur in patients with AIDS. Molecular diagnostic techniques include ribosomal ribonucleic acid (rRNA) or conventional PCR to detect infection.

Treatment

Combination of intravenous amphotericin B and flucytosine remains the standard first-line treatment in non-AIDS and immune competent patients. Alternatively, fluconazole or itraconazole can be used in patients having only focal disease as limited to skin, no serious underlying disease or no systemic spread. In patients with AIDS, intravenous amphotericin B with or without flucytosine is given for initial 10–14 days followed by fluconazole for long-term maintenance and most patients on HAART appear to achieve remission.

SYSTEMIC CANDIDIASIS

The majority of invasive *Candida* infections are due to four pathogenic species: (i) *Candida albicans*, (ii) *Candida glabrata*, (iii) *Candida parapsilosis*, and (iv) *Candida tropicalis*. *C. albicans*, the most common of all, is a commensal of the alimentary tract, cutaneous, and mucocutaneous areas.

Epidemiology

Candidiasis is the most common opportunistic mycosis worldwide. *Candida albicans* is the most common infective species and becomes pathogenic when normal equilibrium between pathogen and the host is disturbed as in immune suppressed individuals. Extremes of age, prolonged treatment with antibiotics, corticosteroids, or other cytotoxic/immunosuppressive agents, diseases like HIV/AIDS, diabetes mellitus and neoplasias and substance abuse are some of the predisposing factors. Esophageal candidiasis is also considered one of the AIDS-defining diseases. Systemic infection via intravenous infusion lines is another important mode of acquiring the disease.

Clinical Features

Systemic *Candida* infection commonly involves liver, spleen, muscle, kidney, retina, and heart valves. Renal involvement is the most common in systemic disease manifesting as diffuse renal abscesses, renal papillary necrosis, urethral obstruction, and progressive renal insufficiency. Prolonged antibiotic treatment of preexisting valvular disease, cardiac valve prosthesis, and drug addiction predispose a patient to *Candida* endocarditis. Tachycardia, hypotension, dyspnea, and high fever in a debilitated patient particularly with indwelling catheters, hyperalimentation and extensive antibiotic therapy suggests systemic *Candida* septicemia. Other manifestations include muscle pain, endophthalmitis, and renal involvement. Cutaneous lesions are uncommon in *Candida* septicemia.

Cutaneous lesions of disseminated candidiasis, mostly in patients with immune suppression, usually present as firm erythematous papules or nodules often with a pale center over trunk and extremities. They may become purpuric in patients with thrombocytopenia. Pustules, abscesses, and ecthyma gangrenosum-like lesions can occur. Among all, *C. tropicalis* is more likely to produce cutaneous lesions.

Diagnosis

The diagnosis is mostly on clinical suspicion especially in immune compromised individuals. Other systemic mycoses, tuberculosis, neoplasms, and bacterial infections need differentiation.

Pathology

Although a biopsy is seldom needed, demonstration of *Candida* cells in the histologic sections of a skin lesion provides a rapid diagnosis even before blood culture is positive. Other features are parakeratosis, spongiosis, subcorneal pustules and fungal pseudohyphae and yeast in stratum corneum. *Candida* in tissue sections is usually identified as small, oval or spherical, thin-walled budding yeast (5–7 μm in diameter) and long delicate aseptate pseudohyphae.

Culture of Causative Fungus

The *Candida* species can be cultured on SDA from clinical samples. Culture from blood samples may be negative because of transient nature of *Candida* septicemia but it will yield positive results when *Candida* colonizes in-dwelling catheters. Demonstration of the budding yeast cells and mycelial elements in KOH or LCB mounts from culture isolates or direct smears will be diagnostic.

Other Diagnostic Methods

Serological tests used for detection of specific circulating candidal antigens, mannan, enolase or Hsp 90, or measuring the metabolites such as arabinitol.

Latex agglutination and immunodiffusion for antibodies of *Candida* species are useful diagnostic techniques for diagnosis of systemic candidiasis in immunocompetent persons. Detection and measurement of *Candida* antigen by latex agglutination is also available. Counter-immunoelectrophoresis detects precipitins. However, the results are liable to misinterpretation as significant number of healthy persons may have antibodies to *Candida* spp. and the infection mostly occurs in immune compromised individuals. *Candida* enolase antigenemia is indicative. Deoxyribonucleic acid (DNA) probes for diagnosis are mainly available for research labs.

Treatment

Amphotericin B remains the first-line treatment in neutropenic patients with candidemia. Liposomal formulations are better tolerated even in higher doses than the conventional preparation. Amphotericin B is combined with flucytosine for treating candidal meningitis. Although resistance to fluconazole and ketoconazole is frequent in certain non-*albicans Candida* spp., fluconazole forms a first-line therapy for deep candidal infections in both immune competent and immune compromised patients. Response to voriconazole and caspofungin is encouraging in invasive candidiasis in neutropenic patients with solid organ transplant.

ASPERGILLOSIS

Aspergillosis is caused by members of the genus *Aspergillus* that is *A. niger*, *A. fumigatus*, and *A. flavus*. These are ubiquitous molds in environment and saprophytes to soil and decaying plant matter. Severe disease may occur from reactivation of endogenous infection in predisposed persons due to immunosuppression from underlying diseases or drug therapy, prolonged neutropenia, organ transplant recipients, chronic graft versus host disease.

Epidemiology

Transmission to humans is via inhalation of fungal spores. Bronchopulmonary aspergillosis, aspergilloma, bronchial asthma due to hypersensitivity reaction, and cerebral aspergillosis are common presentations reported worldwide including India. *Aspergillus fumigatus* is the most common species in both allergic and invasive diseases, while *A. flavus* commonly infect immune compromised patients. *Aspergillus niger* and *A. fumigatus* cause aspergillomas while *A. niger* is frequently reported in otomycosis and primary cutaneous aspergillosis.

Clinical Features

Although aspergillosis can affect any organ system, lungs remain the most frequently affected organ manifesting as allergic bronchopulmonary aspergillosis, chronic necrotizing pulmonary aspergillosis, aspergilloma, and invasive aspergillosis. Hematogenous dissemination beyond lungs occurs in severely immunocompromised potentially causing corneal ulceration, endophthalmitis, rhinosinusitis, fungemia, osteomyelitis, and abscesses in the myocardium, kidney, liver, spleen, and soft tissues.

Hypersensitivity response to the *A. fumigatus* colonizing tracheobronchial tree causes allergic bronchopulmonary aspergillosis manifesting with symptoms similar to those of asthma. However, bronchial plugging is more severe and shows features of lung collapse distal to bronchial occlusion. Pulmonary eosinophilia, episodic airway obstruction, and abundant fungi in culture are constant features.

Chronic necrotizing pulmonary aspergillosis is a subacute form usually seen in patients with some immunosuppression as from chronic alcoholism, underlying lung disease or chronic corticosteroid therapy. It often remains unrecognized for weeks or months and causes progressive pulmonary disease with nodular shadows, halo sign, consolidation, and cavitary changes in chest X-ray.

Invasive aspergillosis is rapidly progressing and often a fatal infection usually in severely immune suppressed individuals including patients with profound neutropenia, bone marrow or solid organ transplant, HIV/AIDS, or chronic granulomatous disease. Dissemination to other organs particularly the central nervous system can occur in about 10% cases. This infection is characterized by invasion of blood vessels resulting in multifocal infiltrates which are often wedge shaped, pleural based, and cavitary.

The aspergilloma or fungus ball develops from colonization of a preexisting lung cavity from tuberculosis or other diseases. Uniform, round, or oval opacity with a radiolucent crescent (Monod's sign) over the upper part and shifting of density with change of position is characteristic. Episodes of severe hemoptysis can occur.

Cutaneous aspergillosis is usually from secondary dissemination and skin lesions begin as small, discrete, erythematous papules that become pustular. *Aspergillus* species can colonize burn wounds. Primary cutaneous Aspergillosis is rare and characterized by polymorphic lesions such as multiple nodules, plaques with pustules, abscesses, folliculitis, ulcers, eschar, or cellulitis with purpuric discoloration.

Diagnosis

Diagnosis is usually on clinical suspicion in predisposed individuals presenting with characteristic systemic signs and symptoms, skin lesions, and unremitting fever not responding to antibiotic therapy. Other systemic mycoses, tuberculosis, neoplasms, and bacterial infections need differentiation.

Pathology

Characteristic branching septate hyphae can be visualized in KOH mounts or histology sections from biopsy material, surgical specimens, sputum or bronchoalveolar lavage, and tissue debris from cases of suspected aspergillosis. Tissue sections stained with methenamine silver staining are better for visualization.

Other Diagnostic Methods

Molecular diagnostic methods are employed for rapid diagnosis of invasive aspergillosis. Detection of precipitins by immunodiffusion test or counter-immunoelectrophoresis is useful and specific diagnostic method for aspergillosis in immunocompetent persons. Enzyme immunoassay for serum galactomannan antigen detection is used for early diagnosis of invasive aspergillosis in immunocompromised hosts.

Treatment

Voriconazole, amphotericin B, and itraconazole are preferred therapeutic agents for invasive aspergillosis that is often associated with significant morbidity and mortality. Posaconazole and amphotericin B are alternatives for patients intolerant to voriconazole. Itraconazole is the current drug of choice for chronic disseminated aspergillosis. Although largely underevaluated, echinocandins possess antifungal activity against *Aspergillus* and combination with azoles is preferred for secondary prophylaxis. Allergic aspergillosis can be effectively treated with corticosteroids and itraconazole. Natamycin as an aerosol 0.25% suspension has been used for pulmonary infection. Surgical resection, when possible, is ideal for aspergillomas.

PENICILLIOSIS

Penicilliosis is an important opportunistic fungal infection caused by dimorphic yeast *Penicillium marneffei* that affects primarily the immune compromised individuals living in endemic areas. *Penicillium marneffei* is the only pathogenic species among more than 200 species described. The characteristic feature of thermal dimorphism is important factor for its virulence. Although *P. marneffei* can infect otherwise healthy individuals, it is one of the common emerging opportunistic infection in patients with AIDS.

Epidemiology

Countries such as Thailand, South China, Hong Kong, Taiwan, and Vietnam in Southeast Asia are particularly endemic for the infection. However, sporadic cases are reported from Japan and other Asian countries including India. Europe and the United States too have reported imported cases. Although the natural source of *P. marneffei* is unknown, infections are known to occur in bamboo rats of the genus *Cannomys*. The infection is most common after the rainy season.

Clinical Features

The systemic infection usually occurs via lungs following inhalation or through traumatic implantation of the fungus. Multiorgan system involvement including cutaneous spread is common from hematogenous dissemination but it is not known whether a primary cutaneous infection exists.

Patients usually present initially with fever, weight loss, respiratory symptoms such as cough and chest pain or with signs of dissemination such as anemia, lymphadenopathy, hepatosplenomegaly, bony, or skin lesions. Skin lesions occur in over 50% cases as multiple small papules, nodules, ulcers, subcutaneous cold abscesses, gumma-like or molluscum-like lesions widely scattered over face, and trunk. Mucosae may also be involved with papules or ulcers.

Diagnosis

The common differentials include other disseminated mycoses such as histoplasmosis and cryptococcosis especially in an endemic area, AIDS patients, tuberculosis, leishmaniasis, and molluscum contagiosum. Biopsy and culture will distinguish between the different causes.

Pathology

The characteristic yeast-like cells of *P. marneffei* that are best visualized intracellularly within macrophages in histopathologic sections of biopsy from a skin lesion, lymph node, spleen, or liver stained with methenamine silver. Although they resemble *H. capsulatum*, they do not show budding but divide by a septum in the middle. However, these small (2–4 µm) yeast cells are difficult to see in direct smears from blood, skin lesions, or bone marrow but can be highlighted with Leishman stain.

Culture of Causative Fungus

In culture on SDA at 27°C, *P. marneffei* produces velvety and folded colonies of green or grayish mold with a characteristic diffusible red pigment. Microscopically, it shows typical fruiting structure or *Penicillium* conidiophores.

Other Diagnostic Methods

Immunofluorescence with monoclonal antibodies for antigen detection and PCR or DNA hybridization techniques have been used in diagnosis or for pathogen identification from cultures. No serologic test is available for routine/commercial use.

Treatment

Intravenous amphotericin B is necessary in severe cases due to high mortality among untreated cases. Itraconazole, miconazole, and voriconazole have shown good therapeutic response particularly in mild disease. Fluconazole and 5-flucytosine have variable efficacy. Itraconazole is continued after initial therapy with amphotericin B to prevent relapses in patients with AIDS or severe infection.

PNEUMOCYSTOSIS

Pneumocystis jirovecii, previously known as *Pneumocystis carinii*, is a common opportunistic fungal pathogen in immune compromised persons, recipients of solid-organ transplant, AIDS patients, and neonates. It was considered a protozoan parasite earlier but recent DNA analysis favors its identity as a nonfilamentous fungus inhabiting the lungs of mammalian hosts. The organism cannot be cultured but it reproduces extracellularly within the lung alveoli.

Clinical Features

The lungs are the most common site of infection manifesting as pneumonia with fever (in >80%), nonproductive cough (in 95%), dyspnea on exertion that is progressive (in 95%), and chest discomfort. Dissemination to liver, spleen, and lymph nodes may occur in less than 3% of patients. Skin involvement is rare and manifesting with erythematous or skin-colored, nontender papules, or nodules sometimes with ulceration. The external ear including the auditory canal is the most common site of involvement.

Diagnosis

Diagnosis of pulmonary *P. jirovecii* infection is usually based on clinical suspicion based on characteristic symptoms of pneumonia in HIV seropositive persons with CD4 cell counts less than 200 cells/μL, hypoxia and diffuse interstitial infiltrates, and warrants empirical treatment with cotrimoxazole (sulfamethoxazole 800 mg + trimethoprim 160 mg) twice daily for 3 weeks.

Microscopic examination of smears prepared from clinical samples and stained with methenamine silver is method of choice for the demonstration of pathogen. *Pneumocystis* organisms is visualized as round, nonbudding structures 5–10 μm in diameter in smears from BAL fluid, induced sputum sample, tracheal aspirate, nasopharyngeal aspirate, trans bronchial and open lung biopsy specimens from pulmonary pneumocystosis cases, and fine needle aspirates from lymph nodes/ extrapulmonary sites. Cysts or trophozoites forms are commonly identified from samples from lungs.

Treatment

Treatment with cotrimoxazole twice daily is the treatment of choice for *P. jirovecii* infection. Parenteral pentamidine or oral atovaquone are other options.

Prophylaxis treatment with oral cotrimoxazole or aerosolized pentamidine, oral dapsone, or oral atovaquone is recommended in the setting of immunosuppression.

PREVENTION

There are no known preventive measures for these infections as most deep mycoses are acquired via inhalation. Immune suppressed individuals must avoid travel to endemic regions to avoid getting infected. Use of adequate protective clothes and masks while involved in activities that predispose individuals for these infections must be stressed. Taking needful care of wounds and injuries against contamination with soil or vegetable material will be preventive for cutaneous infections. Provision for standard biosafety measures like use of masks while working, free airflow and exhaust, and efficient particulate air filters in the labs for persons handling biological material or fungus must be ensured. Patient education for completion of antifungal treatment with recommended doses for a prolonged period to achieve mycologic cure will prevent recurrences. Persons with immunodeficiency must be treated adequately or receive prophylactic antifungal therapy for life to prevent morbidity associated with these infections.

CONCLUSION

The prevalence of systemic mycoses has increased beyond earlier delineated endemic boundaries especially in the present era of immune suppression. Traumatic inoculation and inhalation of pathogen leading to subcutaneous mycoses or systemic mycoses is usual modes of infection. Systemic infection also reflects hematogenous spread of pathogens to other organs systems. Histoplasmosis, blastomycosis, coccidioidomycosis and paracoccidioidomycosis are due to true pathogens seen in immunocompetent. Common opportunistic systemic mycoses in immunocompromized include cryptococcosis, aspergillosis, zygomycosis, systemic candidiasis, penicilliosis, and pneumocystosis. They usually have a protracted clinical course for want of diagnostic tools with short turn-round time and effective treatments leading to poor quality of life and significant morbidity/mortality. Hence, high clinical suspicion particularly remains the key to an early diagnosis.

Editor's Comment

Systemic mycoses are conditions that are not uncommon, and often lead to significant morbidity, poor patient quality of life and even mortality in many cases. In this article, the author has provided a clear background of these conditions, classifying them either endemic or opportunistic, and using the article to help differentiate these infections from superficial and other fungal diseases. Dr Mahajan has also discussed geographic influences, immune system status, and diagnostic features of diseases ranging from blastomycosis, coccidioidomycosis, cryptococcosis and others.

Seemal R Desai, Rashmi Sarkar

REFERENCES

1. Antony S, Dominguez DC, Sotelo E. Use of liposomal amphotericin B in the treatment of disseminated coccidioidomycosis. *J Natl Med Assoc.* 2003;95:982-5.
2. Benard G. An overview of the immunopathology of human paracoccidioidomycosis. *Mycopathologica.* 2008;165:209-21.
3. Bicalho RN, Santo MF, de Aguiar MC, Santos VR. Oral paracoccidioidomycosis: a retrospective study of 62 Brazilian patients. *Oral Dis.* 2001;7:56-60.
4. Bonifaz A, Chang P, Moreno K. Disseminated histoplasmosis associated with acquired immunodeficiency syndrome: report of 23 cases. *Clin Dermatol.* 2008;34:481-6.
5. Capoor MR, Sen B, Varshney P, Verghese M, Shivaprakash MR, Chakrabarti A. Coccidioidomycosis masquerading as skeletal tuberculosis: an imported case and review of coccidioidomycosis in India. *Trop Doct.* 2014;44:25-8.
6. Catanzaro A, Cloud GA, Stevens DA, Levine BE, Williams PL, Mirels LF, et al. Safety tolerance, and efficacy of posaconazole therapy in patients with nonmeningeal disseminated or chronic pulmonary coccidioidomycosis. *Clin Infect Dis.* 2007;45:562-8.
7. Chapman SW, Bradsher RW, Campbell GD Jr, Pappas PG, Kauffman CA. Practice guidelines for the treatment of patients with blastomycosis. *Clin Infect Dis.* 2000;30:679-83.
8. Cleod DS, Mortimer RH, Perry-Keene DA, Allworth A, Woods ML, Perry-Keene J, et al. Histoplasmosis in Australia: report of 16 cases and literature review. *Medicine (Baltimore).* 2011;90:61-8.
9. CramptonTL, Light RB, Berg GM, Meyers MP, Schroeder GC, Hershfield ES, et al. Epidemiology and clinical spectrum of blastomycosis diagnosed at Manitoba hospitals. *Clin Infect Dis.* 2002;34:1310-6.
10. De Rosa FG, Garazzino S, Pasero D, Di Perri G, Ranieri VM. Invasive candidiasis and candidemia: new guidelines. *Minerva Anestesiol.* 2009;75:453-8.
11. DiSalvo AF, Klein BS. Blastomycosis. In: Merz WG, Hay RJ (Eds). Topley and Wilson's Microbiology and Microbial Infections: Medical Mycology, 10th edition. Washington DC: ASM Press; 2005. pp. 479-501.
12. Durkin M, Witt J, LeMonte A, Wheat B, Conolly P. Antigen assay with the potential aid in diagnosis of blastomycosis. *J Clin Microbiol.* 2004;42:4873-5.
13. Gupta D, Thappa DM. Deep fungal infections. In: Singal A, Grover C (Eds) Comprehensive Approach to Infections in Dermatology, 1st edition. New Delhi: Jaypee Brothers Medical Publishers (P) Ltd.; 2015. pp. 158-83.
14. Huston SM, Mody CH. Cryptococcosis: an emerging respiratory mycosis. *Clin Chest Med.* 2009;30: 253-64.
15. Kathuria S, Capoor MR, Yadav S, Singh A, Ramesh V. Disseminated histoplasmosis in an apparently immunocompetent individual from north India: a case report and review. *Med Mycol.* 2013;51:774-8.
16. López-Martínez R, Méndéz-Tovar LJ. Blastomcosis. *Clin Dermatol.* 2012;30:565-72.
17. Mahajan VK. Subcutaneous mycoses. In: Singal A, Grover C (Eds). Comprehensive Approach to Infections in Dermatology, 1st edition. New Delhi: Jaypee Brothers Medical Publishers (P) Ltd.; 2015. pp. 116-57.
18. Marques SA. Paracoccidioidomycosis. *Clin Dermatol.* 2012;30:610-5.
19. Mays SR, Bogle MA, Bodey GP. Cutaneous fungal infections in the oncology patient: recognition and management. *Am J Clin Dermatol.* 2006;7:31-43.
20. Morejon KM, Machado AA, Martinez R. Paracoccidioidomycosis in patients infeted with and not infected with human immunodeficiency virus: a case control study. *Am J Trop Med Hyg.* 2009;80:359-66.
21. Negroni R. Cryptococcosis. *Clin Dermatol.* 2012;30:599-609.
22. Pappas PG, Pottage JC, Powderly WG, Fraser VJ, Stratton CW, MvKenzie S, et al. Blastomycosis in patients with acquired immunodeficiency syndrome. *Ann Int Med.* 1992;116:847-53.
23. Park DW, Sohn JW, Cheong HJ, Ki WJ, Kim MJ, Kim JH, et al. Combination therapy of disseminated coccidioidomycosis with caspofungin and fluconazole. *BMC Infect Dis.* 2006;6:26.
24. Perfect J, Casadevall A. Cryptococcosis. *Infect Dis North Am.* 2002;16:837-74.

25. Perfect JR, Dismukes WE, Dromer F, Goldman DL, Graybill JR, Hamill RJ, et al. Clinical practice guidelines for the management of cryptococcal disease: 2010 update by the Infectious Diseases Society of America. *Clin Infect Dis.* 2010;50:291-322.
26. Poncio Mendes R, Negroni R, Bonifaz A, Pappaqianis D. New aspects of some endemic mycoses. *Med Mycol.* 2000;38:237-41.
27. Powderly WG. Recent advances in the management of cryptococcal meningitis in patients with AIDS. *Clin Infect Dis.* 1996;22:19-27.
28. Prabhu RM, Bonnell M, Currier BL, Orestein R. Successful treatment of disseminated nonmeningeal coccidioidomycosis with voriconazole. *Clin Infect Dis.* 2004;39:e74-7.
29. Randhawa HS, Chowdhary A, Kathuria S, Roy P, Misra DS, Jain S, et al. Blastomycosis in India: report of an imported case and current status. *Med Mycol.* 2013;51:185-92.
30. Subbalaxmi MV, Umabala P, Paul R, Chandra N, Raju YS, Rudramurthy SM. A rare presentation of progressive disseminated histoplasmosis in an immunocompetent patient from a non-endemic region. *Med Mycol Case Rep.* 2013;2:103-7.
31. Thomas I. Superficial and deep candidosis. *Int J Dermatol.* 1993;32:778-83.
32. Ustianowski AP, Sieu TP, Day JN. Penicillium marneffei infection in HIV. *Curr Opin Infect Dis.* 2008;21:31-6.
33. Vanittanakom N, Cooper CR Jr, Fisher MC, Sirisanthana T. Penicillium marneffei infection and recent advances in the epidemiology and molecular biology aspects. *Clin Microbiol Rev.* 2006;19:95-110.
34. Walsh TJ, Gamaletsou MN. Treatment of fungal diseases in the setting of neutropenia. *Hematology Am Soc Hematol Educ Program.* 2013;2013:423-7.
35. Warnock DW. Fungal infections in neutropenia: current problems and chemotherapeutic control. *J Antimicrob Chemother.* 1998;41(Suppl D):95-105.
36. Welsh O, Vera-Cabrera L, Rendon A, Gonzales G, Bnifaz A. Coccidioidomycosis. *Clin Dermatol.* 2012;30: 573-91.
37. Wheat LJ, Freifeld AG, Kleiman MB, Baddley JW, McKinsey DS, Loyd JE, et al. Clinical practice guidelines for the management of patients with histoplasmosis: 2007 update by the Infectious Diseases Society of America. *Clin Infect Dis.* 2007;45:807-25.

World Clin Dermatol. 2016;3(1):110-38.

Subcutaneous Mycoses

Vikram K Mahajan MD

Department of Dermatology, Venereology, and Leprosy,
Dr R.P. Government Medical College, Kangra, Himachal Pradesh, India

ABSTRACT

Human fungal infections are broadly classified as superficial and deep mycosis depending on the tissues/sites involved. Deep mycoses account for almost 1% of the total mycoses and involve the skin, subcutaneous tissue, fascial planes and bones, and/or various organs systems. They are endemic in countries with tropical/subtropical climates and reported frequently among other populations especially travelers/workers returning from endemic areas or following accidental exposure to fungus in nonendemic regions. Increasing prevalence of opportunistic or deep mycosis in current era is attributable to immunosuppression from human immunodeficiency virus infection and immunosuppressive therapy for cancers, autoimmune diseases, or organ transplantation. Sporotrichosis remains the most common subcutaneous mycosis worldwide while chromoblastomycosis and phaeohyphomycosis, mycetomas, subcutaneous zygomycosis (entomophthoromycosis and mucormycosis), and lobomycosis perhaps have their own endemic foci. Rhinosporidiosis, once grouped in fungal infections, is now considered to be due to a parasite belonging to class *Mesomycetozoea*. These infections are acquired mostly following traumatic implantation of the pathogen usually a saprophyte to the soil and decaying plant material. Clinically, the lesions are heterogeneous in morphology manifesting either as nodules, plaques, noduloulcerative, nodulocystic or warty lesions, discharging sinuses, or subcutaneous swellings or masses with a protracted clinical course causing significant morbidity. Treatment in most instances remains unsatisfactory leading to a significant public health problem.

Email: vkm1@rediffmail.com

© 2016 Jaypee Brothers Medical Publishers. All rights reserved.

INTRODUCTION

Fungal infections are broadly classified as superficial and deep mycosis depending on the tissues/sites involved. Superficial mycoses, mostly due to dermatophytes, involve the superficial layers of skin and appendages like hair and nails, and account for more than 99% of the total mycoses cases. Deep mycoses, account for almost 1% of the total mycoses, are a group of infections involving the skin, subcutaneous tissue, fascial planes and bones, and/or other organs systems leading to protracted clinical course and significant morbidity.

The fungi that cause systemic infections belong to two distinct groups: (i) the true pathogens and (ii) the opportunists. The true pathogens include *Histoplasma capsulatum,* and *Coccidioides immitis*, which invade and develop in the tissues of an immunocompetent host without predilection. The opportunistic organisms, *Aspergillus fumigatus*, are less virulent, and well adapted to invade the tissues of an immunocompromised host. Slowly evolving, chronic skin lesions not responding to routine therapy should always arouse strong clinical suspicion of deep mycosis. Other systemic mycoses, such as histoplasmosis, cryptococcosis, and paracoccidioidomycosis, occur worldwide and are not restricted to tropical regions. The zygomycosis and aspergillosis generally present as systemic infections but rarely manifest as localized infections of the skin and subcutis. Subcutaneous mycoses include sporotrichosis, chromoblastomycosis and phaeohyphomycosis, mycetomas, subcutaneous zygomycosis (entomophthoromycosis and mucormycosis), and lobomycosis. Rhinosporidiosis, once grouped in fungal infections, is now considered to be due to a protistan parasite belonging to class *Mesomycetozoea*.

Subcutaneous mycoses are prevalent in tropics/subtropics due to high temperature and humidity conducive for the growth of causative fungi. There has been an increase in the prevalence of opportunistic or deep mycosis in general in the present era, the attributes of which are immunosuppression due to human immunodeficiency virus (HIV) infection, immunosuppressive therapy for cancers, autoimmune diseases, or organ transplantation.

The subcutaneous mycoses are mostly acquired following traumatic implantation of organisms that grow as saprophytes in the soil, and plant detritus. The rural population with agricultural background worldwide is, thus, particularly at risk to get infected. The disease may either remain localized at inoculation site or involve the adjacent tissues. Clinically, the lesions have heterogeneous morphology manifesting either as nodules, plaques, noduloulcerative, nodulocystic or warty lesions, discharging sinuses, or subcutaneous swellings or masses. Widespread hematic or lymphatics dissemination of the infection may occur in a debilitated or immunocompromised host. Serology tests have limited diagnostic use, and most cases are diagnosed clinically and needs confirmation by demonstration/ culture of causative fungus in the laboratory. Treatment in most instances remains unsatisfactory leading to a significant public health problem.

CUTANEOUS SPOROTRICHOSIS

This chronic infection is usually limited to skin and subcutis and may get disseminated occasionally. Usually, the skin lesion(s) develops at the site of traumatic inoculation of the fungus *Sporothrix schenckii*, a dimorphic yeast, saprophyte of soil, decaying wood, hay, and sphagnum moss. *Sporothrix schenckii* is a complex of at least six clinicoepidemiologically important species with significant differences in geographical distribution, biochemical properties (dextrose, sucrose, and raffinose assimilation), degree of virulence, different disease patterns and response to therapy. These include *S. albicans*, *S. brasiliensis* (in Brazil), *S. mexicana* (in Mexico), *S. globosa* (in the United Kingdom, Spain, Italy, China, Japan, the United States of America, and India), and *S. schenckii* sensu stricto.

Epidemiology

Sporotrichosis occurs worldwide mainly in warm and humid regions of the tropical and subtropical countries. Most frequent occurrences are from Japan, China, India, Australia, and Central and South America (Mexico, Brazil, Colombia, and Peru). In India, endemic areas are located in the sub-Himalayan belt that extends from Himachal Pradesh, Uttaranchal, and Uttar Pradesh to Assam and is sporadic in other parts. As the occurrence of infection depends upon the presence of abundant fungus in the environment, and portal of entry, age, gender, and race play no role in its epidemiology. However, the disease frequently occurs in young individual between 20 and 40 years of age coinciding with most active years of life. Only up to 60% of patients would recall history of prior injury as it usually occurs few weeks earlier that may be very innocuous and is mostly forgotten. Professionals such as agriculturists, gardeners, florists, foresters, and nursery workers are particularly at risk of acquiring the disease. Human infections have also been associated with insect bites, fish handling, and bites of birds, dogs, horses, reptiles, squirrels, rats, or cats. Secondary wound contamination is perhaps responsible more often in such cases. A significantly high number of infections and long-lasting outbreaks of cat-transmitted sporotrichosis in Brazil indicate the emergence of other at-risk personnel handling cats within the same geographical area. Human-to-human spread may rarely occur through infected wound dressings.

Clinical Features

The incubation period varies from a few days to a few months with an average of 3 weeks. Clinically, it manifests either as fixed cutaneous sporotrichosis, lymphocutaneous sporotrichosis, or systemic infection involving lungs or joints. Lymphocutaneous sporotrichosis (Figure 1) is the classic form having

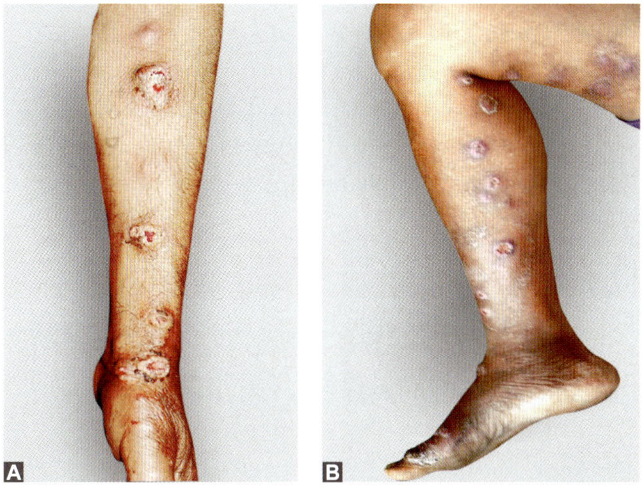

Figure 1: Cutaneous sporotrichosis: lymphocutaneous sporotrichosis involving **A,** upper limb and **B,** lower limb. A string of noduloulcerative lesions appear along the lymphatics proximal to the initial inoculation (injury) site. *Source:* Mahajan VK. Subcutaneous mycoses. Singal A, Grover C, editors. Comprehensive Approach to Infections in Dermatology. 1st ed. New Delhi: Jaypee Brothers Medical Publishers (P) Ltd.; 2015. pp. 116-57, *with permission.*

a characteristic clinical picture, and accounts for 70–80% of the cases. Upper extremities are involved more often than legs or face. Involvement of face is more common with fixed cutaneous variety, and in children. After traumatic inoculation of the fungus, a subcutaneous nodule develops that may ulcerate, the sporotrichotic chancre. Later, a string of similar lesions develop along the lymphatics in lymphocutaneous variety. In fixed cutaneous sporotrichosis, infection remains confined to single skin lesion at the inoculation site (Figure 2). Lesional morphology varies from noduloulcerative or crusted erythematous plaques to an occasional verrucous plaque. Variable morphology of lesions is not uncommon. Treatment is needed in majority of patients as spontaneous resolution occurs as an exception. Most patients will develop lymphocutaneous sporotrichosis while others have fixed cutaneous sporotrichosis variant of the disease. Factors such as size, depth of inoculums, heat resistance of causative strains, and host immune response have been implicated for clinical variability. Fixed cutaneous sporotrichosis seems to be caused by strains that grow best at 35°C whereas lymphocutaneous and extracutaneous disease is associated with strains that grow both at 35°C and 37°C, respectively. Fixed cutaneous sporotrichosis is considered to occur in patients with certain immunity against the fungus. Extracutaneous dissemination may present either in the form of most common osteoarticular, pulmonary, ocular, or central nervous system disease in patients with an immunosuppressive condition such as

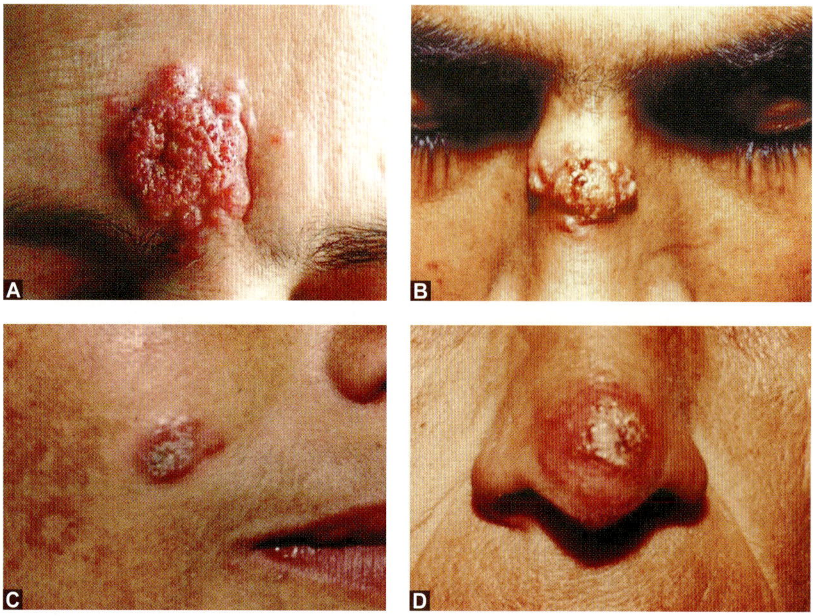

Figure 2: Cutaneous sporotrichosis: fixed cutaneous sporotrichosis. **A,** A large indurated granulomatous plaque over forehead; **B,** Nasal bridge; **C,** Right cheek; **D,** Nose tip. Small papular lesions at the periphery of primary lesion are suggestive of destabilization of the lesion and results from trauma of surgery, or manipulation of lesion. *Source:* Mahajan VK. Subcutaneous mycoses. Singal A, Grover C, editors. Comprehensive Approach to Infections in Dermatology. 1st ed. New Delhi: Jaypee Brothers Medical Publishers (P) Ltd.; 2015. pp. 116-57, *with permission.*

alcoholism, diabetes, acquired immunodeficiency syndrome (AIDS), underlying malignancy, and use of corticosteroids or other immunosuppressive drugs. Recently, extracutaneous sporotrichosis seems to be emerging mycosis in HIV seropositive individuals. Multifocal or disseminated cutaneous sporotrichosis means greater than or equal to three lesions involving two different anatomical sites. Hematologic spread or multiple traumatic implantations of the fungus perhaps underlie cutaneous dissemination, and may even be seen in individuals who apparently have no predisposing factors for immunosuppression.

Diagnosis

The diagnosis of sporotrichosis is often clinical, and need to be differentiated from cutaneous tuberculosis, cutaneous leishmaniasis, other deep mycoses, and atypical mycobacteria.

Culture of Causative Fungus

The direct microscopic examination of tissue sample is mostly unhelpful for paucity of fungal cells. Culture of *S. schenckii* from pus or biopsy specimen on Sabouraud's dextrose agar (SDA) or brain heart infusion agar is diagnostic. Its growth is generally obtained in 2 weeks. Cultures on SDA at 25°C show characteristic colonies of *S. schenckii*, the initial cream-colored colonies turn brown/black after a few weeks (Figure 3). Demonstration of temperature dimorphism; hyphae are seen when *S. schenckii* from a SDA colony is incubated at 37°C in blood glucose-cysteine agar, is highly characteristic and helps in its identification (Figure 4).

Histology

Features are usually nonspecific, and may mimic other deep mycotic infections, cutaneous tuberculosis, leprosy, sarcoidosis, and foreign body granulomas. The spectrum of features varies from acute-on-chronic inflammation with characteristic zonation to chronic epithelioid cell granuloma with foreign body or Langhans giant cells at both ends, and nonspecific chronic granulomatous inflammatory cell infiltration of the dermis in the middle of the spectrum (Figure 5). The yeast is rarely elicited without periodic acid-Schiff (PAS) reaction, Gomori methenamine silver (GMS) stains and its morphology varies from globose budding cells to cigar

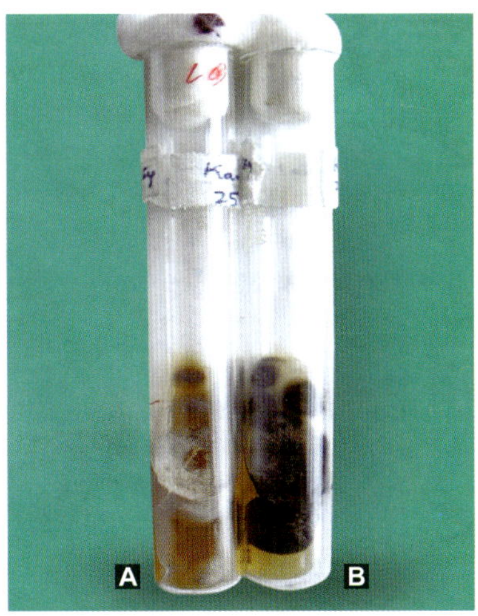

Figure 3: Cutaneous sporotrichosis: *Sporothrix schenckii* colony on Sabouraud's glucose agar. **A,** Initial cream color and **B,** turns brown black as it matures. *Source:* Mahajan VK. Subcutaneous mycoses. Singal A, Grover C, editors. Comprehensive Approach to Infections in Dermatology. 1st ed. New Delhi: Jaypee Brothers Medical Publishers (P) Ltd.; 2015. pp. 116-57, *with permission.*

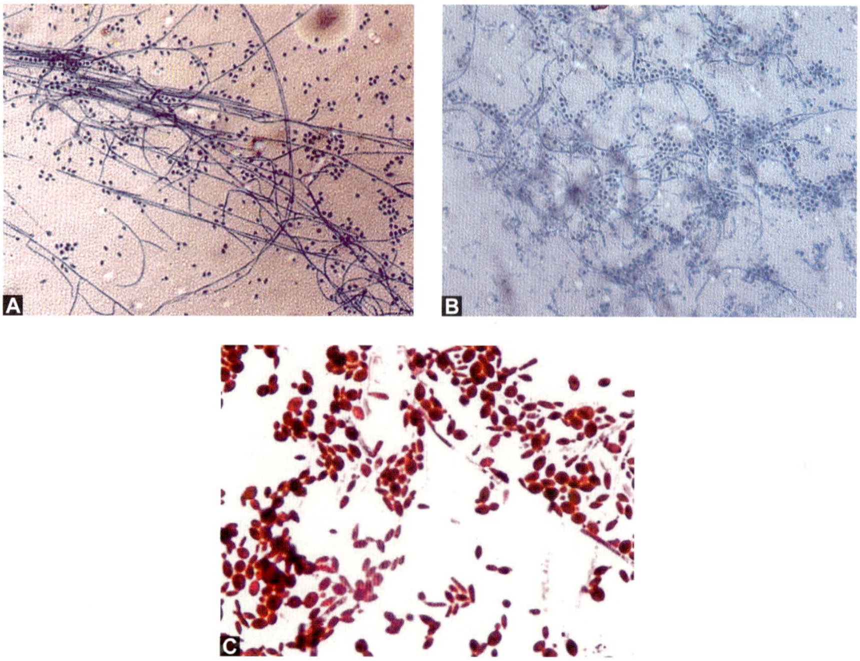

Figure 4: Cutaneous sporotrichosis: *Sporothrix schenckii* in delicate branching, mold form with pyriform conidia in **A,** characteristic flower-like arrangement or **B,** dense sleeve-like pattern. Smears taken from culture in Sabouraud's glucose agar at 25°C (Stain: Lactophenol cotton blue x40). **C,** Yeast form from culture in brain-heart infusion broth at 37°C (Gram stain x40). *Source:* Mahajan VK. Subcutaneous mycoses. Singal A, Grover C, editors. Comprehensive Approach to Infections in Dermatology. 1st ed. New Delhi: Jaypee Brothers Medical Publishers (P) Ltd.; 2015. pp. 116-57, *with permission.*

shaped cells surrounded by a thick radiate eosinophilic substance forming asteroid body the Splendore-Hoeppli phenomenon.

Intradermal Tests

It is performed by using sporotrichin or peptide-rhamnomannan antigen to detect delayed hypersensitivity, and is often positive in healthy people in endemic areas, and in cured patients. It is negative in severe or disseminated sporotrichosis. The diagnostic value of the test, therefore, remains ambiguous.

Molecular Techniques

Analysis of antibody responses by immunoblotting and enzyme-linked immunosorbent assay, agglutination, complement-fixation tests, immunohistochemical, immunofluorescence, immunodiffusion, and immune electrophoresis techniques

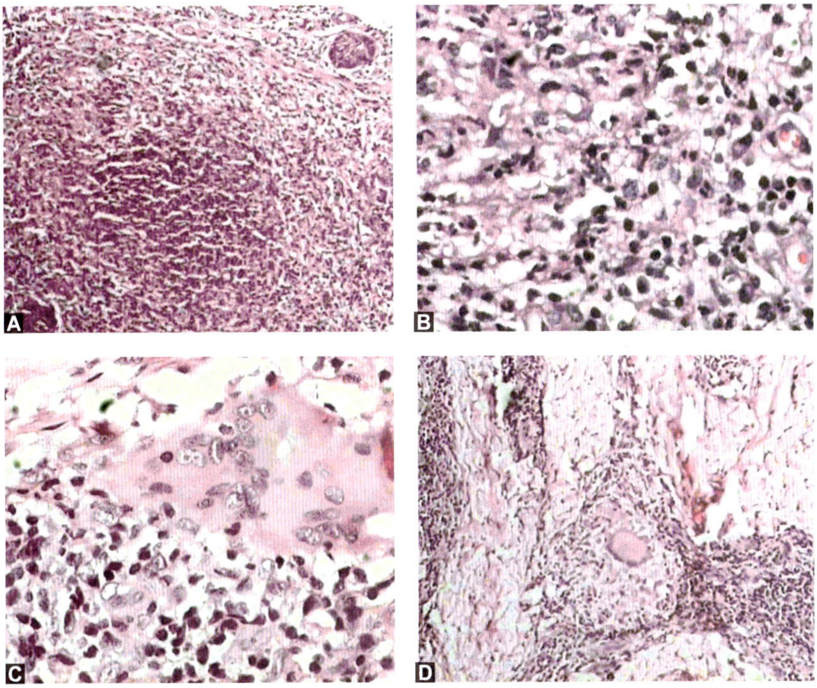

Figure 5: Cutaneous sporotrichosis: Histopathology— **A,** Neutrophilic abscesses in the dermis with lymphoplasmacytic epithelioid cell infiltrate. **B,** Acute-on-chronic inflammation with characteristic central zone of chronic suppuration, middle tuberculoid inflammation zone comprising epithelioid and Langerhans' cells and outer syphilitic zone of lymphoplasmacytic cells, fibroblasts, and capillary proliferation; **C,** Chronic inflammatory cell infiltrate with foreign body giant cell reaction; **D,** Epithelioid cell granuloma with a Langerhans' giant cell. *Source:* Mahajan VK. Subcutaneous mycoses. Singal A, Grover C, editors. Comprehensive Approach to Infections in Dermatology. 1st ed. New Delhi: Jaypee Brothers Medical Publishers (P) Ltd.; 2015. pp. 116-57, *with permission.*

and detection of *S. schenckii* by polymerase chain reaction are useful in diagnosing rarer extracutaneous and disseminated forms. Serological testing using antigenic fraction of the *S. schenckii* that binds concanavalin A represents a more recent diagnostic tool.

Treatment

Oral administration of saturated solution of potassium iodide (SSKI) remains the treatment of choice, for fixed cutaneous sporotrichosis, because it is highly effective and cheap. Its initial starting dose is 5 drops three times a day (TID) which may subsequently be increased, up to a maximum dose of 30–40 drops TID, till the complete regression of the lesion. Itraconazole and terbinafine, the oral antifungal agents, are effective and well tolerated in its management. Itraconazole is administered in the dosage of 200–400 mg/day for a period of 3–6 months. It is an acceptable alternative in patient intolerant to SSKI. Terbinafine in the dosage of 500–1,000 mg/day or fluconazole 400–600 mg/day, used alone or in combination with SSKI are other useful therapeutic options. Treatment is to be continued for at least a period of 4–6 weeks even after complete clinical remission for mycological cure. Amphotericin B can be used safely during pregnancy but should be reserved as a drug of choice for treating disseminated cutaneous, and/or pulmonary sporotrichosis. The use of amphotericin B in the dosage of 0.5–1.0 mg/kg/day is recommended for patients with disseminated and/or pulmonary disease. Local hyperthermia (42–43°C) using wet heat or hand held pocket warmer, infrared or far infrared heater is recommended for the treatment of cutaneous sporotrichosis in pregnant women in particular, pending specific therapy.

CHROMOBLASTOMYCOSIS

This localized chronic infection of skin, and subcutaneous tissue is characterized by slow growing nodular, verrucous, and/or noduloulcerative lesions, affecting primarily the extremities. The disease is worldwide in tropical and subtropical regions of the world including China, Japan, Philippines, Malaysia, and India especially in sub-Himalayan, Eastern and Western coastal areas.

Etiology

Chromomycosis/chromoblastomycosis is caused by various black-pigmented dematiaceous fungi, the most common of which are *Phialophora verrucosa, Fonsecaea pedrosoi, Fonsecaea compacta, Cladosporium carrionii,* and occasionally *Rhinocladiella aquaspersa*. They exist as saprophytes and grow freely in nature. The usual mode of infection is through inoculation of the fungus into the skin or subcutis, following minor injury/trauma from thorns or wooden splinters. The farming community is particularly at risk to acquire the infection due to occupation related trauma, equally affecting both men and women at all ages. *F. pedrosoi* is the most common pathogens, and it accounts for 90% of chromomycosis in humid and tropical regions, while *C. carrionii*, *F. compacta*, *P. verrucose*, and *R. aquaspersa* are the causative organisms in rest of the 10%.

Clinical Features

A small, painless, papule is its initial lesion. It enlarges to form a warty nodule and/or plaque over a period of time at the site of injury/trauma after a long incubation. An established lesion is characterized by multiple, nodular, tumorous,

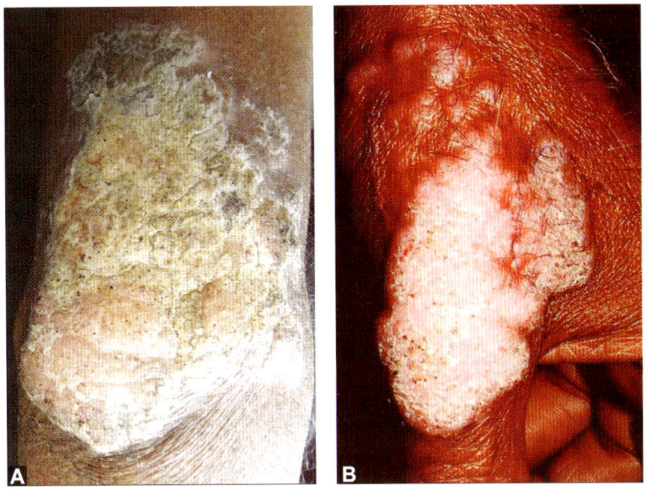

Figure 6: Chromoblastomycosis. **A,** Large, hyperkeratotic, superficial, scaly, verrucous plaque over elbow. **B,** Over dorsal hand, Small, dark aggregations of clotted blood and fungal cells are characteristic and likely to yield fungal cells in smears or histologic sections. *Source:* Mahajan VK. Subcutaneous mycoses. Singal A, Grover C, editors. Comprehensive Approach to Infections in Dermatology. 1st ed. New Delhi: Jaypee Brothers Medical Publishers (P) Ltd.; 2015. pp. 116-57, with permission.

hyperkeratotic verrucous plaque(s) seldom associated with mild pruritus and pain (Figure 6). The exposed body parts like hands and feet are its site of involvement. They are usually unilateral. Satellite lesions can develop around the original lesion, following either autoinoculation or superficial lymphatic spread. Extracutaneous spread to lymph nodes, brain, ileocecal region, tonsils, tracheobronchial tree, lungs, pleural cavity, and bone may occur.

Diagnosis

The lesions of chromomycosis are required to be differentiated from tuberculosis verrucosa cutis and fixed cutaneous sporotrichosis. Demonstration of characteristic small, round, thick-walled, brown-pigmented muriform cells, the sclerotic bodies, in addition to longitudinal and transverse septa are fairly diagnostic. The preceding features are evident in potassium hydroxide (KOH) mounts, prepared from the scrapings taken from the surface of lesions (Figure 7). However, the diagnosis is confirmed by culture of the causative fungus in SDA from skin scraping/ biopsy tissue. Besides, its confirmation through histopathology is imperative. It is marked by pseudoepitheliomatous epidermal hyperplasia, granulomatous inflammation with foreign body giant cells, and areas of microabscess formation. Nevertheless, the presence of fungal cells, the copper penny bodies within giant cells is pathognomic.

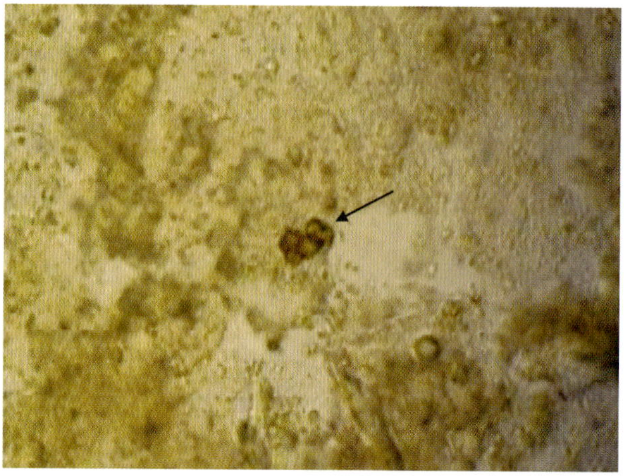

Figure 7: Chromoblastomycosis: Sclerotic bodies, as seen in potassium hydroxide mounts, are 5–13 µm, round, thick-thi walled, brown muriform cells, having longitudinal and transverse septa. *Source:* Mahajan VK. Subcutaneous mycoses. Singal A, Grover C, editors. Comprehensive Approach to Infections in Dermatology. 1st ed. New Delhi: Jaypee Brothers Medical Publishers (P) Ltd.; 2015. pp. 116-57, *with permission.*

Treatment

Small lesions of shorter duration are amenable to surgical excision, local heat therapy, laser, or cryotherapy. Surgical excision should invariably be combined with chemotherapy for chronic lesions, distant cutaneous or extracutaneous dissemination for better therapeutic outcome. Treatment with SSKI alone or in combination with other antifungal agents is prevalent. Currently, itraconazole and terbinafine are recommended for oral administration. Itraconazole in the dosage of 200–400 mg/day or terbinafine in the dosage of 500 mg/day is given for a period of 6–12 months or longer.

Oral flucytosine, 50–150 mg/kg of body weight, divided in four equal doses every 6 hours, or intravenous amphotericin B is also used. Amphotericin B is administered in the dosage of 0.5–1.0 mg/kg/day to a maximum of 1.5 mg/kg.

PHAEOHYPHOMYCOSIS

Prior to the advent of current nomenclature, these cases were described under chromoblastomycosis. It is a rare infection caused by dematiaceous fungi affecting the skin and subcutis, the subcutaneous phaeohyphomycosis. Paranasal sinuses, or central nervous system, may also be affected. The condition is worldwide, and is encountered in all climates. More than 100 different moulds, classified in 60 different genera, have been implicated. The important etiological agents include *Alternaria*, *Cladosporium*, *Phialophora*, *Curvularia*, *Exophiala*, and *Fonsecaea* species, generally saprophytes of soil, wood, and plant detritus.

Clinical Features

Once the organism gains entry into the skin through trauma/injury, a single subcutaneous nodule develops at the site. This nodule slowly increases in size to form a painless cystic abscess containing purulent material (Figure 8). Abscesses, cysts, papulonodules, verrucous or ulcerated plaques, nonhealing ulcers or sinuses, or scaly hyperkerototic lesions are the presenting features. The lesions appear morphologically similar regardless of the implicated organism. They are usually present over the feet, legs, and hands in about 60% of the patients.

Diagnosis

Microscopically, brown, pigmented, septate hyphae with occasional branching are visualized in KOH mounts from the purulent discharge or skin scrapings under light microscope but the confirmation of the etiological agent comes through the recovery of the organism from SDA culture (Figures 9 and 10). However, the presence of brown colored fungal hyphae and yeast-like elements in the background of a granulomatous inflammatory reaction containing central neutrophilic abscess

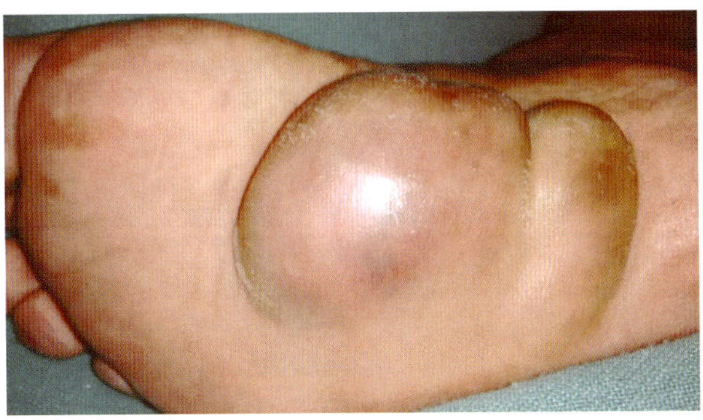

Figure 8: Phaeohyphomycosis: Diffuse induration involving the sole, a painless encapsulated cystic abscess containing purulent material, and no tendency to rupture in a diabetic patient. In contrast, the chromoblastomycosis patients are generally in good health. The lesions of phaeohyphomycosis appear morphologically similar regardless of the implicated organism.

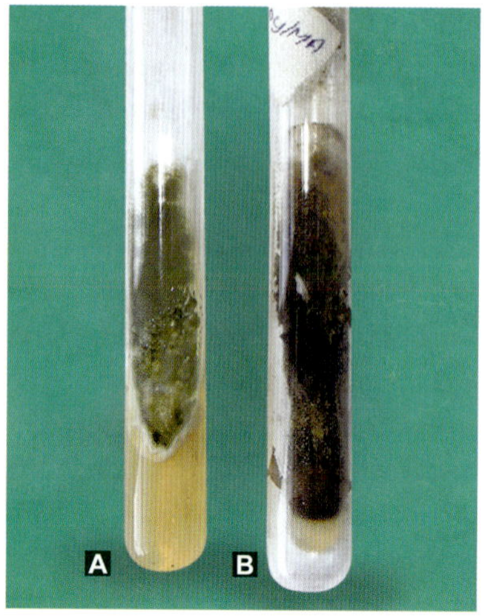

Figure 9: *Fonsecaea pedrosoi*: Colonies of the most common pathogen for chromoblastomycosis/phaeohyphomycosis in Sabouraud's glucose agar are olivaceous-black and velvety in texture. However, clinically the lesions of chromoblastomycosis appear morphologically similar regardless of the implicated organism. *Source:* Mahajan VK. Subcutaneous mycoses. Singal A, Grover C, editors. Comprehensive Approach to Infections in Dermatology. 1st ed. New Delhi: Jaypee Brothers Medical Publishers (P) Ltd.; 2015. pp. 116-57, *with permission.*

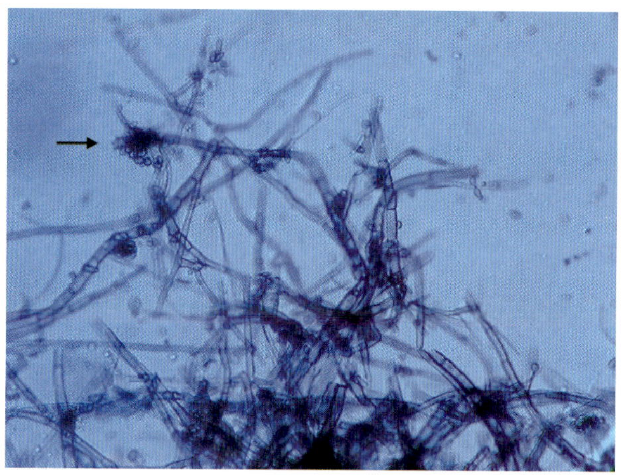

Figure 10: *Fonsecaea pedrosoi*, seen as broad, septate hyphae. Conidia are one-celled and broadly clavate with flat base and arise from the swollen apex of the conidiophore. Source: Mahajan VK. Subcutaneous mycoses. Singal A, Grover C, editors. Comprehensive Approach to Infections in Dermatology. 1st ed. New Delhi: Jaypee Brothers Medical Publishers (P) Ltd.; 2015. pp. 116-57, *with permission.*

on hematoxylin and eosin (H and E) stain section is pathognomic. Fungal cells are prominent in the cyst wall lining.

Treatment

Itraconazole, the oral drug used for the treatment of fungal infections is also advocated for treating phaeohyphomycosis. The drug is administered in the dosage of 200–400 mg/day for a period of 4–6 weeks either alone or in combination with surgical excision of the subcutaneous lesion. Amphotericin B too is used for the purpose. It is given intravenously in the maximum dosage of 0.5–1.0 mg/kg/day. The efficacy of the drug can be improved by combining with surgical excision of the lesions.

MYCETOMAS (MADURA FOOT, MADUROMYCOSIS)

Mycetomas are chronic, localized, destructive infections of the skin, and/or subcutaneous tissue of the foot. Occasionally, the underlying bone may also be affected. They are caused by Gram-positive filamentous bacteria, the actinomycetomas or true fungi, the eumycetomas. It is predominately a disease of geographic regions between latitudes 10°N and 28°N around the Tropic of Cancer with annual rainfall of 50–500 mm and temperature of 15–25°C. It is common in arid tropical and subtropical regions of Africa and Central America known to have low rainfall, pathogen contaminated soil, and abundant thorny bushes. The disease is also endemic in the Indian subcontinent. Actinomycotic mycetoma, resemble those caused by *Actinomyces* species and may contain small particulate granules, such as seen in actinomycosis. It is common across India with the exception of Rajasthan, where eumycetoma is reported more frequently. It is a localized, chronic fungal infection of the skin and subcutaneous tissues, characterized by tumefaction. Rural populations, walking barefoot in the age group of 20–50 years, are in particular at risk. Men are affected almost 4 times more than women.

Clinical Features

Incubation period varies from few weeks to several years. The lesions are located on the feet in 70–85% of cases (Figure 11). Scalp, face, neck, shoulder, upper or lower limbs, buttocks, perineum, and abdomen may be involved (Figure 12). *Nocardia brasiliensis* and *N. asteroides* account for majority of the infection, and follows, mostly forgotten, traumatic implantation or contamination of a wound. Usually, the lesion begins as slowly, enlarging, localized swelling, progress to form multiple nodules and sinuses. The sinuses emitting purulent, seropurulent, or serosanguinous discharge mixed with grains of various color, is cardinal. The triad

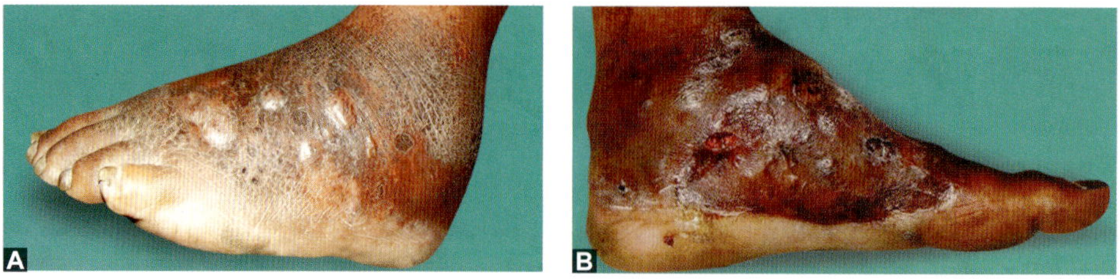

Figure 11: Mycetoma foot. Indurated tumor-like indolent painless swelling (tumefaction) with multiple sinuses discharging "grains" is highly characteristic but actinomycetoma and eumycetoma are sometimes difficult to differentiate clinically. *Source:* Mahajan VK. Subcutaneous mycoses. Singal A, Grover C, editors. Comprehensive Approach to Infections in Dermatology. 1st ed. New Delhi: Jaypee Brothers Medical Publishers (P) Ltd.; 2015. pp. 116-57, *with permission.*

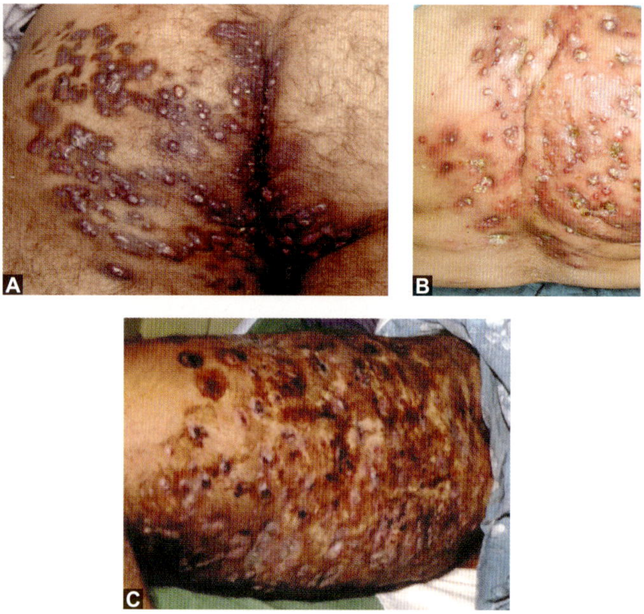

Figure 12: Actinomycetoma due to *Nocardia* spp. Multiple nodules and sinuses discharging profuse purulent, seropurulent material with grains of various colors, and puckered scarring is characteristic. *Source:* Mahajan VK. Subcutaneous mycoses. Singal A, Grover C, editors. Comprehensive Approach to Infections in Dermatology. 1st ed. New Delhi: Jaypee Brothers Medical Publishers (P) Ltd.; 2015. pp. 116-57, *with permission.*

of indurated tumor-like indolent swelling, sinuses and presence of grains in the discharge or within the tissue, is highly characteristic. Regional lymphadenopathy is unusual, and is due to secondary infection. Actinomycetoma and eumycetoma are, therefore, well-recognized clinical entities, the salient features of which are listed in table 1.

Table 1: Comparative Features of Actinomycetoma and Eumycetoma

Features	Actinomycetoma	Eumycetoma
Etiological agents	*Nocardia brasiliensis (most common), N. asteroides, Actinomadura madurae, A. pelletieri, Streptomyces somaliensis*	*Madurella grisea, M. mycetomatis, Leptosphaeria senegalensis, Pyrenochaeta romeroi, Acremonium* species
Incubation period	Short incubation period with faster progression	Long incubation period with slower progression
Morphology of lesions	Ill defined, indurated plaque that tends to merge with surrounding skin. Sinuses are numerous with abundant discharge of pus and grains	Well defined, indurated encapsulated, plaque clearly delineated from surrounding skin. Sinuses fewer with scanty discharge of pus and grains
Inflammation	Signs of inflammation are more pronounced at the sinus orifice	Signs of inflammation are less pronounced
Bone involvement	Bone involvement is early and severely destructive	Bone involvement is late and less destructive
Color of grains (causative agent)	White/yellow (*A. madurae, N. asteroides, N. brasiliensis*), Red (*A. pelletieri*), Yellow/brown (*S. somaliensis*)	Black (*M. grisea, M. mycetomatis, P. romeroi*), White (*Acremonium* species, *A. nidulans*)

Diagnosis

The early tumoral swelling needs differentiation from benign soft tissue tumors and from osteomyelitis of pyogenic or tubercular origin in the late stage. The investigations are directed at identification of causative organism, extent of tissue involvement, and for deciding mode of therapy. The granules in the discharge are actually aggregates of microcolonies of causative organism and identification is possible by their gross and microscopic examination (Table 1). Actinomycotic grains contain very fine filaments of less than 1 μm in diameter, whereas fungal grains have short and broad hyphae of 2–4 μm in diameter. The grains preferably obtained from deeper tissue are subjected to culture, for the recovery of actinomycetes on blood agar or egg-containing media, for aerobic actinomycetes. In addition, the recovery of fungus on SDA and bacteria on Lowenstein-Jensen medium. Pathogenic agents are identified from their colony morphology, optimum temperature requirements, and biochemical characteristics.

The H and E stained sections reveal the presence of a granuloma comprising chronic inflammatory infiltrate, epithelioid cells, Langhans giant cells, and brown, oval, circular or irregular granule, surrounding eumycotic black granules in tissue, the Splendore-Hoeppli phenomenon is pathognomic. Furthermore, the presence of fungi in the granuloma is confirmed by positive PAS and GMS stains. It is imperative to scan the lesions by computerized tomography (CT) in order to define the extent and involvement of deep tissue. It is apparent in the form of soft tissue swelling, widening of intermetatarsal spaces, periosteal reaction, and osteolytic or osteosclerotic boney changes. The bone involvement is diffuse in actinomycotic mycetoma while localized in eumycotic mycetoma.

Treatment

The treatment issues of eumycetoma relate to epidemiology, pathogenesis, clinical manifestations, diagnosis, and prevention. There are several clinical treatments available for this disease. They include radical surgery, amputation, itraconazole, ketoconazole, or voriconazole. Eumycetomas in general is not amenable to antifungal drugs alone, and may need radical surgical removal. Amputation of affected limb is required, if local excision fails.

Oral antifungal drugs, like ketoconazole [200 mg twice a day (BID)] itraconazole (100 mg BID), terbinafine (250 mg once a day), alone or in combination, with/without surgery can be used for small well-localized lesions. The treatment is required to be continued for 12–18 months period, and may be extended for another 6 months after clinical resolution. The preceding medical treatment is usually effective in all cases of mycetoma, except most advanced cases of actinomycetoma. The latter can be treated with cotrimoxazole (sulfamethoxazole 800 mg + trimethoprim 160 mg), dapsone, amikacin, streptomycin, rifampicin, isoniazid, sulfadiazine, sulfadoxine, gentamicin, amoxicillin plus clavulanic acid, either alone or in combination, with variable success. A few useful therapeutic regimens are:

- Dapsone 100–200 mg/day is given for initial 6 months and then maintained at lower dose of (50 mg/day) for 1–2 years
- Combination of dapsone (100 mg/day), cotrimoxazole (sulfamethoxazole 800 mg + trimethoprim 160 mg) BID, and streptomycin (1 g IM daily) given for initial period of 1–2 months, followed by dapsone and cotrimoxazole until clinical cure. Subsequently, the regression of the lesions needs to be maintained with dapsone monotherapy in the dosage of 50–100 mg/day
- Welsh regimen—a combination of amikacin (500 mg intramuscular BID), and cotrimoxazole (BID) may be administered for 3 weeks, followed by cotrimoxazole alone for another 2 weeks. This 5 weeks of therapy constitute one treatment cycle, and most patients require one to three such treatment cycles. Subsequently, only cotrimoxazole monotherapy is continued for another 1–1.5 years. Addition of rifampicin (10 mg/kg/day) as a third drug has improved efficacy and cured 16 of 18 patients with actinomycetoma who had poorly responded to Welsh regimen alone.

New broad spectrum triazole antifungals, namely voriconazole (400–600 mg/day) and posaconazole (800 mg/day) are recommended for use for a period of 16–24 months, with favorable results. Well encapsulated, localized superficial lesions and failure of chemotherapy require surgical intervention.

SUBCUTANEOUS ZYGOMYCOSIS

Zygomycosis infections are caused by pathogenic fungi belonging to Zygomycetes group. They include species of Entomophthorales and Mucorales, the former is incriminated for entomophthoromycosis, and the latter mucormycosis. Entomophthorales usually cause chronic disease of nasal mucosa and subcutaneous tissue, while Mucorales present with more severe form of the disease.

Entomophthoromycosis

The infection in humans is caused by genera *Basidiobolus* and *Conidiobolus* producing two distinct clinical forms, Basidiobolomycosis and Rhinofacial conidiobolomycosis, respectively.

Basidiobolomycosis is a slowly progressive, chronic inflammatory and/or granulomatous infection of the subcutis, seldom involving muscle and fascial planes. It is caused by *Basidiobolus ranarum* (synonym: *B. haptosporus)* that gets inoculated into the skin through minor injury inflicted by thorn prick, insect bites, and scratches. The initial lesion is a well-demarcated subcutaneous nodule that develops over time into a large, firm, rubbery, indurated, painless, and freely mobile plaque. The lesion is attached to the skin that may be pigmented, while it does not ulcerate. A line of demarcation is observed and fingers can be insinuated at the margins. It primarily occurs in children; however, all age groups and both genders are susceptible with male preponderance. The most common sites involved are limbs, chest, back or buttocks, and thighs.

Rhinofacial conidiobolomycosis is a chronic inflammatory or granulomatous localized subcutaneous fungal infection due to *Conidiobolus coronatus* and very rarely *C. incongruus*. It originates, and typically remains localized in the nasal submucosa or to the adjacent subcutaneous tissue of the face. Infections in humans occur mostly in adults with some preponderance for males. The saprophyte is introduced into the nasal mucosa by soiled hands or following inhalation of conidia, and tissue invasion of traumatized mucosa occurs subsequently. The features include unilateral nasal obstruction and development of subcutaneous nodule in the nasal and perinasal regions leading to diffuse swelling on the upper lip or face that may be progressive (Figure 13). Nasal discharge, pain, and sinus tenderness are the other clinical symptoms.

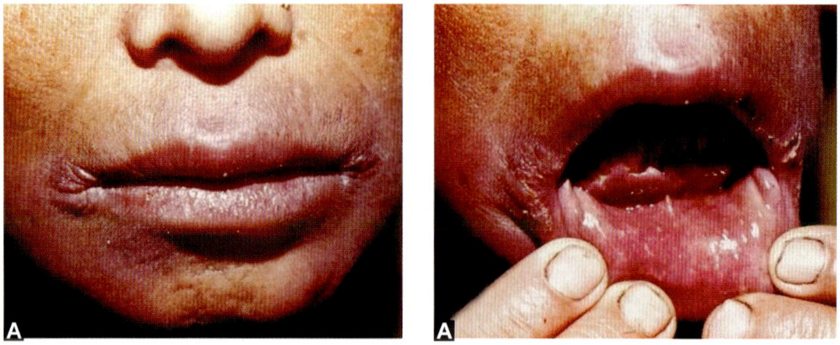

Figure 13: Rhino-orofacial conidiobolomycosis: Erythematous, infiltrated skin, swollen lips, and gingival mucosa.

Diagnosis

Histopathology is identical in all forms of entomophthoromycosis but a skin biopsy is essential and is the most rapid diagnostic method. Presence of broad, 5–15 μm wide, infrequently septate, thin-walled hyphae surrounded by Splendore-Hoeppli phenomenon, and absence of vascular invasion and necrosis in H and E stained sections is pathognomic and will histologically differentiate entomophthoromycosis from mucormycosis. Periodic acid–Schiff and GMS stained sections will demonstrate the causative fungus. Direct microscopic examination of tissue in KOH or calcofluor mounts prepared from the nasal mucosa or skin lesions teased on a glass slide show broad, nonseptate or infrequently septate (coenocytic), irregularly branching hyphae. Culture from a biopsy tissue on SDA containing antibiotics, but without cyclohexamide is useful to identify the fungus.

Treatment

Saturated solution of potassium iodide given for 6–12 months still appears to be first line treatment. Oral itraconazole (200–400 mg/day), ketoconazole (400 mg/day), fluconazole (200 mg/day), or cotrimoxazole, used alone or in combinations have shown variable effectiveness. Amphotericin B or surgical resection is seldom successful. Treatment in conidiobolomycosis is comparatively far less successful.

Mucormycosis

Mucormycosis is caused by saprophytic fungi of the order Mucorales which include *Rhizopus arrhizus, Mucor racemosus, Rhizomucor pusillus,* and *Absidia corymbiform*. Although they are generally considered to be of low virulence, they become pathogenic in patients who are severely debilitated or have uncontrolled diabetes mellitus with ketoacidosis, chronic renal failure on hemodialysis, immunosuppressive therapy, or diseases like AIDS, leukemias, or lymphomas. *Rhizopus* spp. is the most common species in human infections. Common clinical presentations are from rhinocerebral, ocular, pulmonary, gastrointestinal, and cutaneous involvement.

Primary cutaneous mucormycosis is rare and due to direct inoculation of causative fungus into the skin/ulcers of varied etiology via contaminated wound dressings/needles. Most cases are secondary to the disseminated form of disease. The painful lesions enlarge progressively with nodular ecchymotic areas of cutaneous infarction. Necrotizing fasciitis, when occurs has high mortality rate. Cutaneous involvement sometimes occurs in rhinocerebral zygomycosis, which is the most common and fulminating type. The infection spreads from nasal mucosa to turbinate bones, paranasal sinuses, orbit, palate, and brain leading to vascular infarcts ending fatally (Figure 14). The facial lesions are usually swelling and necrotizing ulcers with black eschar. Prognosis in primary cutaneous mucormycosis is better than that in invasive form.

Diagnosis

The acute and fulminant clinical course of the disease in the setting of immuno-suppressive conditions should arouse suspicion. Demonstration of the fungus

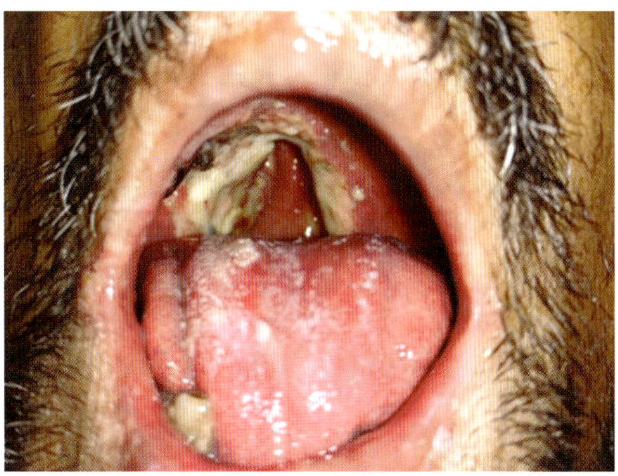

Figure 14: Mucormycosis: Progressive necrotizing infarction involving palate. The infection may spreads from nasal mucosa to turbinate bones, paranasal sinuses, orbit, palate, and brain leading to vascular infarcts ending fatally.

as nonseptate (rarely septate), freely branching hyphae with thin membranous wall in KOH mounts prepared from tissue specimens helps in diagnosis. Isolation by culture in SDA without cycloheximide is confirmatory. Presence of pyogenic inflammatory reaction with presence of polymorphonuclear leukocytes surrounding hyphae, basophilic or amphophilic, broad and aseptate in H and E stained sections, extensive necrosis from vascular invasion, and thrombi with fungal invasion into the vessel wall in histologic sections are hallmark features. A granulomatous inflammation may be seen in chronic infection.

Treatment

It is essential to assess the extent of involvement of the disease by radiologic workup that includes X-ray, CT scan, and magnetic resonance imaging. Treatment with amphotericin B in a dose of 0.5–1.0 mg/kg/day is recommended for about 2 weeks. Avoidance and treatment of predisposing factors is imperative for recovery, and in preventing recurrence.

LOBOMYCOSIS

Lobomycosis (synonyms: keloidal blastomycosis, Lobo's disease) is a rare chronic subcutaneous mycosis that presents with multiple subcutaneous lesions resembling keloids. Geographically, its distribution is mainly limited to tropical zone of South America (Brazil, Ecuador, Bolivia, Colombia, Guyana, Peru, and Suriname) and is sporadically reported from Mexico, Central America (Costa Rica, Panama), France, and the United States. Several names have been used for its pathogen originally named as *Glenosporella loboi* (synonyms: *Glenosporopsis amazonica*, *Paracoccidioides loboi*, *Blastomyces loboi*, *Lacazia loboi*), but *Lacazia loboi* is the most accepted nomenclature. The disease also occurs in fresh water dolphins suggesting that the fungus is perhaps an aquatic saprophyte. Major natural reservoir, however, remains soil and vegetation. Farming, gold mining, fishing, and hunting are high-risk activities for contracting the disease. Most cases appear to be occupational with clear predilection for males between 40 and 70 years. Injuries from a sharp instrument, bite or sting from an insect, snake, and stingray are implicated predisposing factors for the infection. Incubation period is variable, from months to years, and skin lesions develop slowly over time.

The skin lesions often begin as a small papule or pustule, and typical keloid-like lesions appear after several months. Lesions are well-defined, lobulated nodule of variable size, and not attached to underlying structures. The epidermis is smooth, shiny, and has telangiectasias and sometimes "black dots". Any body area is potentially susceptible for the lesions, but these are present mostly over pinna, and lower and upper limbs in that order.

Diagnosis

The important differential diagnosis is from lepromatous leprosy, cutaneous leishmaniasis, keloids, xanthomas, and chromoblastomycosis. Demonstration of causative agent in direct skin smears is quick and easy as the fungus is abundant in the skin lesions. These appear as yeast-like round thick-walled cells, 5–15 μm in diameter arranged in chains of 2–10 cells. Histopathology is pathognomic and shows feature of epidermal atrophy, progressively fibrous, diffuse, inflammatory granulomas composed of histiocytes, and numerous multinucleated giant cells with PAS, GMS positive phagocytosed fungal cells. Attempts to culture *L. loboi* have been unsuccessful.

Treatment

Wide surgical excision of the lesions remains the most successful treatment. Electrodessication for early small lesions is useful. Clofazimine 300 mg/day is the first line drug, and must be given for at least 2 years after initial clinical improvement. Ketoconazole, itraconazole, amphotericin B, and 5-fluorocytosine by and large remain ineffective.

RHINOSPORIDIOSIS

Rhinosporidiosis is caused by *Rhinosporidium seeberi,* an unusual hydrophilic protistan protozoon with phylogenetic features common with microbes infecting fish. It causes a benign chronic granulomatous infection of conjunctiva, nostrils, or other respiratory mucosae.

Epidemiology

Rhinosporidiosis is worldwide especially in tropical and subtropical regions of America, Europe, Africa, and South Asia. Coastal India, Sri Lanka, Argentina, Brazil (Caatinga' region), the United States of America (Texas), and Uganda have high endemicity of rhinosporidiosis. Ocular infections occur in arid conditions where dust acts as a vector while nasal infection is most prevalent among persons bathing in rivers and lakes in tropical areas. Sporadic cases have been reported in travelers returning from endemic areas and nonendemic regions as well.

Clinical Features

Most patients are adult males from poor socioeconomic background while customs and sanitary conditions are considered important factors in disease transmission. The infection is acquired from aquatic source following implantation of endospores into the respiratory mucosa while ocular rhinosporidiosis possibly occurs from dust-borne pathogen. Lesions from autoinoculation may occur from finger contamination or after surgery. Subclinical upper respiratory infection may disseminate via hematogenous route. The incubation period mostly remains undetermined due to slow growth of the evolving papules and hyperplastic polyps involving nasal, nasopharyngeal, or other respiratory mucosae. Ocular rhinosporidiosis is more common in females presenting commonly with the involvement of palpebral and bulbar conjunctiva.

Clinically, the polyp is very friable and its irregular red surface is characteristically studded with yellow-white pinhead sized dots due to numerous mature subepithelial sporangia. While nasal polyp is unilateral, pedunculated and obstructs breathing or cause nasal bleeds, the nasopharyngeal polyps are usually multilobed impairing food intake and speech (Figure 15). Erosion of bone or cartilage, or perforation of nasal septum can occur. Involvement of external ear canal, trachea, bronchial tree, and external genitalia/male urethra is less frequent and dissemination to skin, lymph nodes, lungs, brain, bones, and abdominal viscera

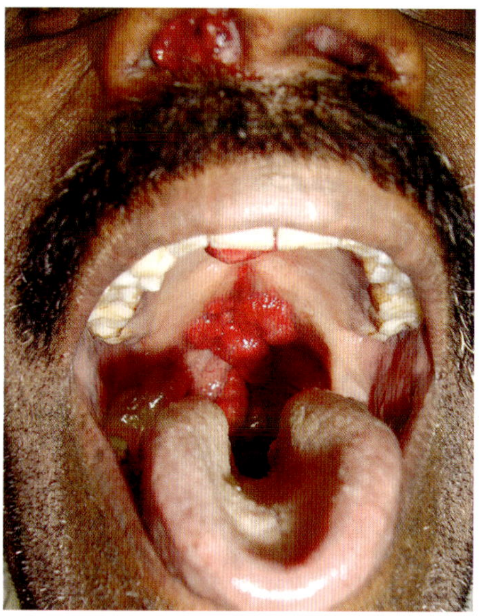

Figure 15: Rhinosporidiosis. Characteristic hyperplastic mucosal polyps of nasal cavity extending into naso-oropharynx and involving the soft palate. Buccal cavity is rarely affected. *Source:* Mahajan VK. Subcutaneous mycoses. Singal A, Grover C, editors. Comprehensive Approach to Infections in Dermatology. 1st ed. New Delhi: Jaypee Brothers Medical Publishers (P) Ltd.; 2015. pp. 116-57, *with permission.*

is extremely rare. Skin lesions are usually subcutaneous nodules, warty growths, or sessile or pedunculated, noninfiltrating polyps.

Diagnosis

Coccidioidomycosis, hemangioma, mucocele, condyloma, neoplasia, granuloma pyogenicum, and subcutaneous myospherulosis, an iatrogenic condition from application of nasal substances, are usual differentials. Osseous lesions may mimic bone tumor.

Pathology

The diagnosis is by demonstration of characteristic thick-walled giant sporangia in histopathologic sections, which may contain numerous endospores in various stages of development. Histologically, wide variation in stroma and cellular infiltrate is observed and subcutaneous myospherulosis and coccidioidomycosis need differentiation. Mild to moderate inflammatory cells infiltrate comprising lymphocytes, plasma cells, histiocytes, and rarely eosinophils or neutrophils (in secondary infected lesions) are observed and especially around endospores. Fibroedematous or fibromyxomatous reactions occur in the subepithelial stroma with few or absent sporangia. Gomori methenamine silver will not stain subcutaneous myospherulosis while large and thick-walled mature stages of *C. immitis* in coccidioidomycosis are smaller than *R. seeberi* sporangia which also contain endospores.

Endospores can also be demonstrated in wet mounts or smears from mucoid material from rhinosporidial polyps and stained with GMS, Papanicolaou's, PAS, Mayer's mucicarmine.

Culture of Causative Organism

The cultivation of the organism in various types of laboratory culture media, with or without nutritional additives, from clinical samples or materials from aquatic sources has remained unsuccessful. The claimed successful growth of *R. seeberi* in monolayers of human rectal epithelioid tumor cell-line remains unsubstantiated. Although sustained propagation and repetition of classic life cycle is not observed on any culture media, laboratory viability and development of endospores has been possible.

Other Diagnostic Methods

The recent molecular techniques based on molecular analysis for 18S small subunit ribosomal ribonucleic acid to identify the organism. There are no serologic tests for diagnosis.

Treatment

Dapsone in adjunct with surgery is the only effective therapy available. Surgical excision of polyp is the treatment of choice despite frequent recurrences as spontaneous remissions are extremely rare. Cauterization of the base of the excised polyp will minimize spillage of endospores, formation of new lesions from autoinoculation, or recurrences while local infiltration of amphotericin B will prevent reinfection and spread of the disease. Povidone-iodine in nasal packs, chlorhexidine and cetrimide-chlorhexidine for skin, and povidone-iodine and silver nitrate for ocular rhinosporidiosis are useful antiseptics in surgery. Small lesions can be treated with cryosurgery but extensive disease may require amputation of the effected part.

OTHER OPPORTUNISTIC SUBCUTANEOUS MYCOSES

Hyalohyphomycosis

A newly recognized mycosis "hyalohyphomycosis" includes infections with hyaline hyphae with no pigment/melanin in the fungal wall (tissue form). The etiologic fungi are saprophytes from class Hyphomycetes and include several organisms from *Acremonium* spp., *Beauveria* spp., *Fusarium* spp., *Paecilomyces* spp., *Penicillium* spp., *Scedosporium* spp., and *Scopulariopsis* spp. causing systemic infections and produce skin lesions in the process of bloodstream dissemination. Clinically, aspergillosis, pseudallescheriasis, fusariosis, and some cases of basidiomycosis form cases of hyalohyphomycosis. They are significant cause of morbidity among immune compromised individuals. However, the nomenclature "hyalohyphomycosis" is not a group of clinical entities or discrete clinical syndrome and the clinical forms are better identified by the actual fungus identified appropriately.

Pythiosis

Pythiosis, an infection caused by *Pythium insidiosum*, is rare in humans but *Pythium* species usually infect animals mainly horses and mules. However, a number of cases have been reported mainly from Thailand in past few years among farmers exposed to swampy areas.

Zoospores are responsible for the infection that usually present with severe ascending gangrene of the lower limbs.

Diagnosis is based on the demonstration of hyaline, sparsely septate, broad (3–20 μm) hyphae in histologic sections stained with methenamine silver and presence of Splendore-Hoeppli phenomenon, an eosinophilic granulomatous reaction around the hyphal elements.

The organism can be cultured from clinical samples on Sabouraud's broth and corn meal agar incubated at 27°C for 5 days.

Amphotericin B in high doses and amputation of affected limb remains the only treatment for want of effective therapeutic agents. Immunotherapy has been tried as an alternative.

Protothecosis

Protothecosis, caused by organisms of genus *Prototheca*, an achlorophilic aerobic algae that occur ubiquitously in nature. Colonization of nails and skin may occur as transients. *Prototheca wickerhamii* and *P. zopfii* are mainly responsible for the human infections that usually follow their traumatic implantation. The clinical presentations vary from cutaneous and subcutaneous lesions to systemic involvement of several internal organs. Protothecal bursitis involving olecranon bursa after injury has been reported. Cutaneous disease usually presents with papules, nodules, ulcers, and multiple granulomatous lesions and the organisms may be found in the epidermis and dermis. Widespread cutaneous, subcutaneous, or deep infection occurs in immunocompromised hosts including AIDS patients.

Small-localized lesions are amenable to surgical excision. Systemic amphotericin B, ketoconazole, or itraconazole are effective.

Fusarium

Fusarium species can cause systemic infection in humans especially in patients with neutropenia, hematological malignancies, and bone marrow or solid organ transplant, often with fatal outcome. *Fusarium* infection may produce widely distributed targetoid lesions with central necrosis, digital cellulitis and superficial white onychomycosis are usual clinical presentations.

Other rare fungi from genera *Scedosporium, Pseudallescheria, Acremonium, Lecythophora, Phialemonium, Phaeoacremonium, Paecilomyces,* and *Emmonsia* causing systemic infections may also produce skin lesions in the process of bloodstream dissemination.

PREVENTION

Since personnel handling plants or plant detritus are at risk of acquiring the disease, use of protective gears and avoiding walking bare feet while working or animal handling will minimize risk for occupational injuries and for acquiring subcutaneous mycotic infections. Making the patients aware of risks of wound contamination from manipulation of skin lesions with thorns and unsterile needles or applying herbal pastes will be preventive. Similarly, contracting lobomycosis and rhinosporidiosis can be escaped by avoiding bathing/swimming in contaminated water bodies. Personal safety measures must particularly be enforced in high-risk occupations like farming, animal husbandry, mining and forestry, aquarium cleaning, fishing, and hunting. Clinicians must also have high index of clinical suspicion for existence of these infections. This will provide an early diagnosis and treatment to prevent chronicity and morbidity. Completion of recommended antifungal therapy for a sufficient period is imperative for mycological cure and to prevent recurrences. Appropriate treatments for immune suppression will prevent severe forms of these infections.

CONCLUSION

Deep mycoses, subcutaneous and systemic, almost account for 1% of the total mycoses and have shown increasing prevalence in this era of immune suppression. These infections are from pathogens which are usually saprophytes to the soil and decaying plant material. Traumatic inoculation of pathogenic fungus leads to involvement of skin, subcutaneous tissue, fascial planes and bones, and infection may disseminate to other organs systems. Sporotrichosis is the commonest subcutaneous mycosis reported worldwide. Chromomycosis (chromoblastomycosis, phaeohyphomycosis), mycetomas (actinomycotic, eumycotic), subcutaneous zygomycosis (entomophthoromycosis, mucormycosis), lobomycosis and rhinosporidiosis have their own endemic foci having tropical/subtropical climates but occur frequently among other populations especially returning travelers/workers from endemic areas. Clinically, the lesions are polymorphic (nodules, plaques, nodulo-ulcerative, nodulo-cystic or warty lesions, discharging sinuses, subcutaneous swellings or masses). Most have protracted clinical course with significant morbidity and poor quality of life for want of diagnostic tools with short turn-round time or effective therapeutic modalities leading to a significant public health problem. High clinical suspicion remains the key to an early diagnosis.

Editor's Comment

Subcutaneous mycoses are a challenging and diverse breadth of infections that can affect both the immunocompetent and immunocompromised host(s). In this article, the author has written a thorough review of infections ranging from chromoblastomycosis, phaeohyphomycosis, mucormycosis, and others. Dr Vikram Mahajan has also commented on therapies as well as prevention items that could help in the management and prevention of these often devastating types of fungal infections.

Seemal R Desai, Rashmi Sarkar

REFERENCES

1. Mahajan VK. Subcutaneous mycoses. In: Singal A, Grover C, editors. Comprehensive Approach to Infections in Dermatology. 1st ed. New Delhi (India): Jaypee Brothers Medical Publishers (P) Ltd.; 2015. pp. 116-57.
2. Arenas R. Sporotrichosis. In: Merz WG, Hay RJ, editors. Topley and Wilson's Microbiology and Microbial Infections: Medical Mycology. 10th ed. Washington DC: ASM Press; 2005. pp. 367-84.
3. Hay R, Ashbee HR. Mycology: subcutaneous mycosis. In: Burns T, Breathnach S, Cox N, Griffiths C, editors. Rook's Textbook of Dermatology. 8th ed. Oxford: Wiley-Blackwell Publishing Ltd.; 2010. pp. 69-79.
4. Gonçalves AP, Canizare O, Hay R, Harman R. Cosmopolitan deep fungal infections of tropical importance. In: Canizare O, Harman R, editors. Clinical Tropical Dermatology. Massachusetts, USA: Blackwell Scientific Publications; 1992. pp. 88-104.
5. Lupi O, Tyring SK, McGinns MR. Tropical dermatology: fungal tropical diseases. *J Am Acad Dermatol.* 2005;53:931-51.
6. Herr RA, Ajello L, Taylor JW, Arseculeratne SN, Mendoza L. Phylogenetic analysis of *Rhinosporidium seeberi's* 18S small-subunit ribosomal DNA groups this pathogen among the members of the protoctistan Mesomycetozoa clade. *J Clin Microbiol.* 1999;37:2750-4.
7. da Rosa AC, Scroferneker ML, Vettorato R, Gervini RL, Vettoreato G, Weber A. Epidemiology of sporotrichosis: a study of 304 cases in Brazil. *J Am Acad Dermatol.* 2005;52:451-9.
8. Gonçalves AP. Sporotrichosis. In: Canizare O, Harman R, editors. Clinical Tropical Dermatology. Massachusetts, USA: Blackwell Scientific Publications; 1992. pp. 88-93.
9. Mahajan VK, Sharma NL, Sharma RC, Gupta ML, Garg G, Kanga AK. Cutaneous sporotrichosis in Himachal Pradesh, India. *Mycoses.* 2005;48:25-31.
10. Mahajan VK, Sharma NL, Shanker V, Gupta P, Mardi K. Cutaneous sporotrichosis: unusual clinical presentations. *Indian J Dermatol Venereol Leprol.* 2010;76:276-80.
11. Gordhan A, Ramdial PK, Morar N, Moodley SD, Aboobaker J. Disseminated cutaneous sporotrichosis: a marker of osteoarticular sporotrichosis masquerading as gout. *Int J Dermatol.* 2001;40:717-9.
12. Esterre P. Chromoblastomycosis. In: Merz WG, Hay RJ, editors. Topley and Wilson's Microbiology and Microbial Infections: Medical Mycology. 10th ed. Washington DC: ASM Press; 2005. pp. 347-55.
13. Sharma NL, Sharma RC, Grover PS, Gupta ML, Sharma AK, Mahajan VK. Chromoblastomycosis in India. *Int J Dermatol.* 1999;38:846-51.
14. Sharma NL, Mahajan V, Sharma RC, Sharma A. Subcutaneous pheohyphomycosis in India: a case report and review. *Int J Dermatol.* 2002;41:16-20.
15. Chowdhary A, Meis JF, Guarro J, de Hoog GS, Kathuria S, Arendrup MC, et al. ESCMID and ECMM joint guidelines for the diagnosis and management of systemic phaeohyphomycosis: diseases caused by black fungi. *Clin Microbiol Infect.* 2014;20(Suppl. 3):47-75.
16. Hay RJ. Eumycetomas. In: Merz WG, Hay RJ, editors. Topley and Wilson's Microbiology and Microbial Infections: Medical Mycology. 10th ed. Washington DC: ASM Press; 2005. pp. 385-95.
17. Sharma NL, Mahajan VK, Aggarwal S, Katoch VM, Das R, Kashyap M, et al. Nocardial mycetoma: diverse clinical presentations. *Indian J Dermatol Venereol Leprol.* 2008;74:635-40.
18. Capoor MR, Khanna G, Nair D, Hasan A, Rajni, Deb M, et al. Eumycetoma pedis due to Exophiala jeanselmei. *Indian J Med Microbiol.* 2007;25:155-7.
19. Loulergue P, Hot A, Dannaoui E, Dallot A, Poirée S, Dupont B, et al. Successful treatment of black-grain mycetoma with voriconazole. *Am J Trop Med Hyg.* 2006;75:1106-7.
20. Resnik BI, Burdick AE. Improvement of eumycetoma with itraconazole. *J Am Acad Dermatol.* 1995;33(5 Pt 2):917-9.
21. Ellis DH. Subcutaneous zygomycosis. In: Merz WG, Hay RJ, editors. Topley and Wilson's Microbiology and Microbial Infections: Medical Mycology. 10th ed. Washington DC: ASM Press; 2005. pp. 345-6.
22. Sharma NL, Mahajan VK, Singh P. Orofacial conidiobolomycosis due to Conidiobolous incongruus. *Mycoses.* 2003;46:137-40.

23. Harman R. Subcutaneous zygomycosis. In: Canizares O, Harman R, editors. Clinical Tropical Dermatology, 2nd edition. Massachusetts: Blackwell Scientific Publications; 1992. pp. 85-7.
24. Talhari S, Pradinaud R. Lobomycosis. In: Merz WG, Hay RJ, editors. Topley and Wilson's Microbiology and Microbial Infections: Medical Mycology. 10th ed. Washington DC: ASM Press; 2005. pp. 430-5.
25. Sterling JB, Heymann WR. Potassium iodide in dermatology: a 19th century drug for the 21st century: uses, pharmacology, adverse effects, and contraindications. *J Am Acad Dermatol.* 2000;43:691-7.
26. Narendranath S, Sudhakar GK, Pai MR, Kini H, Pinto J, Pai MR. Safety and efficacy of oral potassium iodide in chromoblastomycosis. *Int J Dermatol.* 2010;49:341-2.
27. Welsh O, Sauceda E, Gonzalez J, Ocampo J. Amikacin alone and in combination with trimethoprim-sulfamethoxazole in the treatment of actinomycotic mycetoma. *J Am Acad Dermatol.* 1987;17:443-8.
28. Damle DK, Mahajan PM, Pradhan SN, Belgaumkar VA, Gosavi AP, Tolat N, et al. Modified Welsh regimen: a promising therapy for actinomycetmoa. *J Drug Dermatol.* 2008;7:853-7.
29. Barati M, Talebi-Taher M, Nojomi M, Kerami F. Ten-year experience of rhinocerebral zygomycosis in a teaching hospital in Tehran. *Iranian J Clin Infect Dis.* 2010;5:117-20.
30. Yeung CK, Cheng VC, Lie AK, Yuen KY. Invasive disease due to *Mucorales*: a case report and review of the literature. *HKMJ.* 2001;7:180-8.
31. Chambers CJ, Merin MR, Fung MA, Huntley A, Sharon VR. Primary cutaneous mucormycosis at sites of insulin injection. *J Am Acad Dermatol.* 2011;64:e79-e80.
32. Chakrabarti A, Das A, Sharma A, Panda N, Das S, Gupta KL, et al. Ten years experience in Zygomycosis at a tertiary care center in India. *J Infect.* 2001;42:261-6.
33. Ameen M, Arenas R. Developments in the management of mycetomas. *Clin Exp Dermatol.* 2009;34:1-7.
34. Bermudez L, Bressem MV, Reyes-Jaimes O, Sayegh AJ, Paniz-Mondolfi AE. Lobomycosisi man and lobomycosis like disease in bottlenose dolphin, Venezuela. *Emerg Infect Dis.* 2004;15:1301-3.
35. Ajello L. Hyalohyphomycosis: a disease entity whose time has come. *Med Mycol Soc NY (News Letter).* 1982;20:3-5.
36. Matsumoto T, Ajello L, Matsuda T, Szaniszlo PJ, Walsh TJ. Developments in hyalohyphomycosis and phaeohyphomycosis. *J Med Vet Mycol.* 1994;32 Suppl 1:329-49.

World Clin Dermatol. 2016;3(1):139-50.

Overview of Antifungal Therapies

Allen SW Oak BS, *Boni E Elewski MD

Department of Dermatology, University of Alabama
Birmingham, Alabama, USA

ABSTRACT

Superficial fungal infections, such as onychomycosis, that are often nonproblematic in healthy patients can have more significant sequelae in those with primary or secondary immunodeficiency, an underlying malignancy, or diabetes mellitus. Furthermore, the economic burden of treating cutaneous fungal infections is considerable. There has been great interest in understanding the pathogenesis of fungal infections to meet the growing need to develop more efficacious antifungal therapy. Several classes of antifungal agents, including azoles and allylamines, with distinct antifungal mechanisms are currently available. Other miscellaneous agents, such as griseofulvin—a fungal mitotic inhibitor, are also available. An up-to-date mechanistic understanding, indications, adverse effects, pertinent clinical trials findings, and relevant pharmacologic properties are discussed for the following four systemic antifungals that are commonly used to treat cutaneous fungal infections—itraconazole, fluconazole, terbinafine, and griseofulvin.

INTRODUCTION

The global prevalence of cutaneous fungal infections exceeds 984,290,432,[1] and the estimated annual total cost of cutaneous fungal infections is over $1.9 billion in the United States alone.[2] In an immunocompetent host, most superficial mycoses respond adequately to topical antifungal therapy. However, systemic treatment is needed under certain circumstances. Such conditions include hair or nail involvement, failure of topical treatments, extensive cutaneous involvement, significant inflammatory reaction secondary to the superficial mycosis, and chronic or recurrent cases. Furthermore, systemic treatments are required to treat superficial mycoses in immunocompromised hosts.

*Corresponding author
Email: beelewski@gmail.com

© 2016 Jaypee Brothers Medical Publishers. All rights reserved.

AZOLES

Mechanism of Action

Ergosterol, a fungal analog of 7-dehydrocholesterol present in animals, plays a critical role in maintaining permeability and membrane fluidity in fungal cells.[3,4] Ergosterol is also found in various other organelles (e.g., peroxisomes and endoplasmic reticulum).[3] Deletion of genes that encode early steps of ergosterol synthesis is lethal.[3] Azoles target the ergosterol biosynthesis pathway by acting as competitive metalloenzyme inhibitors of 14α-demethylase, a fungal-specific cytochrome P450 (CYP450)-dependent enzyme that facilitates the biosynthesis of ergosterol from lanosterol.[3,4] The resulting inhibition of 14α-demethylase not only depletes ergosterol, but also causes a buildup of its sterol precursors that jeopardize the integrity of the fungal plasma membrane.[4]

Itraconazole

Indications

Itraconazole capsules are Food and Drug Administration (FDA)-approved to treat fingernail or toenail onychomycosis.[5] A pulse regimen (Table 2) is FDA-approved for treating onychomycosis involving only fingernails.[5] Itraconazole tablets, approved to treat toenail onychomycosis caused by *Trichophyton rubrum* or *Trichophyton mentagrophytes*, contain a dose of 2 capsules, and allow once-daily dosing.[6] An oral solution formulation is FDA-approved to treat esophageal/oropharyngeal candidiasis, but not for onychomycosis.

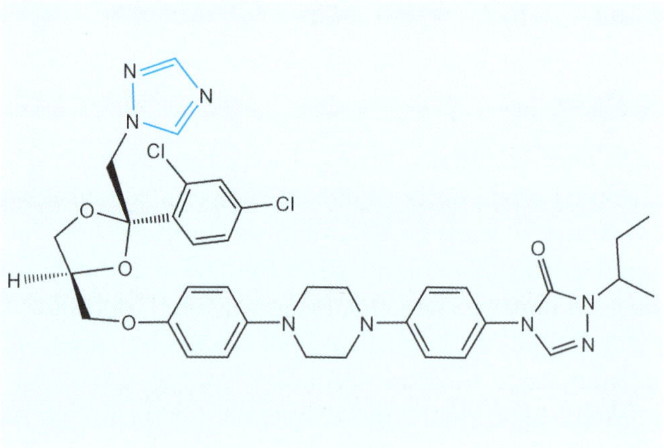

Figure 1: Structure of itraconazole. The characteristic triazole ring in blue.

When evaluating an antifungal agent's efficacy in treating onychomycosis (Table 2), three parameters—clinical cure, mycologic cure (MC), and complete cure (CC)—are used. The attainment of clinical cure indicates that 100% of the nail plate is clear of infection. Mycologic cure is attained when the fungal culture and the potassium hydroxide smear are both negative. Complete cure requires both MC and clinical cure.[7]

Adverse Effects

Itraconazole is tolerated well overall, and only 3% of patients report AEs when it is used to treat onychomycosis.[8] Common AEs include headache (2.2–10%), diarrhea and abdominal pain/discomfort (1.7–4%), rash (4%), and upper respiratory tract infections (6–8%).[5,6] Rare AEs include acute liver injury and acute generalized exanthematous pustulosis (AGEP).[5] Increased bone fragility, reduced activity of bone plates, and increased dental abnormalities have been reported as itraconazole-induced bone defects in animal studies.[5] Such defects make itraconazole treatment, especially over a prolonged period, undesirable in children. Itraconazole exerts a negative inotropic effect and causes QT prolongation.[6] Itraconazole use had been linked to 58 cases of congestive heart failure, 13 of which were fatal, between 1992 and 2001.[9]

Fluconazole

Indications

Fluconazole is approved to treat onychomycosis in European countries, and is widely used off-label to treat onychomycosis in the United States. Pulse fluconazole (Table 2) is a weekly regimen that may potentially increase patient compliance; its

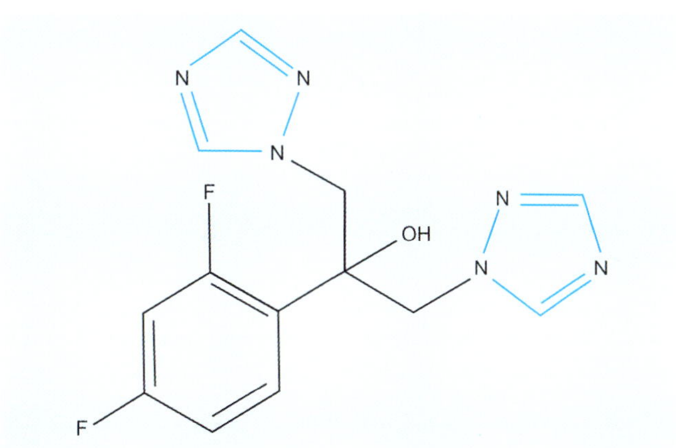

Figure 2: Structure of fluconazole. The characteristic triazole rings in blue.

Table 1: Drug Metabolism, Parameters to Monitor, Contraindications, and Pregnancy Category for Systemic Antifungals

Allylamine	
Terbinafine	• Metabolism: Undergoes extensive hepatic metabolism • Inhibition of CYP enzymes:[40] CYP2D6 (moderate), CYP1A2 (weak) • Parameters to monitor: CBC (when treating immunocompromised patients for >6 weeks) and LFTs (before and during use). Levels and drug-drug interactions between drugs metabolized by CYP2D6 • Contraindications: Prior liver disease (relative contraindication) • Pregnancy category: B
Azoles	
Fluconazole	• Metabolism: Approximately 80% of the administered dose found in urine in unchanged form; 11% found as N-oxide and glucuronide metabolites, both products of hepatic metabolism by CYP3A4 • Inhibition of CYP enzymes:[40,41] CYP3A4 (≥200 mg/day, moderate), CYP2C9 (moderate), CYP2C19 (strong) • Parameters to monitor: Periodic renal function tests and LFTs. Levels and drug-drug interactions between drugs metabolized by CYP2C9, CYP3A4, and CYP2C19 • Contraindications: Concomitant administration of drugs metabolized by CYP3A4 that cause QT prolongation. Severe liver disease • Pregnancy category: D
Itraconazole	• Metabolism: Occurs extensively in the liver. Major substrate of CYP3A4 • Inhibition of CYP enzymes:40 CYP3A4 inhibitor (strong) • Parameters to monitor: Renal function and signs/symptoms of CHF. LFT for those treated >1 month or those with preexisting liver dysfunction • Contraindications: Concomitant administration of certain drugs metabolized by CYP3A4 (e.g., ergot alkaloids), or other drugs that cause QT prolongation. A history of CHF or any evidence of ventricular dysfunction. Strongly discouraged in those with reported liver toxicity with other drugs, or patients with active liver disease • Pregnancy category: C
Miscellaneous	
Griseofulvin	• Metabolism: Occurs extensively in the liver • Parameters to monitor: Periodic LFTs. Hematopoietic and renal function tests, especially with long-term use • Contraindications: pregnancy, liver failure, and porphyria. Male patients advised to wait at least 6 months after completing griseofulvin treatment prior to fathering a child • Pregnancy category: X

Note: All information was retrieved from package inserts unless otherwise noted.
LFT, liver function test; CHF, congestive heart failure; CBC, complete blood count.

efficacy is duration-dependent, but not dose-dependent.[10] Onychomycosis trials evaluating the cure rates of pulse fluconazole, pulse itraconazole, and continuous terbinafine demonstrated that pulse fluconazole was the least efficacious in attaining CC and MC.[11,12] Therefore, fluconazole may have a role as a third line treatment in those unable to tolerate itraconazole and terbinafine. A notable exception is onychomycosis caused by *Candida* species, frequent colonizers of toe webs in diabetic feet.[13] Since terbinafine lacks reliable efficacy against *Candida* onychomycosis, and itraconazole's negative inotropic effect makes its use undesirable in diabetics, fluconazole is the treatment of choice for *Candida* onychomycosis in diabetics.[13]

Fluconazole is also used off-label to treat tinea capitis in the United States and Europe. A randomized controlled trial of pediatric patients with tinea capitis (n = 880, isolated dermatophytes on culture: *Microsporum canis* 11% and *Trichophyton tonsurans* 86%) treated with either fluconazole (6 mg/kg/day for 6 weeks) or griseofulvin (11 mg/kg/day for 6 weeks) demonstrated no significant differences in mycological, clinical, or combined outcomes.[14] A meta-analysis in 2016 reported no significant differences in rates of CC and treatment-related AEs between children treated with fluconazole (2–6 weeks) and griseofulvin (6 weeks) with 8–12 weeks of follow-up.[15] Therefore, fluconazole may be a safe alternative to griseofulvin with comparable treatment efficacy.

Adverse Effects

Most common AEs include nausea (3.7%, 2% in children), headache (1.9%), abdominal pain (1.7%, 3% in children), vomiting (1.7%, 5% in children), and diarrhea (1.5%, 2% in children).[16] Rare AEs include drug eruption, Stevens-Johnson syndrome (SJS), toxic epidermal necrolysis, and AGEP.[16] Telogen effluvium had been associated with prolonged use (400 mg/day for 2 months or longer).[17] The risk of liver injury with fluconazole use is low. However, cases of deadly hepatic necrosis have been reported.[16] Fluconazole causes QT prolongation.[16] Oral fluconazole use should be avoided during pregnancy based on recent epidemiological studies that demonstrate that (i) *in utero* exposure of fluconazole increases the risks of tetralogy of Fallot,[18] cleft lip with cleft palate, and D-transposition of the great arteries[19] and (ii) an increased risk of spontaneous abortion is observed with oral fluconazole use during pregnancy.[20]

ALLYLAMINE

Mechanism of Action

Allylamines act as noncompetitive inhibitors of squalene epoxidase.[8] The resulting deficiency of ergosterol and the intracellular accumulation of squalene interfere with membrane function and the fungal cell wall synthesis.[8]

Terbinafine

Indications

Terbinafine is the most efficacious systemic antifungal currently FDA-approved to treat onychomycosis (Table 2). Terbinafine tablets are approved to treat fingernail or toenail dermatophyte onychomycosis in adults.[21] Prospective, randomized, multicenter, double-blind clinical trials, including the Lamisil vs. Itraconazole in Onychomycosis (LION) study, have previously compared continuous terbinafine (250 mg/day) and continuous (200 mg/day) or pulse (400 mg/day for 1 week, every 4 weeks) itraconazole in treating dermatophyte onychomycosis.[22-25] At the end of outcome assessments that were carried out at up to 40-72 weeks, continuous terbinafine yielded CC and MC of 38–55% and 73–81%, respectively; continuous or pulse itraconazole yielded CC and MC of 23–26% and 38–63%.[22-25] Terbinafine also showed a lower rate of both mycologic and clinical relapse in the LION Icelandic Extension Study that prospectively followed up 144 LION study participants from Iceland for 5 years.[26]

Other desirable properties of terbinafine include (i) its lack of interaction with CYP3A4 (Table 1), hepatic isozyme responsible for metabolizing most drugs currently available and (ii) its fungicidal properties.[21] Such properties make terbinafine a first line agent for treating onychomycosis, except in rare cases caused by *Candida* species or nondermatophyte molds.

Pulse therapy with terbinafine is not FDA-approved, but it still is commonly used.[27] For treating dermatophyte toenail onychomycosis, no significant difference was found between pulse and continuous regimens for achieving CC.[28]

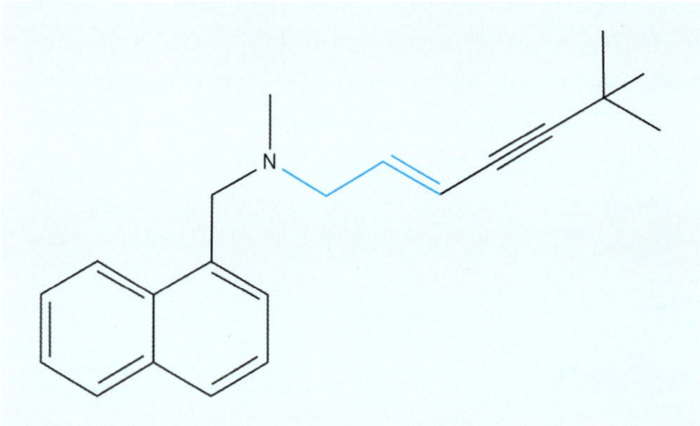

Figure 3: Structure of terbinafine. The characteristic allylamine structure in blue.

Table 2: Reported Cure Rates Against Onychomycosis and the Route of Incorporation into Nails

		Dosage and cure rates		Route of incorporation
Allylamine				
Terbinafine		*Toenails*[*,42]		• Diffuses from the nail plate, as well as the nail matrix[8]
		250 mg/day for 12 weeks	MC: 70% CC: 38%	
		Fingernails[*]		
		250 mg/day for 6 weeks	MC: 79% CC: 59%	
Azoles				
Fluconazole[†]		*Toenails*[10,43]		• Rapidly diffuses from the nail bed, as well as the nail matrix[8] • Detectable in <2 h after a single dose in nails[44]
		150, 300, or 450 mg once weekly for 12–48 weeks	MC: 55–62% CC: 20–36%	
		Fingernails[10]		
		150, 300, or 450 mg once weekly for 12–48 weeks	MC: 90–99% CC: 78–90%	
Itraconazole	C	*Toenails*[†]		• Diffuses from the nail bed, as well as the nail matrix[8]
		200 mg/day for 12 weeks	MC: 54% CC: 14%	
		Fingernails[†]		
		Pulse: 400 mg/day for 1 week, followed by 3 weeks without treatment; 2 pulses recommended	MC: 61% CC: 47%	
	T	*Toenails*[*]		
		200 mg/day for 12 weeks	MC: 44% CC: 22%	
Miscellaneous				
Griseofulvin[‡]		*Toenails*[45-48]		• Taken up by keratin precursor cells[36] • Binds new keratin that subsequently become resistant to fungal invasion[36] • Binds with higher affinity to diseased tissue[36]
		0.5–1 g/day (microsize or ultramicrosize) for ≤18 months	MC: 46–62% CC: 2–56%	
		Fingernails[49]		
		500 mg/day (microsize) for 12 weeks	MC: 63% CC: 39%	

C, capsule; T, tablet; CC, complete cure; MC, mycologic cure.

*Rates reported on the package insert.

†Not Food and Drugs Administration-approved to treat onychomycosis.

‡Not commonly used for dermatophyte onychomycosis since itraconazole and terbinafine have better efficacy, tolerability, and safety profiles.

However, the risk of treatment discontinuation due to AEs was higher for those on continuous therapy [pooled risk: 3.44%, 95% confidence interval (CI): 2.28%–4.61%] than those on pulse therapy (pooled risk: 2.09%, 95% CI: 0%–4.42%).[29] A potential benefit of eradicating newly germinating spores between pulses of treatment provides an additional advantage for using pulse therapy since these structures are thought to be responsible for relapse.[28]

Miniature oral granules of terbinafine hydrochloride are FDA-approved to treat tinea capitis in children older than 4. Terbinafine requires a shorter duration of therapy, typically 4 weeks, than griseofulvin that requires 6 weeks or more.[30] Terbinafine and griseofulvin are both safe to administer with comparable rates of AEs [risk ratio (RR): 1.11, 95% CI: 0.79-1.57], but their relative therapeutic efficacies are species-dependent.[15,30,31] Terbinafine has a higher rate of CC for cases caused by *T. tonsurans* (RR: 1.47, 95% CI: 1.22–1.77).[15,30,31] However, terbinafine has a lower rate of CC for tinea capitis caused by *Microsporum* species (RR: 0.68, 95% CI: 0.53–0.86). Efficacies are comparable for treating cases caused by *T. violaceum*.[15,30,31]

Adverse Effects

Approximately, 10.5% of patients report AEs. Most AEs are mild and transient events that involve either the skin (2.3%) or the gastrointestinal system (4.9%).[32-34] Rare cutaneous AEs include erythema multiforme, SJS, AGEP, and drug reaction with eosinophilia and systemic symptoms (DRESS) syndrome.[21] Cases of terbinafine-induced subacute cutaneous lupus erythematosus (SCLE) are rare, but are well-documented with more than 31 reported cases that account for 26% of all cases of drug-induced SCLE.[35] Rare reversible cases of transient taste disturbance (0.06%) and hepatobiliary events (0.2%) have been reported.[32] Clinically apparent cases of hepatic injury are observed in only 1:50,000–120,000 patients after continuous therapy for 4–6 weeks.[27]

MISCELLANEOUS AGENT

Griseofulvin

Mechanism of Action

Griseofulvin results in mitotic arrest at metaphase by binding microtubules, and inhibiting their assembly and contraction.[36] Consequently, griseofulvin is a fungistatic agent that only exerts its effect on actively dividing cells.

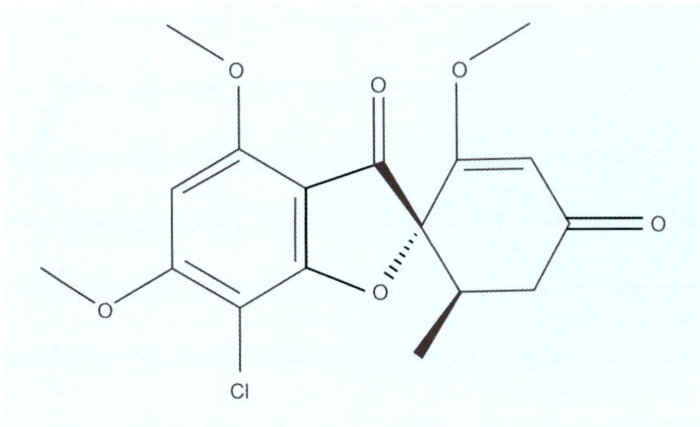

Figure 4: Structure of griseofulvin

Indications

Griseofulvin is available in the United States, but is no longer available in Canada and some European nations (e.g., Belgium, Portugal, and Greece). Griseofulvin is widely used to treat tinea capitis, and remains the treatment of choice for infections caused by *Microsporum* species. *Microsporum* species infections are ectothrix, and thus require the therapeutic agent to reach the hair surface either by sweat or sebum to exert its antifungal effect. However, children have low sebum excretion, and thus require drug delivery via sweat. Griseofulvin can be detected on the body surface several hours after an oral administration since it tends to be secreted in sweat.[37] On the other hand, terbinafine is highly lipophilic, and is not found in sweat.[38] Griseofulvin's ability to utilize sweat as a carrier to the stratum corneum may explain its higher efficacy in treating *Microsporum* species infections.[38]

Adverse Effects

Griseofulvin (10–20 mg/kg) was well-tolerated in pediatric patients (n = 509) for treating tinea capitis for 6 weeks, and no severe AEs were attributed to its use.[31] Common mild or moderate AEs reported with griseofulvin use include nausea (1.2%), vomiting (1.6%), diarrhea (1%), headache (1.4%), and upper abdominal pain (1%).[31]

Rare AEs linked to griseofulvin use include intrahepatic cholestasis, SCLE, and systemic lupus erythematosus exacerbation.[36] Acute intermittent porphyria precipitation in predisposed individuals had been reported with griseofulvin use.[39] Cases of griseofulvin-induced photosensitivity have been reported.[36] Griseofulvin, a spindle poison, is teratogenic and embryotoxic. Cases of conjoined twins had been linked to griseofulvin use during the first trimester of pregnancy.[36]

CONCLUSION

The clinical importance of cutaneous fungal infections led to substantial progress in developing more efficacious systemic antifungal agents, especially over the past two decades. As a result, griseofulvin is no longer considered first line therapy for dermatophyte onychomycosis since itraconazole and terbinafine have better tolerability and efficacy. Fluconazole may have a role as a third line treatment in those unable to tolerate itraconazole and terbinafine. Pulse regimen, which may potentially increase patient compliance, is commonly used in clinical practice.

Griseofulvin and terbinafine hydrochloride are currently FDA-approved to treat tinea capitis. Fluconazole is not FDA-approved for this indication, but it is a safe alternative to griseofulvin with similar treatment efficacy. Griseofulvin requires a prolonged treatment course of at least 6 weeks. Terbinafine hydrochloride offers the advantage of shorter treatment duration, typically 4 weeks. Both are safe with similar rates of AEs, but their relative therapeutic efficacies are species-dependent. Terbinafine is superior to griseofulvin for treating tinea capitis caused by *T. tonsurans*, but is inferior for treating cases caused by *Microsporum* species. Terbinafine and griseofulvin have a similar efficacy for treating cases caused by *T. violaceum*.

Editor's Comment

The authors of this article have addressed a vitally important and equally challenging area of fungal disease management. Without a thorough and comprehensive understanding of antifungal agents, dermatologists and other practioners would find it very difficult to effectively treat patients suffering from these often serious conditions. Dr. Boni Elewski and Allen Oak have eloquently highlighted each drug category, mechanism of action, indications and adverse effects. Through this organized process, the reader will gain invaluable knowledge to aid in the treatment of the patient with fungal disease.

Seemal R Desai, Rashmi Sarkar

REFERENCES

1. Hay RJ, Johns NE, Williams HC, Bolliger IW, Dellavalle RP, Margolis DJ, et al. The global burden of skin disease in 2010: an analysis of the prevalence and impact of skin conditions. *J Invest Dermatol.* 2014;134(6):1527-34.
2. Bickers DR, Lim HW, Margolis D, Weinstock MA, Goodman C, Faulkner E, et al. The burden of skin diseases: 2004 a joint project of the American Academy of Dermatology Association and the Society for Investigative Dermatology. *J Am Acad Dermatol.* 2006;55(3):490-500.
3. Zhang Y-Q, Rao R. Beyond ergosterol: linking pH to antifungal mechanisms. *Virulence.* 2010;1(6):551-4.

4. Barrett-Bee K, Dixon G. Ergosterol biosynthesis inhibition: a target for antifungal agents. *Acta Biochim Pol.* 1995;42(4):465-79.
5. Janssen Pharmaceuticals. SPORANOX (itraconazole) Capsules [package insert]. Beerse, Belgium; 2014 Dec.
6. Merz Pharma. ONMEL (itraconazole) Tablets [package insert]. Greensboro, North Carolina; 2012 Nov.
7. Scher RK, Tavakkol A, Sigurgeirsson B, Hay RJ, Joseph WS, Tosti A, et al. Onychomycosis: Diagnosis and definition of cure. *J Am Acad Dermatol.* 2007;56(6):939-44.
8. Elewski B, Tavakkol A. Safety and tolerability of oral antifungal agents in the treatment of fungal nail disease: a proven reality. *Ther Clin Risk Manag.* 2005;1(4):299-306.
9. Ahmad SR, Singer SJ, Leissa BG. Congestive heart failure associated with itraconazole. *Lancet Lond Engl.* 2001;357(9270):1766-7.
10. Gupta AK, Drummond-Main C, Paquet M. Evidence-based optimal fluconazole dosing regimen for onychomycosis treatment. *J Dermatol Treat.* 2013;24(1):75-80.
11. Havu V, Heikkilä H, Kuokkanen K, Nuutinen M, Rantanen T, Saari S, et al. A double-blind, randomized study to compare the efficacy and safety of terbinafine (Lamisil) with fluconazole (Diflucan) in the treatment of onychomycosis. *Br J Dermatol.* 2000;142(1):97-102.
12. Arca E, Taştan HB, Akar A, Kurumlu Z, Gür AR. An open, randomized, comparative study of oral fluconazole, itraconazole and terbinafine therapy in onychomycosis. *J Dermatol Treat.* 2002;13(1):3-9.
13. Cathcart S, Cantrell W, Elewski B. Onychomycosis and diabetes. *J Eur Acad Dermatol Venereol.* 2009;23(10):1119-22.
14. Foster KW, Friedlander SF, Panzer H, Ghannoum MA, Elewski BE. A randomized controlled trial assessing the efficacy of fluconazole in the treatment of pediatric tinea capitis. *J Am Acad Dermatol.* 2005;53(5):798-809.
15. Chen X, Jiang X, Yang M, González U, Lin X, Hua X, et al. Systemic antifungal therapy for tinea capitis in children. *Cochrane Database Syst Rev.* 2016;5:CD004685.
16. Pfizer. DIFLUCAN (Fluconazole) Tablets and oral suspension [package insert]. New York City, NY;
17. Pappas PG. Alopecia Associated with Fluconazole Therapy. *Ann Intern Med.* 1995;123(5):354.
18. Mølgaard-Nielsen D, Pasternak B, Hviid A. Use of oral fluconazole during pregnancy and the risk of birth defects. *N Engl J Med.* 2013;369(9):830-9.
19. Howley MM, Carter TC, Browne ML, Romitti PA, Cunniff CM, Druschel CM, et al. Fluconazole use and birth defects in the National Birth Defects Prevention Study. *Am J Obstet Gynecol.* 2016;214(5):657.e1-9.
20. Mølgaard-Nielsen D, Svanström H, Melbye M, Hviid A, Pasternak B. Association between use of oral fluconazole during pregnancy and risk of spontaneous abortion and stillbirth. *JAMA.* 2016;315(1):58.
21. Novartis. LAMISIL (terbinafine hydrochloride) Tablets [package insert]. Basel, Switzerland; 2015 Feb.
22. De Backer M, De Vroey C, Lesaffre E, Scheys I, De Keyser P. Twelve weeks of continuous oral therapy for toenail onychomycosis caused by dermatophytes: a double-blind comparative trial of terbinafine 250 mg/day versus itraconazole 200 mg/day. *J Am Acad Dermatol.* 1998;38(5):S57-63.
23. Bräutigam M, Nolting S, Schopf RE, Weidinger G. Randomised double blind comparison of terbinafine and itraconazole for treatment of toenail tinea infection. Seventh Lamisil German Onychomycosis Study Group. *BMJ.* 1995;311(7010):919-22.
24. Evans EG, Sigurgeirsson B. Double blind, randomised study of continuous terbinafine compared with intermittent itraconazole in treatment of toenail onychomycosis. The LION Study Group. *BMJ.* 1999;318(7190):1031-5.
25. Sigurgeirsson B, Billstein S, Rantanen T, Ruzicka T, di Fonzo E, Vermeer BJ, et al. L.I.ON. Study: efficacy and tolerability of continuous terbinafine (Lamisil) compared to intermittent itraconazole in the treatment of toenail onychomycosis. Lamisil vs. Itraconazole in Onychomycosis. *Br J Dermatol.* 1999;141 Suppl 56:5-14.
26. Sigurgeirsson B, Olafsson JH, Steinsson JB, Paul C, Billstein S, Evans EGV. Long-term effectiveness of treatment with terbinafine vs itraconazole in onychomycosis: a 5-year blinded prospective follow-up study. *Arch Dermatol.* 2002;138(3):353-7.
27. Kanzler MH. Reevaluating the need for laboratory testing in the treatment of onychomycosis: safety and cost-effectiveness considerations. *JAMA Dermatol.* 2016;152(3):263-4.

28. Gupta AK, Paquet M, Simpson F, Tavakkol A. Terbinafine in the treatment of dermatophyte toenail onychomycosis: a meta-analysis of efficacy for continuous and intermittent regimens. *J Eur Acad Dermatol Venereol.* 2013;27(3):267-72.
29. Chang C-H, Young-Xu Y, Kurth T, Orav JE, Chan AK. The safety of oral antifungal treatments for superficial dermatophytosis and onychomycosis: a meta-analysis. *Am J Med.* 2007;120(9):791-8.
30. Tey HL, Tan ASL, Chan YC. Meta-analysis of randomized, controlled trials comparing griseofulvin and terbinafine in the treatment of tinea capitis. *J Am Acad Dermatol.* 2011;64(4):663-70.
31. Elewski BE, Cáceres HW, DeLeon L, El Shimy S, Hunter JA, Korotkiy N, et al. Terbinafine hydrochloride oral granules versus oral griseofulvin suspension in children with tinea capitis: Results of two randomized, investigator-blinded, multicenter, international, controlled trials. *J Am Acad Dermatol.* 2008;59(1):41-54.
32. O'Sullivan DP, Needham CA, Bangs A, Atkin K, Kendall FD. Postmarketing surveillance of oral terbinafine in the UK: report of a large cohort study. *Br J Clin Pharmacol.* 1996;42(5):559-65.
33. Hall M, Monka C, Krupp P, O'Sullivan D. Safety of oral terbinafine: results of a postmarketing surveillance study in 25,884 patients. *Arch Dermatol.* 1997;133(10):1213-9.
34. O'Sullivan DP. Terbinafine: tolerability in general medical practice. *Br J Dermatol.* 1999;141 Suppl 56:21-5.
35. Kalińska-Bienias A, Kowalewski C, Woźniak K. Terbinafine-induced subacute cutaneous lupus erythematosus in two patients with systemic lupus erythematosus successfully treated with topical corticosteroids. *Adv Dermatol Allergol.* 2013;4:261-4.
36. Janssen Pharmaceuticals. Grifulvin V [package insert]. Beerse, Belgium; 2011 Sep.
37. Shah VP, Epstein WL, Riegelman S. Role of sweat in accumulation of orally administered griseofulvin in skin. *J Clin Invest.* 1974;53(6):1673-8.
38. Wolverton SE, editor. Comprehensive dermatologic drug therapy. 3rd ed. Edinburgh: Saunders/Elsevier; 2013. p. 826.
39. Hay RJ. Risk/benefit ratio of modern antifungal therapy: Focus on hepatic reactions. *J Am Acad Dermatol.* 1993;29(1):S50-4.
40. Drug Development and Drug Interactions: Table of Substrates, Inhibitors and Inducers [Internet]. U.S. Food and Drug Administration; 2014 Oct [cited 2016 Sep 19]. Available from: http://www.fda.gov/Drugs/DevelopmentApprovalProcess/DevelopmentResources/DrugInteractionsLabeling/ucm093664.htm.
41. Venkatakrishnan K, von Moltke LL, Greenblatt DJ. Effects of the antifungal agents on oxidative drug metabolism: clinical relevance. *Clin Pharmacokinet.* 2000;38(2):111-80.
42. Drake LA, Shear NH, Arlette JP, Cloutier R, Danby FW, Elewski BE, et al. Oral terbinafine in the treatment of toenail onychomycosis: North American multicenter trial. *J Am Acad Dermatol.* 1997;37(5 Pt 1):740-5.
43. Scher RK, Breneman D, Rich P, Savin RC, Feingold DS, Konnikov N, et al. Once-weekly fluconazole (150, 300, or 450 mg) in the treatment of distal subungual onychomycosis of the toenail. *J Am Acad Dermatol.* 1998;38(6):S77-86.
44. Hay R. Pharmacokinetic evaluation of fluconazole in skin and nails. *Int J Dermatol.* 31(Suppl. 2):6.
45. Baran R, Belaich S, Beylot C, Bonnetblanc J, Cribier B, Daniel F, et al. Comparative multicentre double-blind study of terbinafine (250 mg per day) versus griseofulvin (1 g per day) in the treatment of dermatophyte onychomycosis. *J Dermatol Treat.* 1997;8(2):93-7.
46. Faergemann J, Anderson C, Hersle K, Hradil E, Nordin P, Kaaman T, et al. Double-blind, parallel-group comparison of terbinafine and griseofulvin in the treatment of toenail onychomycosis. *J Am Acad Dermatol.* 1995;32(5 Pt 1):750-3.
47. Hofmann H. Treatment of toenail onychomycosis: a randomized, double-blind study with terbinafine and griseofulvin. *Arch Dermatol.* 1995;131(8):919.
48. Korting HC, Schäfer-Korting M, Zienicke H, Georgii A, Ollert MW. Treatment of tinea unguium with medium and high doses of ultramicrosize griseofulvin compared with that with itraconazole. *Antimicrob Agents Chemother.* 1993;37(10):2064-8.
49. Haneke E, Tausch I, Bräutigam M, Weidinger G, Welzel D. Short-duration treatment of fingernail dermatophytosis: a randomized, double-blind study with terbinafine and griseofulvin. LAGOS III Study Group. *J Am Acad Dermatol.* 1995;32(1):72-7.

World Clin Dermatol. 2016;3(1):151-7.

Topical Therapies for Cutaneous Fungal Infections

*Larissa R Leopoldo MD, Tania F Cestari MD PhD

Department of Dermatology, Hospital de Clínicas de Porto Alegre, Porto Alegre, Rio Grande do Sul, Brazil

ABSTRACT

Fungi infect the skin by invading the stratum corneum. The answer to this invasion will depend on the immune defenses of the host against fungal metabolites, the anatomical site of the infection, and the virulence of the strain.[1] The drugs used to treat these infections can act to stop the proliferation of fungi, being called fungistatic, or to eliminate them, as the fungicides. Topical antifungal medications include some classes known as: polyenes, allylamines, azoles, benzylamines, and hidroxypyridones, such as ciclopirox olamine.[2] The most frequently used drugs in clinical practice belong to the classes of allylamines and azoles. Allylamines are preferred in dermatophyte infections, while azoles have a better therapeutic response in infections by *Candida* spp. and *Malassezia* spp., although azoles are used frequently. Antifungal pharmacological agents may be formulated into different vehicles such as creams, lotions, solutions, and nail lacquer. The choice should be based on the location and extent of the area affected by the infection to be treated.[3]

INTRODUCTION

Superficial fungal infections affect the skin and its associated structures as nails and hair.[4] Approximately, 20–25% of the world population will be affected at least once by fungal superficial infections during their lifetime.[5] They are caused mostly by dermatophytes but also occur due to yeasts such as *Candida* spp. and *Malassezia* spp.[1]

*Corresponding author
Email: larileopoldo@gmail.com

© 2016 Jaypee Brothers Medical Publishers. All rights reserved.

Etiologic agents differ according to anatomical region and geographic territory. The species of dermatophytes that cause infections vary from one continent to another. There are species, such as *Trichophyton rubrum, T. interdigitale,* and *T. mentagrophytes,* that affect the entire industrialized world. However, species as *T. schoenleinii., T. soudanense, and T. violaceum* affect mostly the continents of Africa and Asia, whereas *T. concentricum* affects the Pacific Islands and India. In the south of Europe, South America, and countries of Arabia, there is a higher prevalence of zoophilic dermatophytes such as *Microsporum canis* and *Trichosporum verrucosum.*[5]

Topical antifungal agents are, in general, the first choice of treatment for superficial fungal infections, since they have excellent therapeutic results with low potential for adverse effects. They can be formulated into different types of vehicles, such as creams, lotions, and solutions, and are absorbed through the stratum corneum of the skin.[4] They can have either fungicidal effects, leading to the death of fungal cells, or fungistatic effects, not allowing their growth.[6]

CLASSES OF ANTIFUNGAL DRUGS

The major classes of antifungal drugs are polyenes, allylamines, benzylamines, imidazoles, and hydroxypyridones.[4] The characteristics of each of them are described here.

Polyenes

This class of drugs acts by binding to ergosterol on the fungal cell membrane, promoting an increase in its permeability, extravasation of essential intracellular elements, and cell death.[7] The two representatives that are most commonly used in clinical practice are nystatin and amphotericin B.[1] Amphotericin B was not available for topical use, being administered intravenously only. Amphotericin B in gel and nanoparticle form has recently been evaluated for treatment of cutaneous and mucocutaneous funga, infections but more evidence is required. Nystatin is limited to topical use, as it is highly toxic when used intravenously and not effective via oral route, since systemic absorption takes place.[6]

It is produced through the fermentation of *Streptomyces albidus and S. noursei.* Nystatin is fungistatic at low concentrations and fungicidal at high concentrations. It is not effective in fighting infections by dermatophytes, and its main therapeutic indication is the treatment of candidiasis.[6] It is available for clinical use in creams, ointments, powders, suspensions, and tablets. Its dosage indication for skin infections is twice a day for about 2 weeks in the form of creams or ointments. In the treatment of oral candidiasis, suspensions or tablets can be applied five times a day, also for 2 weeks.[6]

Allylamines and Benzylamines

This group comprises terbinafine, naftifine, and butenafine, the latter being the only marketed representative of benzylamines. The mechanism of action of these two drug groups occurs through the inhibition of an enzyme called squalene epoxidase, which forms ergosterol, the main component of the fungal cell membrane.[8] Due to the accumulation of the metabolite squalene within the cell, the permeability of the membrane is increased, leading to cell death.[1,8]

Allylamines have an anti-inflammatory action by inhibiting neutrophil chemotaxis and the proinflammatory pathway of 5-lipoxygenase. Studies have shown an antibacterial effect associated with this class as well.[9]

These are lipophilic drugs and, therefore, their absorption through the stratum corneum and hair follicles is excellent, being found there for long periods of time. This ability to persist in the stratum corneum gives this class of drugs an advantage in their therapeutic efficiency, because they keep producing effects even after their administration has been discontinued.[10]

Butenafine has a fungicidal action *in vitro* and on animal models against dermatophytes, dimorphic fungi, and *Aspergillus* spp.[11] Allylamines are fungicidal against dermatophytes such as *T. rubrum, T. mentagrophytes, T. tonsurans,* and *Epidermophyton floccosum. M. canis, M. audouinii, and M. gypseum* are more resistant to allylamines. However, they have a fungistatic activity against *Candida* spp.[6]

Topical terbinafine 1% used 1–2 times a day for more than 2 weeks was effective in curing tinea corporis, tinea cruris, tinea versicolor, and intertrigo by *Candida* spp. in a study with 629 patients.[12]

Butenafine cream used once a day was effective for the treatment of tinea cruris, tinea pedis, and tinea corporis caused by dermatophytes, in addition to tinea versicolor caused by *Malassezia furfur*.[6] Butenafine shows good treatment results and may be an alternative off-label treatment for cutaneous candidiasis.

Cochrane's systematic review of the treatment for tinea cruris and tinea corporis, both caused by dermatophytes, showed satisfactory therapeutic effects and a good safety profile for most of the commonly used topical antifungal drugs. No treatment was found to stand out from the others in the study.[13]

Azoles

These agents are divided into two groups: (i) triazoles and (ii) imidazoles, the difference being the presence of three nitrogen atoms in the former and two in the latter. The mechanism of action of this drug group is the inhibition of the synthesis of ergosterol, the main component of the fungal cell membrane. However, there is no deposition of a metabolite capable of causing the death of the fungal cell. Due to this mechanism of action, azole drugs have only a fungistatic capacity and are not fungicides like the allylamines. In general, the fungistatic activity associated with skin peeling is enough to achieve therapeutic success.

The following topical drugs are part of this class: clotrimazole, ketoconazole, miconazole, sertaconazole, oxiconazole, and econazole. Azole compounds exhibit an anti-inflammatory activity by inhibiting neutrophil chemotaxis and the synthesis of leukotrienes and prostaglandins, in addition to reducing the release of histamine by mastocytes.

Clotrimazole was the first representative of this class to be discovered in 1960. It is a broad spectrum medication used for tinea corporis, tinea pedis, tinea versicolor, and oral and cutaneous candidiasis. Clotrimazole cream must be applied twice a day.

Econazole cream is effective for the treatment of skin infections caused by *T. rubrum, T. mentagrophytes, T. tonsurans, M. canis, M. audouinii, M. gypseum,* and *E. floccosum,* in addition to cutaneous candidiasis and tinea versicolor.

Ketoconazole is the most used imidazole around the world and was discovered in 1977, being approved by the Food and Drug Administration (FDA) in 1981. It has low systemic absorption through the skin and is well absorbed by the gastrointestinal mucosa and is available for use in creams, shampoos, and tablets. It is used in the treatment of tinea pedis, tinea manuum, tinea corporis, tinea cruris, and cutaneous candidiasis and also treats tinea versicolor and seborrheic dermatitis, in view of its activity against *Malassezia* spp.

Miconazole is an imidazole medication with optimal absorption through the stratum corneum. It is available for use in creams and intravaginal suppositories. It can be used to fight cutaneous dermatophyte infections, *Candida* spp., and *M. furfur*.

Oxiconazole was approved by the FDA in 1989 for the treatment of dermatomycoses. It is available in creams and lotions and is active against dermatophytosis, cutaneous candidiasis, and tinea versicolor. The dosage for tineas pedis, cruris, and corporis is twice a day and once a day for tinea versicolor.[6]

Hydroxypyridones

Its main representative is ciclopirox olamine, which inhibits the entry of essential nutrients into the fungal cell and impairs the function of the membrane and cellular respiration. It has antifungal, antibacterial, and anti-inflammatory properties. Its anti-inflammatory action occurs by inhibiting cyclooxygenase and 5-lipoxygenase, in addition to inhibiting leukotrienes and prostaglandins.[14]

Ciclopirox has rapid absorption through the stratum corneum, easily penetrating the sebaceous glands and hair follicles.

It has a broad fungicidal and fungistatic spectrum for dermatophytes such as *Trichophyton* spp., *Microsporum* spp., and *E. floccosum*, as well as yeasts such as

Candida spp., *Malassezia* spp., and *Cryptococcus neoformans*, dimorphic fungi, such as *Blastomyces dermatitidis* and *Histoplasma capsulatum*, eumycetes, actinomycetes, and various other fungi—*Aspergillus* spp., *Penicillium* spp., *Phialophora* spp. and *Fusarium* spp.[6]

The use of ciclopirox olamine cream is indicated for skin infections twice a day for at least 2 weeks, when symptoms disappear, the medication should be kept for 1 or 2 weeks.

The ciclopirox olamine nail lacquer 8% is a medication approved by the FDA for the treatment of onychomycosis, being applied once a week to the nails. Its indication for the topical treatment of onychomycosis is quite limited because the results are not good. It has been used in mild cases and in patients who do not tolerate oral medication or those for whom systemic treatment is contraindicated due to clinical comorbidities.[15]

Antifungal drugs are formulated into topical creams, lotions, solutions, gels, and even foams. The most important feature of a topical drug is being lipophilic, because, when applied to the skin, it should be absorbed through the lipidic stratum corneum and delivered to the deeper layers of the skin, epidermis, and dermis.[16] The vehicles play a key role in this important absorption task because they have ingredients capable of breaking the skin barrier, crossing the lipid channels between the corneocytes.[3]

ADVERSE EFFECTS

The most common adverse effects of topical medications are local irritations. They may cause symptoms such as burning, itching, redness, scaling and even blisters at the site.[17]

DRUG INTERACTIONS

There are no reports of significant interactions with topical antifungal medications.[6]

USE IN PREGNANCY AND LACTATION

Topical imidazoles do not show risks during pregnancy or breastfeeding. There are no adequate studies with ciclopirox olamine in pregnancy and breastfeeding.[2,4]

CONCLUSION

Topical antifungal drugs are indicated for the treatment of superficial fungal infections. These medications exhibit excellent therapeutic results once they have been absorbed through the stratum corneum, and they also have good tolerability and safety in their application.[2]

In the treatment of cutaneous candidiasis, imidazole drugs and ciclopirox olamine show better healing results than allylamines and benzylamines, being the best choices for the treatment of these infections.[5]

Rotta et al. conducted a systematic review to compare the various treatments established for dermatomycoses. One of the findings in their study is that topical antifungal medications have better results than the placebo in the treatment of dermatomycoses and that there is no difference between drugs as regards the healing of short-term infections.[17,18] However, allylamines maintain the mycological cure for longer periods compared to azoles.[18] The same study found a very good tolerability and safety profile among all antifungal classes, having mild and local adverse effects on only 1–3% of users.[17]

Editor's Comment

The most frequently used topical antifungal drugs in clinical dermatology practice belong to the classes of allylamines and azoles. Currently, in India and elsewhere dermatophytic infections are becoming increasingly recalcitrant to topical antifungal therapy, especially when used alone. This is addressed in the follow up articles. Nevertheless, authors Dr Leopoldo and Dr Cestari have well delineated the topical antifungal therapies in a simplified manner.

Rashmi Sarkar, Seemal R Desai

REFERENCES

1. Kyle AA, Dahl MV. Topical therapy for fungal infections. *Am J Clin Dermatol.* 2004;5(6):443-51.
2. Bologna JL, Jorizzo JL, Rapini RP. Dermatology. 2nd ed. London: Mosby; 2010.
3. Kircik LH. Advancements in topical antifungal vehicles. *J Drugs Dermatol.* 2016;15(2 Suppl):s44-8.
4. Wolff K, Goldsmith AL, Katz SI, Gilchrest BA, Paller AS, Leffel DJ. Fitzpatrick's Dermatology in General Medicine. 8th ed. New York: McGraw Hill; 2008.
5. Rosen T. Mycological considerations in the topical treatment of superficial fungal infections. *J Drugs Dermatol.* 2016;15(2 Suppl):s49-55.
6. Zhang AY, Camp WL, Elewski BE. Advances in topical and systemic antifungals. *Dermatol Clin.* 2007;25(2):165-83, vi.
7. Georgopapadakou NH. Antifungals: mechanism of action and resistance, established and novel drugs. *Curr Opin Microbiol.* 1998;1(5):547-57.
8. Ryder NS. Squalene epoxidase as a target for the allylamines. *Biochem Soc Trans.* 1991;19(3):774-7.
9. Choi TS, Solomon B, Nowakowski M, Lee WL, Geen S, Suntharalingam K, et al. Effect of naftifine on neutrophil adhesion. *Skin Pharmacol.* 1996;9(3):190-6.
10. Monk JP, Brogden RN. Naftifine: a review of its antimicrobial activity and therapeutic use in superficial dermatomycoses. *Drugs.* 1991;42(4):659-72.

11. Maeda T, Takase M, Ishibashi A, Yamamoto T, Sasaki K, Arika T, et al. Synthesis and antifungal activity of butenafine hydrochloride (KP-363), a new benzylamine antifungal agent. *Yakugaku Zasshi.* 1991;111(2):126-37.
12. Kagawa S. Clinical efficacy of terbinafine in 629 Japanese patients with dermatomycosis. *Clin Exp Dermatol.* 1989;14(2):114-5.
13. van Zuuren EJ, Fedorowicz Z, El-Gohary M. Evidence-based topical treatments for tinea cruris and tinea corporis: a summary of a Cochrane systematic review. *Br J Dermatol.* 2015;172(3):616-41.
14. Abrams BB, Hänel H, Hoehler T. Ciclopirox olamine: a hydroxypyridone antifungal agent. *Clin Dermatol.* 1991;9(4):471-7.
15. Gupta AK, Joseph WS. Ciclopirox 8% nail lacquer in the treatment of onychomycosis of the toenails in the United States. *J Am Podiatr Med Assoc.* 2000;90(10):495-501.
16. Bseiso EA, Nasr M, Sammour O, Abd El Gawad NA. Recent advances in topical formulation carriers of antifungal agents. *Indian J Dermatol Venereol Leprol.* 2015;81(5):457-63.
17. Rotta I, Sanchez A, Gonçalves PR, Otuki MF, Correr CJ. Efficacy and safety of topical antifungals in the treatment of dermatomycosis: a systematic review. *Br J Dermatol.* 2012;166(5):927-33.
18. Rotta I, Otuki MF, Sanches AC, Correr CJ. Efficacy of topical antifungal drugs in different dermatomycoses: a systematic review with meta-analysis. *Rev Assoc Med Bras (1992).* 2012;58(3):308-18.

World Clin Dermatol. 2016;3(1):158-67.

Topical Therapies for Onychomycosis

Casey L Wang MD, Theresa N Canavan MD, *Boni E Elewski MD

Department of Dermatology, University of Alabama
Birmingham, Alabama, USA

ABSTRACT

Treatment of onychomycosis continues to be a challenge for physicians given the low cure rates associated with older antifungal therapies. In the last decade, more effective topical therapies have been developed for onychomycosis. While topical therapies are often preferable to systemic therapies due to their superior side effect profile, the long duration of therapy required of these new formulations can be an impediment to their use. Drug delivery has been a major challenge for both topical and systemic therapies, but significant advances have been made in the last decade with the development of newer topical antifungal agents. Combination therapy with topical plus systemic agents may be a valuable option in some patients.

INTRODUCTION

Onychomycosis is both a commonly seen dermatologic condition and a therapeutic challenge for physicians. While onychomycosis is typically an indolent infection, it is often difficult to cure even with systemic agents. Even with a lengthy and sometimes expensive treatment course, cure rates tend to be low. When left untreated, onychomycosis negatively impacts patients' quality of life. Patients with onychomycosis can suffer from emotional distress due to the unsightly appearance of the toenails, pain secondary to nail dystrophy and trauma, and predisposition to more serious infections, particularly in diabetics and those with compromised circulation.

*Corresponding author
Email: beelewski@gmail.com

© 2016 Jaypee Brothers Medical Publishers. All rights reserved.

Historically, onychomycosis required systemic therapy with oral antifungals. However, oral therapy is sometimes not possible or desirable due to the potential side effects such as hepatotoxic effects, drug-drug interactions, or associated allergic reactions. Furthermore, laboratory monitoring can be cumbersome to some patients. In the past decade, several topical antifungal agents have been developed for treating onychomycosis, thus making it possible to circumvent some of the undesirable aspects of treatment that are associated with systemic therapy.

Treatment with topical antifungals can also have disadvantages, and these disadvantages may be particularly relevant in the elderly population where onychomycosis is most prevalent. For example, slow nail growth in elderly patients may necessitate over 12 months of continuous treatment. Furthermore, application of a topical toenail medication may be difficult for those with limited mobility. Finally, the high cost of newer formulations can be an impediment to using these treatments.

OVERVIEW OF ANTIFUNGAL THERAPIES FOR ONYCHOMYCOSIS

Not every dystrophic nail is a result of a dermatophyte infection, thus it is important to confirm the diagnosis of onychomycosis prior to starting therapy with either a positive potassium hydroxide (KOH) microscopy examination, a nail clipping with periodic acid–Schiff stain-positive hyphae on histology, or a positive fungal culture. One of the first clinical decisions that needs to be made in treating onychomycosis is whether to treat with a systemic or topical agent. Many factors need consideration, including patient factors and nail factors (Table 1). Systemic treatment may be preferred over topical treatment for immunosuppressed patients, those with uncontrolled diabetes mellitus, moderate to severe peripheral vascular disease, or those with limited mobility. Similarly, systemic treatment may be indicated in patients with matrix (lunula) involvement, dermatophytomas, infection that extends close to the proximal nail fold, nail plates greater than 2 mm in thickness, or those with over 65% of nail surface area involved.

Table 1: Conditions Requiring Oral Therapy of Onychomycosis

Patient factors	Nail factors
• Immunosuppression (primary or iatrogenic)	• Matrix involvement
• Body habitus	• Nondermatophyte mold infection
• Limited mobility	• Concurrent fingernail and toenail infection
• Moderate to severe peripheral vascular disease	• Thick nail plate
• Psoriasis	• Area of involvement >65%
• Uncontrolled diabetes mellitus	

Table 2: Topical Therapies for Onychomycosis		
Agents	**Class**	**Availability**
Solutions		
Tioconazole 28%	Imidazole	United Kingdom, Europe
Efinaconazole 10%	Triazole	United States, Canada
Tavaborole 5%	Oxaborole	United States, Canada
Lacquers		
Amorolfine 5%	Morpholine	Europe
Ciclopirox 8%	Hydroxypyridone	United States, Canada, Europe
Creams		
Bifonazole 1% with urea	Imidazole	Europe, Australia

There are several classes of systemic antifungal agents available to treat onychomycosis: griseofulvin, azoles, and terbinafine (an allylamine). Griseofulvin is now rarely used due to its narrow spectrum of activity, undesirable toxicity profile, and low efficacy. The first line oral agent for dermatophyte nail infections is terbinafine, which is dosed daily for twelve weeks. *Candida* and nondermatophytic mold infections can be treated with triazoles such as itraconazole and fluconazole.

The remainder of this article will focus on the scope of topical therapies for onychomycosis, including the relative efficacies of the newer agents. When applicable, data from phase III studies will be reviewed. The majority of studies use the following end point definitions: mycological cure implies a negative KOH microscopy examination of subungual debris plus a negative fungal culture, clinical cure implies a normal appearing nail, and complete cure implies both mycological and clinical cure. Not all studies adhere to these definitions, thus clinical trial results must be reviewed with caution.

TOPICAL THERAPY OF ONYCHOMYCOSIS

Azoles

Tioconazole is currently available in the United Kingdom and Europe as a 28% solution for topical use for onychomycosis. It demonstrated modest efficacy for treating onychomycosis in a small study that included both fingernail and toenail onychomycosis. Overall, only 22% of subjects achieved a clinical cure after 3 months of treatment.[1]

Bifonazole, when applied after nail avulsion, has also shown some efficacy in treating onychomycosis. Nonsurgical nail avulsion is achieved via daily application of 40% urea cream or paste for 2-4 weeks.[2] In a large double-blind and placebo-controlled trial, daily bifonazole application was used for 4 weeks following nail ablation. Cure rates in the bifonazole group were superior when compared to placebo at 2 weeks post-treatment. However, by 6 months following treatment cessation, there were no statistically significant differences between the cure rates of the two groups. Another study has shown that bifonazole may be beneficial in subjects with thick toenails that preclude the use of alternate topical antifungals as this treatment regimen can reduce nail thickness.[3] Currently, bifonazole is available over the counter in Australia and Europe as a kit containing 1% bifonazole cream plus 40% urea cream, an occlusive plaster, and a debriding tool.

Amorolfine

Amorolfine is a derivative of morpholine and is available as a 5% lacquer for the treatment of onychomycosis. Several studies attest to its efficacy in treating onychomycosis, with the majority of subjects using amorolfine either once or twice weekly achieving mycologic cure (range 71–76%). These studies also reported relatively high rates of "complete cure" (46–52%). However, it is important to note that these studies defined complete cure less stringently than later onychomycosis trials. In these studies, patients with up to 10% residual nail involvement at the trials end were considered to be a "complete cure".[4,5] These studies also demonstrated that there was no statistically significant difference in outcome between once and twice weekly application.

Ciclopirox

Ciclopirox is a hydroxyl-pyridone derivative which is used in many formulations (cream, gel, shampoo, solution, powder).[6] For onychomycosis, it is delivered as an 8% lacquer. Phase III studies included patients aged 18–70 with distal lateral subungual onychomycosis of a target great toenail caused by a dermatophytes. Infection severity ranged from 20 to 65% involvement of the target nail. Pertinent exclusion criteria included the presence of white superficial onychomycosis, proximal subungual onychomycosis, fungal spikes extending to the cuticle (although dermatophytomas were not specifically excluded), and significant concomitant nail and foot conditions that could interfere with evaluation (Table 3). Treatment involved daily application of ciclopirox lacquer to both the nail plate plus 5 mm of surrounding epidermis for 48 consecutive weeks. Ciclopirox cure rates were as follows: mycologic cure of 29–36%, complete cure of 5.5–8.5%, and clinical success of 6.5–12%, which was defined as a negative fungal culture plus less than or equal to 10% nail involvement (Table 3).[7,8] Eight percent of ciclopirox lacquer is approved for use in both North America and Europe where the approved treatment regimen includes daily application for 48 weeks plus removal of the lacquer residue once per week.

Efinaconazole 10%

Efinaconazole is a recently approved topical triazole that was developed specifically for treating onychomycosis. Efinaconazole exhibits two properties that allow for excellent nail permeation and subungual spreading—low keratin affinity and low surface tension.[9,10] Indeed, efinaconazole has been shown to concentrate on the nail bed after application to the nail surface.[11]

In two parallel phase III clinical trials, daily application of efinaconazole 10% solution was found to be well tolerated and safe (Table 3). These studies included subjects aged 18–70 with onychomycosis diagnosed by positive KOH microscopy examination from a sampling of subungual debris plus culture of a dermatophyte or dermatophyte plus *Candida*. Pertinent exclusion factors were nail thickness greater than 3 mm, infection within 3 mm of the proximal nail fold, history of immunosuppression, poorly controlled diabetes, nondermatophytic nail infections, severe moccasin tinea pedis, previous target nail surgery, and other concomitant nail abnormalities (Table 3). Patients were treated with either efinaconazole 10% solution or vehicle daily for 48 weeks, and then followed up at 4 weeks post-treatment.

From these studies, efinaconazole 10% solution demonstrated complete cure rates of 17.8 and 15.2%. Mycologic cure rates were 55.2 and 53.4%, while clinical cure rates were 21 and 18%. Treatment success, which was defined as less than or equal to 10% of target nail involvement, was achieved by 35.7 and 31% of subjects (Table 3).[12,13] Cure rates were noted to be augmented when concurrent tinea pedis was also treated.[14] Additionally, a post hoc analysis showed that efinaconazole efficacy was similar in patients with well controlled diabetics. [15] This is significant given that diabetic patients are especially vulnerable to poor outcomes secondary to onychomycosis, such as infection and nonhealing wounds.

Tavaborole

Tavaborole is the first in its class of Food and Drug Administration-approved oxaboroles, which are boron containing molecules. Tavaborale, which was recently approved for treating onychomycosis, has demonstrated excellent nail penetration due to its low molecular weight. [16-19]

Tavaborole 5% solution has completed several phase III clinical trials in which it was applied once daily to the nail plate for 48 weeks. Compared to the efinaconazole studies, the tavaborole phase III trials did not apply an upper age limit (the oldest participant was 88 years old) and included patients with more severe disease (up to 60% target nail involvement) (Table 3). Only purely dermatophytic infections were included, whereas the efinaconazole trials included mixed infections of dermatophyte and *Candida* species.[16]

Table 3: Comparison of Phase III Trial Design and Results

Agents	Ciclopirox 8%	Tavaborole 5%	Efinaconazole 10%
Inclusion criteria	• Age 18–70 • DLSO of great toenail • 20–65% nail involvement • KOH+ • Culture dermatophyte	• Age ≥18 • DLSO of great toenail • 20–60% nail involvement • Nail thickness <3 mm • Unaffected length >3 mm • KOH+ • Culture dermatophyte	• Age 18–70 • DLSO of great toenail • 20–50% nail involvement • Nail thickness <3 mm • Unaffected length >3 mm • Evidence of nail growth • KOH+ • Culture dermatophyte or dermatophyte/*Candida*
Exclusion criteria	• Superficial white disease • Proximal subungual disease • Other nail abnormalities • Foot/nail deformity • Spikes extending to cuticle • Immunosuppression	• Immunosuppression • Uncontrolled diabetes • Proximal subungual disease • Superficial white disease • Severe onychomycosis • Dermatophytoma • Exclusively lateral disease • Yellow/brown spikes • Coinfection with non-dermatophyte • Active tinea pedis requiring treatment • History of chronic moccasin-type tinea pedis • Psoriasis • Lichen planus • Peripheral vascular disease • Structural heart disease	• Immunosuppression • Uncontrolled diabetes • Nondermatophyte infection • Severe moccasin tinea pedis • Prior target nail surgery • Other nail abnormalities • Dermatophytoma • Matrix (lunula) involvement
Mycologic cure rate (%)	• 29–36%	• 31.1–35.9	• 53.4–55.2
Complete cure rate (%)	• 5.5–8.5	• 6.5–9.1	• 15.2–17.8
Clinical success rate (%)	• 6.5–12	• 26.1–27.5	• 31.0–35.7

In the phase III trials, tavaborale demonstrated mycologic cure rates that were superior to the complete clinical cure rates (31.1–35.9%, 6.5–9.1%, respectively). Clinical success, which was defined as less than or equal to 10% of nail involvement, was found to be 26.1 and 27.5%. Of note, most subjects who met the criteria for clinical success also had a negative fungal culture.[16]

Topical Antifungals in Development

Several new topical antifungals have shown promising results as potential therapies for onychomycosis. K101 nail solution is a combination of urea, propylene glycol, and lactic acid, and has demonstrated activity against dermatophytes as well as *C. albicans*. K101 nail solution's mechanism of action has been suggested to be via a nonspecific degradative effect, and thus it may be less susceptible to dermatophyte resistance.[20] A few pilot studies have been completed including a placebo-controlled trial in which K101 nail solution was applied daily for 24 weeks and demonstrated a mycologic cure rate of 17%. This is promising given that cure rates may be higher if patients are treated with a 48–52 week course.[21] Furthermore, the majority of subjects in a smaller study noted significant improvement in nail appearance.[22]

ME1111 is another topical antifungal agent with activity against *T. rubrum* and *T. mentagrophytes* that is currently being investigated in several clinical trials. With its novel mechanism of action and small size that allows for excellent nail penetrance, ME1111 shows great promise for treating onychomycosis.[23]

Luliconazole 10% solution is a novel imidazole with a broad spectrum of activity that has been found to be safe and well tolerated in several studies, including a large phase II trial that enrolled more than 300 subjects.[24]

Topical Therapy in Combination with Systemic Agents

Topical antifungals can play an adjunctive role in treating patients who require oral therapy. Combination regimens have several notable advantages over monotherapy. Combination therapy may allow for a shorter duration of systemic treatment, thereby reducing the risk of adverse effects associated with systemic treatment. Efficacies may also be enhanced with combination treatment. Several studies attest to the value of topical antifungals when combined with systemic therapy for onychomycosis. In a randomized control trial, oral griseofulvin was combined with daily application of 1% bifonazole following urea-induced nail avulsion. This study demonstrated that cure rates with combination topical and oral therapy were superior to those reported for either associated monotherapy cure rate.[25]

Another study investigated the combination of ciclopirox 8% lacquer plus oral terbinafine for moderate to severe onychomycosis, including those cases with matrix involvement. Subjects were treated with either pulsed oral terbinafine therapy (250 mg daily for 4 weeks on, 4 weeks off, then 4 weeks on) plus daily ciclopirox lacquer application, a 12-week course of oral terbinafine 250 mg daily plus daily ciclopirox, or a 12 week course of terbinafine alone. At the end of the study, mycologic cure and effective cure, which was defined as mycologic cure plus greater than 90% reduction in disease, were similar for all three treatment groups.[26]

Topical antifungals may also have a role in prevention of relapse after a cure has been achieved with an oral antifungal agent. Every other week application of amorolfine nail lacquer has been shown to reduce the recurrence rate at 12 months and extend the time to recurrence in patients previously cured with either oral terbinafine plus topical amorolfine or oral terbinafine alone.[27]

CONCLUSION

Topical therapies for onychomycosis is an exciting and expanding field with several new attractive treatment options and many promising new medications currently in clinical development. With the synthesis of new potent antifungals, improved drug delivery, and a greater number of options, the therapeutic outcomes of onychomycosis is likely to improve. This is good news for patients with onychomycosis.

Editor's Comment

Onychomycosis represents a very large portion of outpatient dermatology visits that are centered on fungal diseases. In fact, treatment of this condition continues to be a challenge due to very low mycological and clinical cure rates with many of the currently available therapies. In this article, world-renowned dermatologist and fungal disease expert, Dr Boni Elewski and her co-author, provided a thorough and well-outlined review centering on the topical treatment of fungal nail disease. The authors have outlined risk factors for systemic therapies, and when to initiate those in patients who fail topical treatments. In addition, the data that is shown in this article will help the reader to better understand newer available formulations and therapies.

Seemal R Desai, Rashmi Sarkar

REFERENCES

1. Hay RJ, Mackie RM, Clayton YM. Tioconazole nail solution - an open study of its efficacy in onychomycosis. *Clin Exp Dermatol.* 1985;10:111-5.
2. Tietz H-J, Hay R, Querner S, Delcker A, Kurka P, Merk HF. Efficacy of 4 weeks topical bifonazole treatment for onychomycosis after nail ablation with 40% urea: a double-blind, randomized, placebo-controlled multicenter study. *Mycoses.* 2013;56(4):414-421.
3. Piraccini BM, Bruni F, Alessandrini A, Starace M. Evaluation of efficacy and tolerability of four weeks bifonazole treatment after nail ablation with 40% urea in mild to moderate distal subungual onychomycosis. *G Ital Dermatol Venereol.* 2016;151(1):32-36.
4. Reinel D, Clarke C. Comparative efficacy and safety of amorolfine nail lacquer 5% in onychomycosis, once-weekly versus twice-weekly. *Clin Exp Dermatol.* 1992;17 Suppl 1:44-49.
5. Zaug M, Bergstraesser M. Amorolfine in the treatment of onychomycoses and dermatomycoses (an overview). *Clin Exp Dermatol.* 1992;17 Suppl 1:61-70.
6. Tabara K, Szewczyk AE, Bienias W, Wojciechowska A, Patuszka M, Oszukowska M, et al. Amorolfine vs. ciclopirox - lacquers for the treatment of onychomycosis. *Postepy Dermatol Alergol.* 2015;32(1):40-5.
7. Gupta AK, Fleckman P, Baran R. Ciclopirox nail lacquer topical solution 8% in the treatment of toenail onychomycosis. *J Am Acad Dermatol.* 2000;43(4 Suppl):S70-S80.
8. Gupta AK, Joseph WS. Ciclopirox 8% nail lacquer in the treatment of onychomycosis of the toenails in the United States. *J Am Podiatr Med Assoc.* 90(10):495-501.
9. Zeichner JA, Stein Gold L, Korotzer A. Penetration of ((14)C)-Efinaconazole Topical Solution, 10%, Does Not Appear to be Influenced by Nail Polish. *J Clin Aesthet Dermatol.* 2014;7(9):34-36.
10. Elewski BE, Rich P, Pollak R, Pariser DM, Watanabe S, Senda H, et al. Efinaconazole 10% solution in the treatment of toenail onychomycosis: Two phase III multicenter, randomized, double-blind studies. *J Am Acad Dermatol.* 2013;68(4):600-8.
11. Elewski BE, Pollak RA, Pillai R, Olin JT. Access of efinaconazole topical solution, 10%, to the infection site by spreading through the subungual space. *J Drugs Dermatol.* 2014;13(11):1394-8.
12. Tschen EH, Bucko AD, Oizumi N, Kawabata H, Olin JT, Pillai R. Efinaconazole solution in the treatment of toenail onychomycosis: a phase 2, multicenter, randomized, double-blind study. *J Drugs Dermatol.* 2013;12(2):186-92.
13. Rodriguez DA. Efinaconazole Topical Solution, 10%, for the Treatment of Mild and Moderate Toenail Onychomycosis. *J Clin Aesthet Dermatol.* 2015;8(6):24-29.
14. Markinson BC, Caldwell BD. Efinaconazole Topical Solution, 10%: Efficacy in Patients with Onychomycosis and Coexisting Tinea Pedis. *J Am Podiatr Med Assoc.* 2015. doi:10.7547/14-088.1.
15. Vlahovic TC, Joseph WS. Efinaconazole topical, 10% for the treatment of toenail onychomycosis in patients with diabetes. *J Drugs Dermatol.* 2014;13(10):1186-90.
16. Elewski BE, Aly R, Baldwin SL, Gonzalez Soto RF, Rich P, Weisfeld M, et al. Efficacy and safety of tavaborole topical solution, 5%, a novel boron-based antifungal agent, for the treatment of toenail onychomycosis: Results from 2 randomized phase-III studies. *J Am Acad Dermatol.* 2015;73(1):62-9.
17. Rock FL, Mao W, Yaremchuk A, Tukalo M, Crepin T, Zhou H, et al. An antifungal agent inhibits an aminoacyl-tRNA synthetase by trapping tRNA in the editing site. *Science.* 2007;316(5832):1759-61.
18. Hui X, Baker SJ, Wester RC, Barbadillo S, Cashmore AK, Sanders V, et al. In vitro penetration of a novel oxaborole antifungal (AN2690) into the human nail plate. *J Pharm Sci.* 2007;96(10):2622-31.
19. Elewski BE, Tosti A. Tavaborole for the treatment of onychomycosis. *Expert Opin Pharmacother.* 2014;15(10):1439-48.
20. Hultenby K, Chryssanthou E, Klingspor L, Rensfeldt K, Strömbeck L, Faergemann J. The effect of K101 Nail Solution on Trichophyton rubrum and Candida albicans growth and ultrastructure. *Mycoses.* 2014;57(10):630-8.

21. Emtestam L, Kaaman T, Rensfeldt K. Treatment of distal subungual onychomycosis with a topical preparation of urea, propylene glycol and lactic acid: results of a 24-week, double-blind, placebo-controlled study. *Mycoses*. 2012;55(6):532-40.
22. Faergemann J, Gullstrand S, Rensfeldt K. Early and Visible Improvements after Application of K101 in the Appearance of Nails Discoloured and Deformed by Onychomycosis. *J Cosmet Dermatological Sci Appl*. 2011;01(03):59-63.
23. Tabata Y, Takei-Masuda N, Kubota N, Takahata S, Ohyama M, Kaneda K, et al. Characterization of Antifungal Activity and Nail Penetration of ME1111, a New Antifungal Agent for Topical Treatment of Onychomycosis. *Antimicrob Agents Chemother*. 2015;60(2):1035-9.
24. Jones T, Tavakkol A. Safety and Tolerability of luliconazole solution 10-percent in patients with moderate to severe distal subungual onychomycosis. *Antimicrob Agents Chemother*. 2013;57(6):2684-9.
25. Friedman-Birnbaum R, Cohen A, Shemer A, Bitterman O, Bergman R, Stettendorf S. Treatment of onychomycosis: a randomized, double-blind comparison study with topical bifonazole-urea ointment alone and in combination with short-duration oral griseofulvin. *Int J Dermatol*. 1997;36(1):67-69.
26. Gupta AK. Ciclopirox topical solution, 8% combined with oral terbinafine to treat onychomycosis: a randomized, evaluator-blinded study. *J Drugs Dermatol*. 2005;4(4):481-5.
27. Sigurgeirsson B, Olafsson JH, Steinsson JT, Kerrouche N, Sidou F. Efficacy of amorolfine nail lacquer for the prophylaxis of onychomycosis over 3 years. *J Eur Acad Dermatol Venereol*. 2010;24(8):910-5.

World Clin Dermatol. 2016;3(1):168-77.

Physical Modalities for the Treatment of Onychomycosis

*,[1]Aditya K Gupta MD PhD, [2]Sarah G Versteeg MSc PhD

[1]Department of Medicine, University of Toronto, Toronto, Ontario, Canada
[2]Mediprobe Research Inc., London, Ontario, Canada

ABSTRACT

Onychomycosis is a chronic fungal nail infection, most commonly caused by dermatophytes. Treatment of this fungal infection is necessary as onychomycosis can affect quality of life. Treatment options vary and include oral treatments, topical therapy, and physical modalities. Published literature suggests that lasers can effectively increase the amount of clear nail, supporting its Food and Drug Administration-approved use. Other physical modalities that have shown potential include iontophoresis, ultraviolet radiation, and ultrasound technologies.

INTRODUCTION

Onychomycosis is a fungal infection of the nail, commonly caused by dermatophytes, a fungus that can thrive on skin, hair, and nails.[1] Other causative organisms include nondermatophyte molds (NDMs) and yeasts.[1] Characteristic symptoms of this infection include nail crumbling, thickening of the nail plate, and discoloration.[2] If left untreated, onychomycosis can lead to depression, anxiety, discomfort, and other health complications (e.g., secondary infection).[3] Risk factors for onychomycosis include age, diabetes, human immunodeficiency virus status, and previous foot trauma.[4]

Current treatments available for this infection include oral treatments, topical therapies, and physical modalities. In drug trials, onychomycosis treatments strive to obtain complete cure, which is characterized by mycological cure (negative microscopy and negative culture) and clinical cure (100% clear nail). Complete cure

*Corresponding author
Email: publications@mediproberesearch.com

© 2016 Jaypee Brothers Medical Publishers. All rights reserved.

ensures the underlying cause of onychomycosis is addressed (through mycological examination) and takes into account the health of the new nail (complete clearance).[5] To allow for easy comparisons across onychomycosis treatments, physical modalities [e.g., lasers and photodynamic therapy (PDT)] should also be evaluated with these endpoints. The modalities that will be examined in this article include lasers, nail debridement, PDT, iontophoresis, ultraviolet (UV) radiation, ultrasound technology, and the combination thereof.

CURRENT AND FUTURE PHYSICAL MODALITIES FOR TREATMENT OF ONYCHOMYCOSIS

Lasers

Laser treatment is performed in pulses (300–650 μs) with moderate energy, enabling fungal cell damage and death.[6] Lasers can be used to decrease fungal mass, thin infected nails, and add aesthetic value.[7] The United States Food and Drug Administration (FDA) has approved the use of lasers to "temporary increase the amount of clear nail" in onychomycosis patients, a cosmetic and temporary outcome.[8] This indicated use does not require elimination of the fungus itself (mycological cure), so it should not be presumed that lasers are approved to cure onychomycosis.[8]

In order to determine the efficacy of lasers for treatment of onychomycosis, a critical review of the literature was performed (PubMed, Clinicaltrials.gov, Medline, and Embase databases). Inclusion and exclusion criteria were developed based on a modified version of a Cochrane protocol.[9] Twenty-one clinical trials evaluating laser therapy for onychomycosis confirmed by mycology (e.g., positive culture and/or positive microscopy) were selected (Table 1).[5,10-30] In these clinical trials, lasers were used in monotherapy (19/21 = 90%), in combination studies with antifungal treatments (1/21 = 5%) and other physical modalities (1/21 = 5%). It should be noted that randomization (9/21 = 43%), use of placebo/sham, untreated or comparative controls (9/21 = 43%), and large sample sizes were not common characteristics of these laser trials. In order to avoid biased results (e.g., selection bias, performance bias, and detection bias), randomization, blinding, and proper controls should be incorporated.

The selected laser studies were then compared to standard onychomycosis endpoints (e.g., complete cure, mycological cure, etc.). Complete cure (mycological cure and clinical cure) was reported in 1 of 21 laser trials with a rate of 50% using nails as the unit of analysis.[28] Mycological testing of any kind (e.g., microscopy and/or culture) was performed in 67% (14/21) of laser studies. Mycological cure (microscopy and culture) found across laser studies in the literature is 11%[15,29] using patients as a unit of analysis and 63%[12,15,23] using nails as the unit of analysis. Clinical cure, defined as 100% clear nail, was reported in half of the studies,

Table 1: Clinical Trials Conducted with Lasers for Treatment of Onychomycosis

Study	1,064 nm laser	Randomized study	Controlled study	Investigator blind	Mycological cure	Clinical cure	Clinical improvement
Hollmig et al.[10]	√	√	√	–	√*	√	√H
Kimura et al.[5]	√	–	–	–	–	√	–
Landsman et al. (2010)[11]	Near-infrared diode	√	√	√B	√* **	√	√I
Landsman et al. (2012)[12]	Near-infrared diode	√	√	√B	√*	√	–
Stanford University[13]	√	√	√	–	√*	–	√H
Noguchi et al.[14]	√	–	–	–	–	√	–
Carney et al.[15]	√	–	–	–	√	√	–
Hees et al.[16]	√	–	–	√A	√* **	–	–
Moon et al.[17]	√	–	–	–	√**	–	–
Erchonia Corporation[18] (Sullivan)[19]	Erchonia LUNULA	–	–	–	–	–	√H
Harris et al.[20]	√	√	√	√A	–	–	√H
Weiss et al.[21]	√	–	–	–	–	–	–
Renner et al.[22]	√	–	–	–	–	–	–
Li et al.[23]	√	√	√	–	√	–	–
Waibel et al.[24]	√	√	√	–	√*	–	–
Ortiz et al.[25]	1,320 nm Nd:YAG	√	√J	√A	√*	–	√H

Continued

Continued

Table 1: Clinical Trials Conducted with Lasers for Treatment of Onychomycosis

Study	1,064 nm laser	Randomized study	Controlled study	Investigator blind	Mycological cure	Clinical cure	Clinical improvement
Gupta and Paquet[26]	√	–	–	–	–	√	√F
Hochman [27]	√	–	–	–	√*	–	–
Lim et al.[28]	Fractional CO_2	–	–	–	√**	√	–
Karsai et al.[29]	√	√	√	√A	√	–	–
de Oliveira et al.[30]	Fractional CO_2 laser	–	–	–	√**	–	–

A—assessor blinded.
B—patients blinded to real or sham treatment, independent examiners also blinded.
F—Clinical improvement as defined as <10% affected nail plate.
H—Clinical improvement as evaluated based on measurements of nail bed/plate clearance (mm).
I—Clinical improvement as evaluated as ≥3 mm clear nail growth.
J—sham and laser treatment used on the same individual.
Controlled = placebo, no treatment group, or active comparator.
Mycological cure = defined as negative potassium hydroxide (KOH) microscopy and negative fungal culture.
Clinical cure = defined as no nail plate involvement (0%).
Clinical improvement = evaluated as clear nail growth as measured in mm (with results).
Combination with antifungals agents can include oral/topical drugs as adjunctive therapies, are used for concomitant, tinea pedis and/or help against infection.
*Mycological cure as evaluated with culture only.
**Mycological cure as evaluated with microscopy (KOH) only.
CO_2, carbon dioxide; Nd:YAG, neodymium-doped yttrium aluminum garnet.

with 48% (10/21) of studies using this endpoint. Based on the number of nails evaluated, the weighted average for clinical cure using lasers in monotherapy is 13%.[5,10,11,12,15,17]

Based on FDA guidelines, a treatment responder is defined as a patient whom achieves at least 6 mm of clear nail growth, an additional 60 mm^2 of clear nail, or complete clearance 6 months after their first treatment.[31-33] One study, thus far, has directly compared the clear nail growth achieved post-treatment to a growth rate similar to the FDA's recommendation (≥3 mm in 3 months).[11] It was found that, 180 days following treatment with a near-infrared diode laser, more than 3 mm of clear nail growth was observed in 65.4% (17/26) of nails, which was significantly greater than the sham control treated nails (1/11 = 9.1%, $p = 0.0112$).[11] Additionally, a few trials (5/21 = 24%) have measured the amount of clear nail growth (mm). The average amount of nail bed or plate clearance among these lasers used as monotherapy was 2.6 mm by week 12. Clear nail growth and nail clearance can be directly related to the FDA-approved use of lasers.[31] Consequently, based on their approved use, lasers may be an effective physical modality to improve the appearance of nails in onychomycosis patients.[32]

Nail Debridement

Another modality that could be used to treat onychomycosis patients is nail debridement. Nail debridement can help remove infected nail material which can be used in diagnosing onychomycosis.[34-36] This modality is unlikely to cure onychomycosis as it does not combat the underlying cause (e.g., fungus).[37] Nail abrasion can increase patient comfort by thinning the infected nail and decreasing fungal mass.[7] Nail filing prior to application of topical therapies can enhance efficacy rates of topical antifungals (e.g., amorolfine and ciclopirox).[35,36] Nail drilling has also been used to create holes or passages through the nail that also allow easy entry of topical treatments.[38] This has been found in a recent open comparative study, where nail drilling was combined with an antifungal agent (oral and topical terbinafine) to treat mild and moderate onychomycosis.[38] Significant improvement in the amount of clear nail in patients, with 51–75% nail involvement, was discovered when nail drilling (two horizontal lines drilled 2 mm apart) was combined with oral (250 mg) and topical (1% spray) formulations of terbinafine ($p = 0.038$). It has been recommended that use of nail debridement be restricted to aid topical treatments only for functional improvement in nail appearance.[31]

Photodynamic Therapy

Photodynamic therapy is a physical modality that could also be used to treat onychomycosis. Photodynamic therapy requires three things to interact simultaneously in order to be successful—a photosensitizer, a light source, and available oxygen.[39,40] Photosensitizers, once applied to the infected nail, are absorbed by fungal cells located within the infected nail bed.[40] Once these fungal cells are illuminated with light of a specific wavelength, fungal cell death can occur.[40]

Although there are no photosensitizers specifically approved for treatment of onychomycosis, several have been researched for their potential use.[41] Small, uncontrolled trials make up most PDT research with pain, a common side effect.[8] Methyl aminolevulinate, 5-aminolevulinic acid, and methylene blue (MB) are photosensitizers that have been tested with some success in onychomycosis patients with several case studies resulting in mycological cure (70–100%).[42-44] Photodynamic therapy has also been compared to topical therapy for treatment of onychomycosis.[45] In a randomized, 24-week, parallel, placebo-controlled, single blind study, MB-PDT showed significantly higher clinical cure rates (complete replacement of the infected nail) as compared to fluconazole ($p < 0.002$).[45] Further research incorporating control groups and larger sample sizes are needed before this physical modality should be frequently used in clinical practice for treatment of onychomycosis.

Iontophoresis

Iontophoresis might also be a promising future physical modality for the treatment of onychomycosis. Iontophoresis is a process that enables the transport of hydrophilic charged molecules across a membrane through applying electricity.[46] This delivery method could be of assistance to topical therapies by increasing the concentration of the drug at the site of infection. Preclinical models have been used to examine iontophoresis delivery of topical antifungals for treatment of onychomycosis. In an *in vitro* iontophoresis model, terbinafine was released into and through the nail plate at concentrations necessary to inhibit *Trichophyton rubrum*, a common causative organism.[47] The drug delivery of terbinafine can be enhanced (7–13-fold higher) with iontophoresis as compared to passive delivery as seen in an *ex vivo* cadaver nail model.[48] Similar results were also found using cadaver drug release studies and permeation studies of onychomycotic nails.[49]

Ultraviolet Radiation

To be an effective onychomycosis treatment, the chosen therapy should have antifungal capabilities.[8] Ultraviolet radiation (UV) exhibits antifungal capabilities as it can cause mutations through interacting with cellular deoxyribonucleic acid, as evident with UV-C radiation.[50] UV-C radiation, at higher intensities, can inhibit fungal isolates (*Trichophyton mentagrophytes* and *T. rubrum*) taken from onychomycosis patients.[50] Ultraviolet radiation can also be used in a UV-curable gel formulation to create a long-lasting glossy film on the nail. This property could enhance the efficacy of topical antifungals as demonstrated in an *in vitro* study.[51] The UV-cured formulation (containing terbinafine) was found to have a higher drug presence in disease-free nail clippings as compared to the positive control (Curanail 32% amorolfine hydrochloride).[51]

Ultrasound Technologies

Different ultrasonic frequencies and intensities can be used to target infected tissues through the creation of hydroxyl radicals.[52] Hydroxyl radicals can produce high antifungal activity against common dermatophytes that cause onychomycosis. For instance, when a 1.6-MHz ultrasound was used, a majority (80%) of fungal strains (e.g., *T. mentagrophytes* and *T. rubrum*) tested after 10 minutes in 50°C water were eradicated.[53]

Ultrasound technologies can also be used for drug delivery to the skin and eyes.[54] Ultrasound delivery increased nail permeability in canine nail models.[55] When canine nails underwent ultrasound exposure for 30 seconds, 60 seconds, and 120 seconds, significantly higher nail penetration occurred as compared to the control ($p = 0.03$, $p = 0.02$, and $p = 0.003$).[55] Clinical research using onychomycosis patients is needed before ultrasound technologies should be put into clinical practice.

Combining Physical Modalities for Treatment of Onychomycosis

Combining physical modalities could also be an effective treatment option. For example, laser therapy combined with PDT has been used successfully to treat onychomycosis.[30] Onychomycosis patients ($n = 7$) received two sessions of fractional carbon dioxide laser treatment, immediately followed by 15 minutes of PDT with a 60-day interval between treatments.[30] Efficacy was measured one year after cessation of treatment with 43% of participants demonstrating clinical success (lightening of lesions) and 100% of patients demonstrating mycological cure (defined as negative microscopy).[30]

CONCLUSION

To conclude, onychomycosis is a fungal infection that can be caused by dermatophytes, NDMs, and yeast.[1] Lasers and nail debridement, when used in monotherapy, may not address the underlying cause of onychomycosis, but paired with topical therapies these physical modalities can be enhanced.[35,36,56] Photodynamic therapy, iontophoresis, ultrasound technologies, and UV radiation show promising results with further research needed to establish applicability in onychomycosis patients.[42,49,50,55] With an increase in risk factors such as our aging population and increased rates of diabetes, the need for physical modalities in treating onychomycosis may increase.

Editor's Comment

The globally reknowned authors, Dr Aditya Gupta and Dr Sarah Versteeg have given good detail of the various physical modalities that can be useful in onychomycosis with the vital stress on the use of lasers. The article is concise, conversant and educational. More than curbing the infection,it is the cosmetic appearance of the nails which severely affects a patient's quality of life. The article touches upon lasers and several innovative physical therapies which will help the clinician to attain optimum management benefits for the patient.

Rashmi Sarkar, Seemal R Desai

REFERENCES

1. Gupta AK, Nakrieko KA. Molecular determination of mixed infections of dermatophytes and nondermatophyte molds in individuals with onychomycosis. *J Am Podiatr Med Assoc.* 2014;104:330-6.
2. Scher RK, Tavakkol A, Sigurgeirsson B, Hay RJ, Joseph WS, Tosti A, et al. Onychomycosis: diagnosis and definition of cure. *J Am Acad Dermatol.* 2007;56:939-44.
3. Elewski BE. The effect of toenail onychomycosis on patient quality of life. *Int J Dermatol.* 1997;36:754-6.
4. Gupta AK, Jain HC, Lynde CW, Macdonald P, Cooper EA, Summerbell RC. Prevalence and epidemiology of onychomycosis in patients visiting physicians' offices: a multicenter Canadian survey of 15,000 patients. *J Am Acad Dermatol.* 2000;43:244-8.
5. Kimura U, Takeuchi K, Kinoshita A, Takamori K, Hiruma M, Suga Y. Treating onychomycoses of the toenail: clinical efficacy of the sub-millisecond 1,064 nm Nd:YAG laser using a 5 mm spot diameter. *J Drugs Dermatol.* 2012;11:496-504.
6. PathoLase, Inc. (2010). PinPointe FootLaser for the treatment of onychomycosis. [online] Available from: http://clinicaltrial.gov/ct2/show/NCT00935649. [Accessed December, 2016].
7. Di Chiacchio N, Kadunc BV, de Almeida ART, Madeira CL. Nail abrasion. *J Cosmet Dermatol.* 2003;2:150-2.
8. Gupta AK, Simpson FC. New pharmacotherapy for the treatment of onychomycosis: an update. *Expert Opin Pharmacother.* 2015;16:227-36.
9. Gupta AK, Simpson F, Daigle D, Villanueva E, John D, Foley K. Cochrane Database Syst Rev Online. (2016). Topical and device-based treatments for fungal infections of the toenails. [online] Available from: http://onlinelibrary.wiley.com/doi/10.1002/14651858.CD012093/full. [Accessed December, 2016].
10. Hollmig ST, Rahman Z, Henderson MT, Rotatori RM, Gladstone H, Tang JY. Lack of efficacy with 1064-nm neodymium:yttrium-aluminum-garnet laser for the treatment of onychomycosis: A randomized, controlled trial. *J Am Acad Dermatol.* 2014;70:911-7.
11. Landsman AS, Robbins AH, Angelini PF, Wu CC, Cook J, Oster M, et al. Treatment of mild, moderate, and severe onychomycosis using 870- and 930-nm light exposure. *J Am Podiatr Med Assoc.* 2010;100:166-77.
12. Landsman AS, Robbins AH. Treatment of mild, moderate, and severe onychomycosis using 870- and 930-nm light exposure: some follow-up observations at 270 days. *J Am Podiatr Med Assoc.* 2012;102:169-71.

13. Stanford University (2012). Treatment of onychomycosis using a 0.65 millisecond pulsed Nd:YAG 1064 nm laser. [online] Available from: http://clinicaltrials.gov/show/NCT01666002. [Accessed December, 2016].
14. Noguchi H, Miyata K, Sugita T, Hiruma M, Hiruma M. Treatment of onychomycosis using a 1064nm Nd:YAG laser. *Med Mycol J.* 2013;54:333-9.
15. Carney C, Cantrell W, Warner J, Elewski B. Treatment of onychomycosis using a submillisecond 1064-nm neodymium:yttrium-aluminum-garnet laser. *J Am Acad Dermatol.* 2013;69:578-82.
16. Hees H, Jäger MW, Raulin C. Treatment of onychomycosis using the 1 064 nm Nd:YAG laser: a clinical pilot study. *J Dtsch Dermatol Ges.* 2014;12:322-9.
17. Moon SH, Hur H, Oh YJ, Choi KH, Kim JE, Ko JY, et al. Treatment of onychomycosis with a 1,064-nm long-pulsed Nd:YAG laser. *J Cosmet Laser Ther.* 2014,16:165-70.
18. Erchonia Corporation. (2012) Study of the use of low level laser light therapy to treat toenail fungus. [online] Available from http://clinicaltrials.gov/ct2/show/NCT01534689. [Accessed December, 2016].
19. Sullivan R, O'Flynn D. Erchonia Laser Therapy in the Treatment of Onychomycosis: A preliminary report on an ongoing clinical trial. *Podiatry Rev.* 2014;71:6-9.
20. Harris DM, McDowell BA, Strisower J. Laser treatment for toenail fungus. *Proc SPIE.* 2009;7161:1-7.
21. Weiss D. Weiss Foot and Ankle Center. (2011). 3 month clinical results using sub-millisecond 1064 nm Nd:YAG laser for the treatment of onychomycosis. [online] Available from http://conejofeet.com/wp-content/uploads/2011/06/David-Weiss-DPM-report.pdf. [Accessed December, 2016].
22. Renner R, Grüsser K, Sticherling M. 1,064-nm diode laser therapy of onychomycosis: results of a prospective open treatment of 82 toenails. *Dermatol Basel Switz.* 2015;230:128-34.
23. Li Y, Yu S, Xu J, Zhang R, Zhao J. Comparison of the efficacy of long-pulsed Nd:YAG laser intervention for treatment of onychomycosis of toenails or fingernails. *J Drugs Dermatol.* 2014;13:1258-63.
24. Waibel J, Wulkan AJ, Rudnick A. Prospective efficacy and safety evaluation of laser treatments with real-time temperature feedback for fungal onychomycosis. *J Drugs Dermatol.* 2013;12:1237-42.
25. Ortiz AE, Truong S, Serowka K, Kelly KM. A 1,320-nm Nd: YAG laser for improving the appearance of onychomycosis. *Dermatol Surg.* 2014;40:1356-60.
26. Gupta AK, Paquet M. A retrospective chart review of the clinical efficacy of Nd:YAG 1064-nm laser for toenail onychomycosis. *J Dermatolog Treat.* 2015;26:376-8.
27. Hochman LG. Laser treatment of onychomycosis using a novel 0.65-millisecond pulsed Nd:YAG 1064-nm laser. *J Cosmet Laser Ther.* 2011;13:2-5.
28. Lim EH, Kim HR, Park YO, Lee Y, Seo YJ, Kim CD, et al. Toenail onychomycosis treated with a fractional carbon-dioxide laser and topical antifungal cream. *J Am Acad Dermatol.* 2014;70:918-23.
29. Karsai S, Jäger M, Oesterhelt A, Weiss C, Schneider SW, Jünger M, et al. Treating onychomycosis with the short-pulsed 1064-nm-Nd:YAG laser: results of a prospective randomized controlled trial. *J Eur Acad Dermatol Venereol.* 2016 Aug 13.
30. de Oliveira GB, Antonio JR, Antonio CR, Tomé FA. The association of fractional CO2 laser 10.600nm and photodynamic therapy in the treatment of onychomycosis. *An Bras Dermatol.* 2015;90:468-71.
31. US Food and Drug Administration. (2015). Medical devices and clinical trial design for the treatment or improvement in the appearance of fungally-infected nails. [online] Available from: http://www.fda.gov/downloads/MedicalDevices/DeviceRegulationandGuidance/GuidanceDocuments/UCM431312.pdf. [Accessed December, 2016].
32. Gupta AK, Foley KA, Daigle D. Clinical trials of lasers for toenail onychomycosis: The implications of new regulatory guidance. *J Dermatolog Treat.* 2016;1-7.
33. Gupta A, Simpson F. Device-based therapies for onychomycosis treatment. *Skin Ther Lett.* 2012;17:4-9.
34. Mochizuki T, Kawasaki M, Tanabe H, Ishizaki H. A nail drilling method suitable for the diagnosis of onychomycosis. *J Dermatol.* 2005;32:108-13.
35. MHRA. (2016). Curanail 5% nail lacquer (Amorolfine hydrochloride) PL 10590/0049 [online] Available from: http://www.mhra.gov.uk/home/groups/l-unit1/documents/websiteresources/con2023787.pdf.[Accessed December, 2016].

36. Valeant. (2012). Product monograph penlac (ciclopirox topical solution, 8% w/w) nail lacquer. [online] Available from: http://webprod3.hc-sc.gc.ca/dpd-bdpp/info.do?lang=eng&code=73535. [Accessed December, 2016].
37. Gupta AK, Paquet M, Simpson FC. Therapies for the treatment of onychomycosis. *Clin Dermatol.* 2013;31:544-54.
38. Shemer A, Gupta AK, Amichai B, Farhi R, Baran R, Daniel CR, et al. An open comparative study of nail drilling as adjunctive treatment for toenail onychomycosis. *J Dermatolog Treat.* 2016;27:480-3.
39. Zhu Z, Tang Z, Phillips JA, Yang R, Wang H, Tan W. Regulation of singlet oxygen generation using single-walled carbon nanotubes. *J Am Chem Soc.* 2008;130:10856-7.
40. Demidova TN, Hamblin MR. Effect of cell-photosensitizer binding and cell density on microbial photoinactivation. *Antimicrob Agents Chemother.* 2005;49:2329-35.
41. Wan MT, Lin JY. Current evidence and applications of photodynamic therapy in dermatology. *Clin Cosmet Investig Dermatol.* 2014;7:145-63.
42. Aspiroz C, Fortuño-Cebamanos B, Rezusta A, Gilaberte Y. Photodynamic therapy with methyl-aminolevulinate can be useful in the management of Scytalidium infections. *Actas Dermosifiliogr.* 2013;104:725-7.
43. Souza LW, Souza SV, Botelho AC. Distal and lateral toenail onychomycosis caused by Trichophyton rubrum: treatment with photodynamic therapy based on methylene blue dye. *An Bras Dermatol.* 2014;89:184-6.
44. Sotiriou E, Koussidou-Eremonti T, Chaidemenos G, Apalla Z, Ioannides D. Photodynamic therapy for distal and lateral subungual toenail onychomycosis caused by Trichophyton rubrum: Preliminary results of a single-centre open trial. *Acta Derm Venereol.* 2010;90:216-7.
45. Figueiredo Souza LW, Souza SVT, Botelho AC. Randomized controlled trial comparing photodynamic therapy based on methylene blue dye and fluconazole for toenail onychomycosis. *Dermatol Ther.* 2014;27:43-7.
46. Kalia YN, Naik A, Garrison J, Guy RH. Iontophoretic drug delivery. *Adv Drug Deliv Rev.* 2004;56:619-58.
47. Nair AB, Kim HD, Chakraborty B, Singh J, Zaman M, Gupta A, et al. Ungual and trans-ungual iontophoretic delivery of terbinafine for the treatment of onychomycosis. *J Pharm Sci.* 2009;98:4130-40.
48. Nair AB, Kim HD, Davis SP, Etheredge R, Barsness M, Friden PM, et al. An ex vivo toe model used to assess applicators for the iontophoretic ungual delivery of terbinafine. *Pharm Res.* 2009;26:2194-201.
49. Nair AB, Vaka SRK, Murthy SN. Transungual delivery of terbinafine by iontophoresis in onychomycotic nails. *Drug Dev Ind Pharm.* 2011;37:1253-8.
50. Nematollahi AR, Badiee P, Nournia E. The Efficacy of Ultraviolet Irradiation on Trichophyton Species Isolated From Nails. *Jundishapur J Microbiol.* 2015;8:e18158.
51. Kerai LV, Hilton S, Murdan S. UV-curable gel formulations: Potential drug carriers for the topical treatment of nail diseases. *Int J Pharm.* 2015;492:177-90.
52. Kushner J, Blankschtein D, Langer R. Heterogeneity in skin treated with low-frequency ultrasound. *J Pharm Sci.* 2008;97:4119-28.
53. Iwasawa A, Saito K, Mokudai T, Kohno M, Ozawa T, Niwano Y. Fungicidal Action of Hydroxyl Radicals Generated by Ultrasound in Water. *J Clin Biochem Nutr.* 2009;45:214-8.
54. Zderic V, Clark JI, Vaezy S. Drug delivery into the eye with the use of ultrasound. *J Ultrasound Med.* 2004;23:1349-59.
55. Abadi D, Zderic V. Ultrasound-mediated nail drug delivery system. *J Ultrasound Med.* 2011;30:1723-30.
56. Kim MS, Jung JY, Cho EB, Park EJ, Kim KH, Kim KJ. The effectiveness of 1,064-nm long-pulsed Nd:YAG laser in the treatment of severe onychomycosis. *J Cosmet Laser Ther.* 2016;18:317-22.

World Clin Dermatol. 2016;3(1):178-88.

Future Therapies for Cutaneous Fungal Infections

*Devinder M Thappa MD DHA FRCP FAMS FIMSA
Malathi Munisamy MD DNB

Department of Dermatology and STD,
Jawaharlal Institute of Postgraduate Medical Education and Research,
Puducherry, India

ABSTRACT

Cutaneous fungal infections continue to be one of the major healthcare problems worldwide affecting 20–25% of the population. These cutaneous infections might result in severe disseminated infections and sometimes can even cause invasive systemic infections in high-risk immunosuppressed individuals. Despite the availability of an armamentarium of old and newer topical and systemic antifungals to tackle these infections, the emerging problems of antifungal resistance, inefficiency of treatment especially in high risk groups, poor compliance, systemic toxicity, and drug interactions, there is an emerging need for effective and safe antifungals with improved drug delivery systems in the future. Though the first step towards the discovery and development of future broad-spectrum antifungals relies on the identification of conserved fungal genes, the successful development of such agents requires knowledge and research beyond the identification of these conserved fungal genes. Recent understanding of the molecular mechanisms involved with virulence, drug resistance, and identification of newer potential targets has provided insights into the development of novel compounds with potent antifungal properties that act against these pathways. Though the development of newer antifungals are challenging, the ever-expanding knowledge coupled with interdisciplinary research involving chemical, molecular, and clinical expertise and ongoing efforts to move from preclinical compound testing to true clinical trials, new exciting possibilities, especially with innovative formulations for the treatment of cutaneous fungal infections, hold promise in the near future.

*Corresponding author
Email: dmthappa@gmail.com

© 2016 Jaypee Brothers Medical Publishers. All rights reserved.

INTRODUCTION

Cutaneous fungal infections continue to be one of the major healthcare problems worldwide affecting 20–25% of the population with a steadily increasing incidence and prevalence over the last three decades.[1] These cutaneous infections might result in severe disseminated infections and sometimes can even cause invasive systemic infections in high risk immunosuppressed individuals like those affected with acquired immunodeficiency syndrome, those on immunosuppressive therapy like organ transplant recipients and cancer patients. Despite the availability of an armamentarium of old and newer topical and systemic antifungals to tackle these infections, the emerging problems of antifungal resistance, inefficiency of treatment especially in high risk groups, poor compliance, systemic toxicity, and drug interactions, there is an emerging need for effective and safe antifungals with improved drug delivery systems in the future.

EXISTING AGENTS AND THE NEED FOR BETTER NEWER THERAPIES

The currently available topical and systemic antifungals can be broadly grouped into eight categories based on their mechanism of action as follows:

1. Azoles: Inhibit ergosterol synthesis of fungal plasma membrane by inhibiting two cytochrome P450 enzymes, lanosterol 14 α-demethylase, and Δ22-desaturase
2. Allylamines
3. Thiocarbamates: Inhibit early stage of ergosterol synthesis by inhibiting squalene epoxidase
4. Polyene macrolides: Interact with ergosterol to form complexes which result in formation of pores in the plasma membrane
5. Fluorinated pyrimidines: Interfere with deoxyribonucleic acid (DNA), ribonucleic acid (RNA), and protein synthesis in fungal cells
6. Candins: Inhibit synthesis of glucan in fungal cell wall by inhibiting β-1,3-D-glucan synthase
7. Griseofulvin: Inhibits microtubules necessary for mitosis
8. Oxaboroles: Inhibit fungal cytoplasmic leucyl-tRNA synthetase, thereby inhibiting fungal protein synthesis.[2]

Among these, nystatin and griseofulvin have been used for five decades now with good safety profile, however, with limited activity against yeasts and dermatophytes, respectively. Similarly, the broad spectrum agents like allylamines and azoles have also proven their efficacy and safety for more than two decades now. In the recent years, no new therapeutic groups have been introduced but newer generations of existing group of antifungals have been developed. In order to enhance the therapeutic efficacy, safety profile, and to improve patient compliance, extensive vehicles and delivery systems have also been developed.

Despite the improved spectrum of activity, efficacy, and improved toxicity profile, the newer generation of antifungals, however, are still associated with limitations like limited spectrum of activity, pharmacokinetic drug interactions, and unusual toxicities with prolonged use. To add to this, increasing reports of clinical resistance to antifungal agents and better understanding of the molecular mechanisms responsible for the development of drug resistance warrant the need for better newer therapeutic strategies.

RESEARCH GOALS FOR FUTURE ANTIFUNGAL AGENTS

The characteristics of an ideal antifungal agent, which are largely unmet, include the following: fungicidal activity that targets the dormant spores thereby preventing reinfection, broad spectrum including activity against resistant strains, rapid relief with a shorter duration of treatment without adverse effects to improve compliance, and affordable price. Hence, the key areas of research in the development of antifungals that need to be explored in the near future should focus on the following:[2-4]

- Enhanced fungicidal action: Future drugs should be more potent that would effectively control the infection attaining optimal drug concentrations at the site of infection
- Greater selectivity for inhibiting fungal enzymes: This is a crucial area to be targeted to reduce the toxicities owing to the evolutionarily smaller differences between the fungus and human
- Broad spectrum of activity: Future antifungals should have a wider spectrum of activity targeting multiple species of fungi including the ones that have developed drug resistance and are inherently resistant
- Reduced incidence of resistance: The future antifungals should act on a wider range of novel potential cellular targets to prevent the development of resistance
- Good pharmacokinetic profile: With the increasing use of drugs for various comorbidities, the future antifungals should have favorable drug interaction profile and reduced dosing to enhance patient compliance
- Better formulations: The future therapies should focus on improved formulations and drug delivery systems that ensure adequate concentration of the drug at the required site of infection that is acceptable by the patients, thereby improving their compliance
- Safer and more effective antifungal therapy in children: Owing to the dramatic differences between children and adults in antifungal pharmacokinetics,

dosing, antifungal drug exposure targets, and increase in interindividual pharmacokinetic variability with decreasing developmental age, the future of antifungal drugs should also focus on pediatric antifungal drug development taking into consideration the above mentioned factors.[5]

STRATEGIES FOR FUTURE THERAPIES FOR CUTANEOUS FUNGAL INFECTIONS

Antifungal research and development is highly challenging and clinical development is hampered by challenges in timely and definitive diagnosis of the less common or more resistant fungi. Despite these issues, some novel products are progressing in development.[6] With the emergence of multidrug-resistant fungi and the limited choice of selective antifungal targets sparing human, current research focuses mostly on bioactive antifungal compounds from natural sources with modifications or their synthetic analogs. Though the first step towards the discovery and development of future broad spectrum antifungals relies on the identification of conserved fungal genes, the successful development of such agents requires knowledge and research beyond the identification of these conserved fungal genes.[7] The strategies to discover novel antifungal scaffolds include high throughput screening of compound library; drug repurposing using marketed drugs as compound library, antifungal natural products, new antifungal targets' identification by genome-scale analysis, comparative genomics, and bioinformatics; medicinal chemistry studies such as structure-activity relationship, chemical genetics approach, new screening models, structural biology, and rational drug design.[8,9]

Drugs under Clinical Trials

Newer second-generation extended-spectrum triazoles with activity against emergent and resistant fungi with extended half-lives and reduced drug interactions with good tolerance are currently under clinical trials. These include ravuconazole, pramiconazole, and albaconazole. Similarly, aminocandin, a newer echinocandin with extended half-life to enable less frequent dosing, is under trial. However, licensure and their role in clinical practice will be determined only based on results of well-conducted, randomized clinical trials.[6,10,11]

Antifungals under Development[10,11]

- SPK-843: A polyene antifungal with activity against *Candida* spp.
- Arylamidine T-2307: An aromatic diamidine associated with the inhibition of mitochondrial function of the fungal cell with activity against *Candida* spp.

- Icofungipen: β-amino acid, a derivative of cispentacin targeting isoleucyl-tRNA synthetase with activity against *Candida* spp.
- Pyridobenzimidazole 75-4590: A specific inhibitor of β-1,6-glucan synthase with activity against *Candida* spp.
- PHS11A and PH11B: Inhibitors of fatty acid synthase active against *Trichophyton rubrum*
- Pradimicins and benanomicins: Bind to C-mannan which is a cell wall glycoprotein that combats the host immune response through disruption of cytokine response and T lymphocyte action.

Experimental Therapies that need to be Explored

- Plant derivatives: With the emergence of resistance to synthetic antifungal agents, the search for cheaper and readily available alternative agents has turned the focus on naturally available plant derivatives which have demonstrated antifungal properties. These include aloe vera juices;[12] green tea catechins;[13] flavonoids like rutin and quercetin from the fruits of *Terminalia chebula*; apigenin from stem of *T. chebula*;[14] tannins from *Arrabidaea chica, Rosmarinus officinalis, Syzygium cumini,* and *Punica granatum*; terpenes and phenolic compounds from *Lippia sidoides;* essential oil and vegetable extracts from *Mentha piperita, Tabebuia avellanedae, Casearia sylvestris,* and *Arctium lappa*, and oil of *Achillea millefolium*; *Mikania glomerata,* and *Stachys byzantina.*[15] Further research is needed to identify the most suitable agent that will target a specific organism at the appropriate dosage among a host of these agents available
- Traditional Chinese medicine: With recent research on natural products with potential antifungal properties, traditional Chinese medicine has gained interest as potential antifungal agents. These include crude extracts of *Rhizoma coptidis* and *Cortex Phellodendri chinesis, Melaphis chinensis, Polygonum cuspidatum, P. granatum,* and *Schisandra chinensis.* Berberine, the active alkaloid obtained from these extracts was effective against *Trichophyton mentagrophytes, T. rubrum, Microsporum canis,* and *Microsporum gypseum.* Another agent pseudolaric acid B, extracted from "tujingpi" or *Cortex pseudolaricis* is active against *Candida* spp. Ginseng stem-leaf saponins comprising of ginsenosides were also found to be effective against *Candida albicans*[16]
- Broad spectrum antimicrobial peptides and antifungal peptides: These small cationic and amphipathic molecules fewer than 50 amino acids are the first line of defense between the host and its environment with direct (increasing permeability of fungal membrane) and indirect (immunostimulatory) antifungal properties. These peptides with primarily antifungal properties include 1,3-β-glucan synthesis inhibitors like echinocandins, pneumocandins,

molundocandins, papulacandins, aculeacins, and WF11899; inhibitors of chitin in the cell wall like nikkomycins, polyoxins, and aureobasidins; membrane-active selective antimicrobial peptides like Rs-ARF2 (plant defensin), drosomycin (insect defensin), and iturins (from *Bacillus subtilis*); histidine-rich peptides like histatins; and chitin-cleaving enzymes like chitotriosidase. The antifungal peptides with wide spectrum of antimicrobial activity include cecropins, magainins, dermaseptins, bombinin-H and bombinin-like peptides, metchnikowin, cathelicidins [indolicidin, tritrpticin, LL-37(CAMP18)], penetratin-like hexapeptide (PAF26), thanatin, protegrins, macrocyclic peptides, syringomycins lactoferrin, bactericidal and permeability-increasing protein, lysozyme, antileukoprotease, ribonucleases, calprotectin, and glyceraldehyde-3-phosphate dehydrogenase-derived peptide from human placental tissue. Synthetic peptides include kaxins, aurein 1.2, citropin 1.1 A, uperin 3.6, VS2, VS3, and KSL-W. A better understanding of antifungal peptides would result in discovery of novel microbial targets and help in designing new antifungal strategies that are more potent, specific, and nontoxic to combat resistant strains. These agents can be synthesized by peptide synthesis methodology, recombinant engineering, or molecular dynamics methods for antimicrobial peptidomimetics[17,18]

- Agents targeting the fungal virulence factors: Use of inhibitors of fungal virulence factors is another attractive strategy in the development of newer antifungals. These include biofilm disruption with plant peptide Tn-AFP1 obtained from fruits of *Trapa natans*, or reducing the adhesion capabilities of the fungus by causing mutations in secreted aspartic proteinases (SAP) coding genes or using pepstatin A, which is an SAP inhibitor, or using antibodies against SAP[18]
- Marine natural product as antifungal agent: Marine products such as cyano-bacteria, algae dinoflagellates, marine sponges, and marine microorganism are also being investigated to isolate and characterize bioactive metabolites from these marine organisms with potential antifungal properties and the main targets identified so far include lanosterol 14-α-demethylase (CYP51) and ribose-5-phosphate isomerase B[19]
- Mycoviruses: These refer to viruses that specifically target and destroy the fungi, and hence, can be used as biological control agents that can cure infections in humans. They can either be generated as chimeric mycovirus or can be used as gene insertion vectors. Genetic engineering of existing mycoviruses is also possible and these might be considered as a promising direction for future research[20]
- Sodarins: These belong to the semisynthetic natural products that target elongation factor 2 involved in fungal protein biosynthesis. They had been demonstrated to have antifungal properties as early as 1970 but no progress

from animal models had been done after 2002 until recently when they have regained interest and *in vivo* experiments in models of candidiasis are being undertaken[6]

- Bromodomain and extraterminal inhibitors: These agents target the fungal bromodomain and extraterminal proteins that belong to a specific family of transcriptional regulators, which bind chromatin through their two bromodomains, which specifically recognize histones acetylated on lysine residues[21]
- Photodynamic therapy: It can be considered as an alternative therapy for drug-resistant patients. With limited data and reports of higher aggravation rates, alternative protocols without usage of photosensitizers, using combinations of visible to near-infrared (VIS-NIR) laser beams in association with broadband beams of ultraviolet B and R-light-emitting diodes are being tried.[6]

Newer Topical Formulations

The main stay of therapy with regards to cutaneous fungal infections is topical therapy owing to its advantage of targeting of drugs to the site of infection, thereby reducing the risk of systemic side effects. However, the efficiency of the drug depends on the drug concentration attained at the site of infection which in turn depends on its effective penetration through the various layers of the skin, especially through the stratum corneum which is dependent on the physicochemical characteristics of the drug and its formulations.[22] Thus, an ideal formulation should be optimized with respect to the drug and structural and biophysical properties of site of administration. Hence, the future of cutaneous antifungal therapies depends a whole lot on the various formulation strategies in addition to novel antifungal agents.

- Nano carriers for antifungals: Nanoparticles have revolutionized the antifungal drug delivery by solving issues like toxicity, solubility, and availability of optimal drug concentration at sites of infection. These novel colloidal systems with a solid lipid matrix function as controlled release carriers and are of two types: (i) solid lipid nanoparticles (SLN); (ii) nanostructured lipid carriers. Nanostructured lipid carriers have high liquid lipid content, support high drug loads, higher entrapment efficiency, and faster release rate compared to SLN. These particles are stable even up to storage for 3 months. Nanoparticle formulations that are currently being investigated include amphotericin B, itraconazole, and topical silver[6,22-24]
- Vesicles: These act as depot formulations which enable sustained release of active compounds modulating the systemic absorption by acting as rate-limiting barrier membrane for transdermal formulations. Rigid vesicles like

liposomes and niosomes are predominantly for epidermal delivery as they get trapped in the superficial layers of stratum corneum while the elastic or ultra-deformable vesicles like transferosomes and ethosomes are effective at enhancing dermal and transdermal delivery of both lipophilic and hydrophilic drugs[22-24]

- Amphiphilic gels: The drugs are solubilized in nonionic surfactants, which act as permeation enhancers that deliver the drugs into and through the skin[22-24]
- Polymeric micelles: Aqueous polymeric micelle solutions of the drugs are prepared with novel amphiphilic methoxy-poly(ethylene glycol)-hexyl substituted polylactide block copolymers to enhance the penetration[22-24]
- Emulgels: Gellified emulsions or emulgels are dual release control system with increased stability[22-24]
- Microsponges: These macroporous beads of diameter of 10–25 μm provide controlled release of topical agents with improved stability in response to stimuli such as rubbing, temperature, pH, etc.[22-24]
- Foams: Hydroalcoholic foams or emollient foams can carry a broad variety of topical drugs, including water-soluble, oil-soluble, and suspended active agents with the advantages of improved compliance, safety, controllable drug delivery, skin barrier build-up, hydration, and enhanced clinical efficacy[22-24]
- Microemulsions: These isotropic formulations of size 20–200 nm, composed of oil, water, surfactant, and cosurfactant, have the advantage of thermodynamical stability, enhanced drug solubility, and optical clarity[22-24]
- Targeted prodrug approach: Prodrugs refer to inactive or less active pharmacological substances that get converted by metabolic or physicochemical transformation into the pharmacologically active agents after administration. A prodrug, thus, increases the drug selectivity to the intended target, facilitates the ease of formulation, and delivers a cytotoxic agent in a nontoxic form to the specific site where it is metabolized to its active form. Many topical antifungal agents currently available use solvents with irritant potential to deliver the drugs owing to poor aqueous solubility of these drugs. Hence, water-soluble prodrugs that would get converted to the active form at the site of infection would be a promising approach in the future. One such example is the use of plant-derived polyphenolic compounds, coumarins as topical agents for superficial fungal infections. The inactive water-soluble coumarin glycoside "esculin" gets converted to the active antifungal coumarin "esculetin" by the β-glucosidase enzyme produced by the target dermatophytes or the dermal commensal microbiota[25]
- Charged lipid submicron emulsions: Positively-charged submicron emulsions containing stearylamine and negatively-charged submicron emulsions containing deoxycholic acid have been investigated as vehicles for drug delivery. It was found that the penetration of positively-charged droplets was more

when compared to the negatively-charged agents due to skin's net negative superficial charge and binding between surfactants and keratin in the stratum corneum which prolonged the retention time in the skin, thereby contributing to the enhanced transport of positively-charged submicron emulsions[26]
- Liquid crystal cream: These topical delivery systems provide optimal drug delivery rate owing to modulation of their nanostructure. Topical itraconazole liquid crystal cream in a ternary water/nonionic surfactant/oil formulation has been studied as a topical agent owing to its high lipophilicity.[26]

Future Strategies to Prevent Antifungal Resistance

- Combination therapy and adjunctive immunomodulatory therapy: Immunosuppressive compounds, like cyclosporine and D-octapeptides, have been found to counteract antifungal resistance due to efflux pumps and chemosensitization of drug-resistant and drug-sensitive fungi to antifungals with specific chemical substances have been demonstrated.[27] Cytokines may be combined with antifungals for immunostimulatory effects, especially in immunocompromised individuals. Transfusion of specific type of leukocytes after priming based on specific type of fungal infection can also be attempted as adoptive transfer of leukocytes has the advantage of increasing the activity of specific components of either innate or adaptive immunity resulting in robust immune response[6,27]
- Newer targets for combating drug resistance: These include heat shock protein 90 (Hsp90) and efflux pumps, especially adenosine triphosphate-binding cassette transporters[27]
- Antifungal vaccines: The possibility of recombinant or DNA antifungal vaccines need to be explored, and the various candidate antigens isolated from fungus that mediate excellent antibody-mediated immune response include β-glucan, cell wall glycoprotein, Hsp-90, aspartyl proteinase, phosphoglycerate kinase, melanin, glucosylceramide, and glucuronoxlymannan.[6,27]

CONCLUSION

The rising global burden associated with fungal infections and significant failure rates associated with the management of fungal infections indicate an unmet need for improved antimycotic therapy, thereby mandating continued efforts to identify new strategies for potent and effective therapy. Recent understanding of the molecular mechanisms involved with virulence, drug resistance, and identification of newer potential targets has provided insights into the development of novel compounds with potent antifungal properties that act against these pathways. Though the development of newer antifungals are challenging, the ever-expanding knowledge coupled with interdisciplinary research involving chemical, molecular, and clinical expertise and ongoing efforts to move from preclinical compound testing to true clinical trials, new exciting possibilities, especially with innovative formulations for the treatment of cutaneous fungal infections, hold promise in the near future.

Editor's Comment

In this article, the author tackles a vitally important topic in the world of fungal diseases. As has been documented in global literature, and nicely in this article, newer therapies for fungal diseases are needed to continue ensuring our success as treating dermatologists. Drug resistance, access to care, and cost, are just three of the very important factors that continue to make fungal disease therapeutics challenging. Dr Thappa has succinctly presented and commented on this topic, and the editors hope that this reading will continue to promote interest in awareness of future directions.

Seemal R Desai, Rashmi Sarkar

REFERENCES

1. Jaulim Z, Salmon N, Fuller C. Fungal skin infections: current approaches to management. *Prescriber.* 2015;26:31-5.
2. Minnebruggen GV, Francois JA, Cammue PA, Thevissen K, Vroome V, Borgers M, et al. A general overview on past, present and future antimycotics. *The Open Mycology J.* 2010;4:22-32.
3. Pianalto KM, Alspaugh JA. New horizons in antifungal therapy. *J Fungi.* 2016;2:1-24.
4. Kurtz MB. New antifungal targets: A vision for the future. [online] Available from: http://www.asm.org. [Accessed December, 2016].
5. Watt KM, Cohen-Wolkowiez M, Ward RM, Benjamin DK. Pediatric antifungal drug development: lessons learned and recommendations for the future. *Pediatr Infect Dis J.* 2012;31:635-7.
6. Ostrosky-Zeichner L, Casadevall A, Galgiani JN, Odds FC, Rex JH. An insight into the antifungal pipeline: selected new molecules and beyond. *Nat Rev Drug Discov.* 2010;9:719-27.
7. Liu M, Healy MD, Dougherty BA, Esposito KM, Maurice TC, Mazzucco CE, et al. Conserved fungal genes as potential targets for broad-spectrum antifungal drug discovery. *Eukaryot Cell.* 2006;5:638-49.
8. Liu N, Wang C, Su H, Zhang W, Sheng C. Strategies in the discovery of novel antifungal scaffolds. *Future Med Chem.* 2016;8:1435-54.
9. Amaral AC, Fernandes L, Galdino AS, Felipe MS, Soares CM, Pereira M. Therapeutic targets in Paracoccidioides brasiliensis: post-transcriptome perspectives. *Genet Mol Res.* 2005;4:430-49.
10. Türel O. Newer antifungal agents. *Expert Rev Anti Infect Ther.* 2011;9:325-38.
11. Eldridge ML, Chambers CJ, Sharon VR, Thompson GR 3rd. Fungal infections of the skin and nail: new treatment options. *Expert Rev Anti Infect Ther.* 2014;12:1389-405.
12. Mosunmola OJ, Remi RR, Abayomi BT, Olaosebikan MS, Charles N, Afolabi O. Susceptibility of dermatophytes to Aloe vera juices using agar diffusion and broth dilution techniques. *Am J Res Commun.* 2013;1:53-62.
13. Hirasawa M, Takada K. Multiple effects of green tea catechin on the antifungal activity of antimycotics against Candida albicans. *J Antimicrob Chemother.* 2004;53:225-9.

14. Singh G, Kumar P, Joshi SC. Treatment of dermatophytosis by a new antifungal agent "apigenin". *Mycoses.* 2014;57:497-506.
15. Anibal PC, de Cássia Orlandi Sardi J, Peixoto IT, de Carvalho Moraes JJ, Höfling JF. Conventional and alternative antifungal therapies to oral candidiasis. *Braz J Microbiol.* 2010;41:824-31.
16. Tseung KS, Zhao J. Update on the fungal biofilm drug resistance and its alternative treatment. *J Biosci Med.* 2016;4:37-47.
17. Matejuk A, Leng Q, Begum MD, Woodle MC, Scaria P, Chou ST, et al. Peptide-based antifungal therapies against emerging infections. *Drugs Future.* 2010;35:197.
18. Mehra T, Köberle M, Braunsdorf C, Mailänder-Sanchez D, Borelli C, Schaller M. Alternative approaches to antifungal therapies. *Exp Dermatol.* 2012;21:778-82.
19. Terra L, Abreu PA, Teixeira VL, Paixão CP, Pereira R, Leal B, et al. Mycoses and Antifungals: reviewing the basis of a current problem that still is a biotechnological target for marine products. *Front Mar Sci.* 2014;1:1-12.
20. van de Sande WW, Lo-Ten-Foe JR, van Belkum A, Netea MG, Kullberg BJ, Vonk AG. Mycoviruses: future therapeutic agents of invasive fungal infections in humans? *Eur J Clin Microbiol Infect Dis.* 2010;29:755-63.
21. Muller S, Filippakopoulos P, Knapp S. Bromodomains as therapeutic targets. *Expert Rev Mol Med.* 2011;13:e29.
22. Güngör S, Erdal MS, Aksu B. New formulation strategies in topical antifungal therapy. *Journal of Cosmetics, Dermatological Sciences and Applications.* 2013;3:56-65.
23. Bseiso EA, Nasr M, Sammour O, Abd El Gawad NA. Recent advances in topical formulation carriers of antifungal agents. *Indian J Dermatol Venereol Leprol.* 2015;81:457-63.
24. Glujoy M, Salerno C, Bregni C, Carlucci AM. Percutaneous drug delivery systems for improving antifungal therapy effectiveness: a review. *Int J Pharm Pharm Sci.* 2014;6:8-16.
25. Mercer DK, Robertson J, Wright K, Miller L, Smith S, Colin S, et al. A prodrug approach to the use of coumarins as potential therapeutics for superficial mycoses. *PLoS One.* 2013;8:e80760.
26. Robert EM, Kalia YN. New developments in topical antifungal therapy. *Am J Drug Deliv.* 2006;4:231-47.
27. Nigam PK. Antifungal drugs and resistance: Current concepts. *Our Dermatol Online J.* 2015;6:212-21.

World Clin Dermatol. 2016;3(1):189-206.

Rising Resistance in Cutaneous Fungal Infections and Strategies to Combat It

Brijesh Nair MD

Department of Dermatology, INHS Sanjivani Hospital
Kochi, Kerala, India

ABSTRACT

Drug resistance in pathogenic fungi, particularly dermatophytes, has become a public health menace. The study of antifungal resistance has lagged behind that of antibacterial resistance. The factors leading to resistance and variants of resistance are variegate with certain aspects being matter of conjecture. The pharmacological efficacy of various antifungals are governed by host hygiene, drug pharmacokinetics, both cutaneous and systemic, drug interactions, host immunity, fungal loco-regional variants, and topical steroid abuse The lean development line in new antifungal systemic and topical agents is a matter of great concern for the practising dermatologist.Various measures to tackle this menace by use of antifungal combinations acting on different mycological targets, antifungal stewardship, therapy based on antifungal pharmacokinetics, efflux pump inhibitors, studying the pharmacogenetics of resistance, and evolving suitable strategies to tackle these barriers. The thought process has to be flexible and inclusive of emerging scientific evidence and should be synergistic between dermatologists, internists, geneticists, and microbiologists to effectively tackle this emergent problem of antifungal resistance.

INTRODUCTION

Drug resistance in pathogenic fungi, including dermatophytes, is gaining importance of late due to the many cases of persistent dermatophytic infections in spite of adequate prescription of antifungal therapy. The increased use of antifungal agents in recent years has resulted in the development of resistance

Email: meshugah12@rediffmail.com

© 2016 Jaypee Brothers Medical Publishers. All rights reserved.

to these drugs. The menace of antifungal resistance and recalcitrance of chronic dermatophytosis, candidiasis, and pityriasis versicolor are on the rise. The study of antifungal resistance has lagged behind that of antibacterial resistance for several reasons. Perhaps, most importantly, fungi were not considered as important pathogens until relatively recently. The approval of the imidazole- and triazole-based antifungals in late 1980s and early 1990s was an important step that greatly advanced the ability to safely and effectively treat local and systemic fungal infections. The high safety profile of the triazoles, particularly fluconazole, led to their extensive, sometimes prophylactic, use. The extensive use of fluconazole has resulted in the development of resistance.[1]

PHENOMENON OF CHRONIC DERMATOPHYTOSES

The dermatological practitioner is facing an onslaught of chronic and recurrent dermatophytosis in volumes never encountered previously. Chronic dermatomycoses are defined as patients who have suffered from the disease for more than 6 months to 1 year duration, with or without recurrence, in spite of being treated. Recurrent dermatophytosis refers to the reoccurrence of the dermatophyte infection within few weeks, after completion of treatment. These cases make up at least 5–10% of new cases seen in the dermatology clinic at a tertiary center in North India.[2,3] Chronic and recurrent dermatophytic infections cause significant distress to the patients socially, emotionally, and financially. Dermatophytic infections are predominant in the tropical countries such as India where the hot and humid weather is favorable for the acquisition and maintenance of the disease. There is a phenomenon described as *Trichophyton rubrum* syndrome which is characterized by involvement of at least four body sites such as feet, hands, nails as well as one another site with the exclusion of inguinal area with microscopic fungal detection from all four sites, and positive culture from at least three of the four sites.[4]

TYPES OF ANTIFUNGAL RESISTANCE

Resistance can be divided into following four types.[5] The major factors governing resistance are tabulated in table 1.

1. Primary (intrinsic) resistance: Without prior exposure to drug where all normal members of a species tolerate a particular drug. In this case, a specific characteristic responsible for resistance is inherent to the species and has arisen through the process of evolution
2. Secondary (acquired) resistance: Is a term used when a resistant strain emerges from a population that was previously drug-sensitive after exposure; considering a low frequency of gene mutation, the selective pressure exerted by the constant use of antifungal agents selects eventual resistant strains that

Table 1: Principal Factors Affecting Antifungal Clinical Resistance

- Net state of immunosuppression
- The changing epidemiology of *Candida* infection manifested by a change from the albicans to the non-albicans *Candida*
- Strain acquisition of increased virulence
- High burden of fungus at initiation of treatment
- Strain acquisition of increased virulence
- Pharmacokinetics and/or pharmacodynamics of drug
- Site of infection (e.g., nail)
- Length of treatment and/or compliance to treatment
- Long-term drug administration
- Underlying disease
- Inadequate patient compliance
- Lifestyle: poor hygiene, tight-fitting clothes, sharing of clothes
- Fomites, family history
- Rampant use of over the counter antifungal agents without clinician's consent
- Regular use of antifungal agents via soaps, shampoos, or creams may incur selective pressure
- Increased immunocompromised status: use of steroids, diabetes
- Human genetic factors
- Personal habits: tight clothes, sharing clothes, inadequate frequency of ablution, fomites, overcrowding, infected socks, etc.
- Pharmacokinetics, pharmacodynamics, drug interaction
- Biofilm formation

will become predominant in the population. Secondary resistance develops among previously susceptible strains after exposure to the antifungal agent and is usually dependent on altered gene expression.

3. Clinical resistance is when the pathogen is inhibited by antimicrobial concentration higher than could be safely achieved with normal dosing. Clinical resistance has been defined as the persistence or progression of an infection despite appropriate antimicrobial therapy. In other words, it is the failure to eradicate a fungal infection despite the administration of an antifungal agent with *in vitro* activity against the organism. Such failures can be attributed to incorrect diagnosis, immunosuppression, and suboptimal dose or duration of therapy
4. Microbiologic resistance: Growth of pathogen is inhibited by antimicrobial concentration higher than the range seen for the wild type strains.

FACTORS GOVERNING DRUG RESPONSE AND ANTIFUNGAL RESISTANCE

It has been time and again stated and proven that a successful clinical response to antimicrobial therapy depends not only on the susceptibility of the pathogenic organism, but also relies on the host immune system, drug penetration and distribution, patient compliance, and absence of a protected or persistent focus of infection.[5,6]

Microbial Factors

Dermatophytes are pathogenic fungi that belong to three genera:. (i) *Epidermophyton*, (ii) *Microsporum*, and (iii) *Trichophyton*, and are classified as anthropophilic, zoophilic, and geophilic species on the basis of their primary habitat associations. Ringworm may be a consequence of the inflammatory reaction of the host to the enzymes secreted by the fungus during its invasive process.[7] The adherence capability has been attributed to the presence of glycoproteins containing mannans in the cell wall of these fungi, which is presumed to correlate with virulence. Mannans produced by *T. rubrum* work by inhibiting the critical steps in antigen processing and presentation. In addition, for dermatophytes to be successful in their installation in the host, the arthroconidia must germinate very rapidly and the hyphae must penetrate the body surface; otherwise they will be eliminated by the continuous desquamation of the epithelium. Once installed, the dermatophytes must scavenge nutrients for growth. Penetration of spores rivalling the desquamation rates of skin is achieved by fungal proteases which aids in rapid expansion of the dermatophytes. Proteases with an optimal activity at acidic pH are important virulence factors of dermatophytes. The keratinolytic proteases secreted by *T. rubrum*, apparently required to its complete installation and to remain in the host, are somehow regulated by PacC protein.[8,9] The conidia are primarily killed by neutrophils and monocytes which is countered by fungal catalase and superoxide dismutase, which act as defense against phagocytic free radicals.

Host Factors

The dermatophytic clearance from the skin is secondary to the activation of cell-mediated immunity and is T helper (Th)-1/Th17 T lymphocyte cell dependent. Acute dermatophytosis is associated with Th1 response, whereas in cases of chronic dermatophytosis, the immunity is skewed toward Th2 cytokines with high levels of immunoglobulin E (IgE) and immunoglobulin G4 antibodies. It has been observed that the free radicals and nitric oxide release have been found to be 20–30% lower than that of controls in patients of chronic dermatophytosis, indicating a defective killing mechanism. The cellular milieu has decreased inflammatory cytokines such as interleukin (IL)-1, IL-6, IL-8, and tumor necrosis factor-α, and increased anti-inflammatory cytokines such as IL-10. The down-regulation of toll-like receptor 4 by *T. rubrum* further decreases the inflammatory response by decreasing pro-inflammatory cytokine production and recruitment of neutrophils.[10]

Patients with immunocompromised status, diabetes mellitus, atopy, and intake of systemic corticosteroids are also predisposed to chronic dermatophytosis. There is an increased prevalence associated with the disorders of keratinization such as ichthyosis vulgaris where retained keratin often acts as a nidus for infection. Recurrent dermatophytosis was more frequent in low socioeconomic group, and tinea corporis and cruris were found to be the most common clinical forms associated with chronicity.[11] Antibodies are not protective against dermatophytes and elevated serum IgE level is associated with chronicity as in cases of tinea imbricate. Reinfection from the contacts or fomites may also be a contributing factor, as majority of patients with chronic or recurrent dermatophytosis have multiple affected family members. Overcrowding, sharing of clothes and footwear, poor hygiene, tight clothes, and migration are also some predisposing factors in Indian scenario.[2]

In vivo resistance is also correlated with antifungal misuse because patients often fail to complete the full course of therapy. Thus, the inadequate use or dosage of drugs contributes to the failure in eliminating the fungus completely, encouraging growth of the most resistant strains, which may lead to hard-to-treat fungal infections. Even considering a low frequency of gene mutation, the selective pressure exerted by the constant use of antifungal agents eventually selects a resistant strain that will become predominant in the population. *T. rubrum* develops resistance on prolonged exposure to itraconazole and fluconazole. In addition, cross-resistance between both the azoles has been observed in the same study. Overexpression of *ERG11* and *CDR1* were associated with increased cross-resistance to ketoconazole and itraconazole but not amphotericin B. The subsequent repeated treatment courses ultimately result in subjecting *Candida* spp. to multiple exposures of the drug. Thus, concomitant with the long term, repeated usage of fluconazole was the emergence of fungal strains exhibiting resistance to this drug as well as cross-resistance to other azoles.[5,12]

Environmental Factors

There is a school of thought and rightly so that the rampant abuse in the environment of antifungals in agriculture causes cross-resistance to medical triazoles.[13]

REPORTS OF ANTIFUNGAL DRUG RESISTANCE

Studies around the world are noticing an increasing rise in resistance to common antifungal drugs used for the treatment of dermatophytic infections. In 2002, a

T. rubrum strain exhibiting primary resistance to terbinafine was detected. This resistance was attributed to a single missense amino acid substitution at *L398F*, which made *T. rubrum* resistant to all antifungals that act on squalene epoxidase enzyme.[14] In a study of 100 isolates of onychomycosis, Sarifakioglu et al. found itraconazole and fluconazole having the greatest variation in minimum inhibitory concentration (MIC).[15] Azambuja et al. found high MIC values for fluconazole and itraconazole (66.7% and 25%, respectively) in 100 isolates of *T. rubrum* from patients with onychomycosis.[16] A study from North India showed that there were nonresponders to gold standard drug griseofulvin among the tinea capitis patients.[17] It is also observed that clinical resistance which is observed is not correlated well with microbiologically proven resistance in practice. The acquired immune deficiency syndrome (AIDS) epidemic has created a nidus for resistant candidiasis. Prior to the introduction of antiretroviral therapy, there was an increase in the prevalence of fluconazole-resistant *Candida albicans* among human immunodeficiency virus-infected patients with oropharyngeal or esophageal candidiasis. Up to one-third of patients with advanced AIDS in one study harbored fluconazole-resistant *C. albicans* in their oral cavities. According to data from the Artemis Global Antifungal Surveillance Program, the incidence of fluconazole resistance in *Candida glabrata* increased from 7% in 2001 to 12% in 2004.[18,19]

MECHANISMS OF DRUG RESISTANCE IN MYCOSES

The most frequent ones involve a decrease in drug uptake, structural alterations in the target site, and an increase in drug efflux or in intracellular target levels. These biochemical changes can result from gene amplification, gene transfer, gene deletion, point mutations, loss of cis- and trans-acting regulatory elements, and transcriptional activation. The five main mechanisms for azole resistance which has been studied most in *Candida* are:

1. Decreased drug concentration:[20] The development of active efflux pumps results in decreased drug concentrations at the site of action. Fungi possess at least two types of efflux pumps; those belonging to the adenosine triphosphate-binding cassette (ABC) and the major facilitator (MF) superfamilies of proteins. The MF efflux pumps are associated with fluconazole resistance. Of the MF superfamily, PDR5, CFTR/MRP, and MDR subfamilies contain genes that encode proteins known to confer azole resistance. However, the most notable ABC efflux pumps in *Candida* spp. are encoded by members of the PDR5 subfamily. These genes have been named *CDR* for *Candida* drug resistance, and are the only ones characterized so far that have been associated with azole resistance. The results of several molecular and genetic studies indicate that

at least 10 *CDR* genes exist in the *C. albicans* genome.[5] Among the *MDR* genes of the MF class, *T. rubrum TruMDR1* gene has been identified, which encodes an ABC transporter

2. Target site alteration:[21] It has been demonstrated that mutations in *ERG11*, the gene encoding for the target enzyme lanosterol C14α-demethylase, prevents binding of azoles to the enzymatic site
3. Upregulation of target enzyme:[22] Some *Candida* isolates with reduced susceptibility to azoles have higher intracellular concentrations of ERG11p than do azole-susceptible strains. The antifungal agent is, therefore, overwhelmed, and routine therapeutic concentrations can no longer effectively inhibit ergosterol synthesis. Target enzyme upregulation can be achieved through gene amplification, increased transcription rate, or decreased degradation of the gene product. For example, overexpression of several genes of the ergosterol biosynthetic pathway has been observed in response to ketoconazole in *T. rubrum*. Azoles inhibit the lanosterol 14α-demethylase, encoded by the *ERG11* gene that showed a 3.6-fold induction in response to ketoconazole
4. Development of bypass pathways:[23] Exposure to azole compounds results in depletion of ergosterol from the fungal membrane and accumulation of the toxic product 14α-methyl-3,6-diol, leading to growth arrest. Mutation of the *ERG3* gene prevents the formation of 14α-methyl-3,6-diol from 14α-methyl fecosterol. Replacement of ergosterol with the latter product leads to functional membranes and negates the action of azoles on the ergosterol biosynthetic pathway
5. Stress response of dermatophytes: Antifungal drugs induce cell stress responses that are required to overcome the toxic effects of these drugs allowing fungal survival. For example, the electrophoretic pattern of the intracellular esterases of *T. rubrum* is altered when the fungus is cultured in the presence of subinhibitory concentrations of tioconazole or griseofulvin. The exposure of *T. rubrum* to sub-MIC of amphotericin B increased the transcription of genes that encode stress-response-related proteins, including heat shock protein (Hsp) 70, Hsp104, and ubiquitin, and oxidative-stress proteins such as glutathione synthase.[5] The mechanisms of resistance against various antifungals including azoles are enumerated in table 2.

There have been recent reports of increasing MICs to amphotericin B among *Candida krusei* and *C. glabrata* isolates. Resistance breakpoints for polyenes have not been determined. Most clinicians use an MIC of more than 1.0 μg/mL to indicate resistance to amphotericin B. Defects in the *ERG3* gene involved in ergosterol biosynthesis lead to accumulation of other sterols in the fungal membrane. Consequently, polyene-resistant *Candida* isolates have relatively low ergosterol content, compared with that of polyene-susceptible isolates.[24]

Table 2: Mechanisms of Drug Resistance

Antifungal agent	Mode of action	Resistance mechanism
Polyenes	Binding to ergosterol	• Absence of ergosterol (ERG3 and ERG6 mutation) • Decreased ergosterol content in cells
Azoles	Inhibition of cytochrome p450 function: lanosterol 14α-demethylase, Sterol Δ_{22}-desaturase	• Efflux mediated by multidrug transporters • Decrease of affinity in ERG11p by mutations • Upregulation of ERG11 • Alterations in the ergosterol biosynthetic pathway • Overexpression of lanosterol 14α-demethylase (ketoconazole) • Tru MDR1 and Tru MDR2 ABC-type multidrug transporter mutations
Allylamines (terbinafine, butenafine, naftifine)	Inhibition of squalene epoxidase (ERG1)	• Modification of target enzyme by mutation • Increased drug efflux • Stress adaptation • Overexpression of salicylate monooxygenase • ABC-type multidrug transporter
Morpholines (amorolfine)	Inhibition of sterol reductase (ERG24)	• Unknown
Griseofulvin	Microtubule assembly	• Increased drug efflux • Stress adaptation • ABC-type multidrug transporter
Echinocandins	Inhibition of β-1,3-glucan synthase (FKS1 and 2)	• Alteration of affinity of echinocandins to β-1,3-glucan synthase
Oxaboroles/ hydroxamic acid ciclopiroxolamine	Iron chelator	–

CLINICAL RESISTANCE

It has been time and again observed by clinical dermatologists that *in vitro* susceptibility testing alone is not sufficient to predict clinical success. There is a need for correlating MICs *in vitro* resistance with clinical resistance, and such studies should be carried out in various parts of the country to find locoregional patterns of resistance and to confirm if clinical resistance is indeed associated with high MICs. Many postgraduate thesis dissertations and research projects on chronic or recurrent dermatophytosis are underway at many centers in India. An unpublished study showed Trichophyton mentagrophytes as the commonest isolate with increased MICs of terbinafine against dermatophytes (Poojary et al., unpublished observation). In an Indian study of MIC determination by broth microdilution method, *Trichophyton mentagrophytes* was the commonest isolate and is found to be more susceptible to itraconazole and ketoconazole (MIC 50–0.125 μg/mL for itraconazole, 0.0625 μg/mL for ketoconazole and 0.5 μg/mL for terbinafine).[25] *Candida* resistant to terbinafine and azoles but sensitive to voriconazole, clotrimazole, itraconazole, and amphotericin B has been reported of late.[26] In almost all major regional and national conferences in India, a dedicated session is being devoted on chronic or recurrent dermatophyte infections.[2] More such studies, discourses, and discussions and further ensuing multicentric studies with standard MIC90 testing correlated with clinical response are the need of the future.

OVER THE COUNTER MENACE

Topical and oral antifungals in suboptimum and irrational regimens are the most often misused medications in India, which are prescribed by various general practitioners, quacks, and specialists who tend to label a majority of skin lesions as "fungal infections". The availability of such over the counter medications is adding to the current situation. Cost of these medications may also be a factor for nonadherence or poor compliance. The differential pricing with OTC steroid antifungal combination is believed to be driving more patients to apply such irrational combinations. There are no precise bioavailability studies for most of these formulations.[2] Newer preparations like sprays, powders, etc. might also be contributing to resistance, but there are no studies to support this theory. Whether this local cutaneous cytokine and immunological milieu of the human resistance mechanism can be aggravated by the proliferating market of improper prescription of steroid antifungal combinations proliferating under the Indian drug price regime needs to be systematically studied. Many of the market preparations are irrational combinations of steroids, and antifungal and antibacterial agents. It is well known that topical steroids reduce number of Langerhans cells as well as Langerhans cell-dependent allostimulatory capacity of epidermal cells. This leads to a deficiency in Langerhans cell-mediated T lymphocyte activation and the effects have been proven to be dependent on potency of the corticosteroid determined by the vasoconstrictor assay.[27,28] This is further proven by the fact that chronic infections are associated with poor T lymphocyte-mediated response to specific fungal antigens, suggesting depression of responses is responsible for poor clinical response.[29] It may be theorized that the combination of ineffective phagocytosis and killing of the hyphae in the presence of anti-inflammatory milieu deviates the immunity from Th1 response to Th2 and leads to chronicity, but same needs to be substantiated.

GENETICS OF CHRONIC DERMATOPHYTOSES

Ethnic susceptibility has also been noted in dermatophytes, especially in tinea capitis.[30] *CARD9* gene mutation, which is involved in the regulation of multiple downstream pathways having antifungal response, is known to be associated with severe fungal infections of varied clinical presentations ranging from candidal meningitis to recurrent dermatophytic infection of skin and nails. In light of these findings, genetics of patients resistant to conventional antifungals might also hold relevance in the future.[31]

NUANCES OF MINIMUM INHIBITORY CONCENTRATION

Antifungal-drug resistance is usually quantified using the MIC, in which growth in the presence of a range of drug concentrations is measured over a defined time period according to a standard protocol. The lowest drug concentration that results in a significant reduction of growth [usually either 50% (MIC 50) or 90% (MIC 90) reduction of growth compared with growth in the absence of the drug] is called the MIC. In 1983, the National Committee for Clinical Laboratory Standards (NCCLS) established a subcommittee to standardize fungal MIC determination. As an outcome of a consensus effort in 1997, the NCCLS adopted the M27 protocol for the susceptibility testing of yeasts. For the azoles, in particular, there is a prominent trailing effect, which results in growth at all drug concentrations regardless of susceptibility. Determination of the MIC depends on a difficult visual assessment of 50–80% reduction in growth relative to the drug-free control. It is important to emphasize the arbitrary nature of all breakpoint determinations and the absence of controlled, evaluative prospective trials. The NCCLS document M38-P proposes methods and guidelines for resistance testing of filamentous fungi. There is currently no susceptibility standard for dermatophytes and M38-A has been adapted to study dermatophyte *in vitro* resistance. *In vitro* demonstration of resistance does not necessarily equate to *in vivo* resistance.[32-35] The correlation between the *in vitro* dermatophyte MICs and the clinical outcomes remains unclear. Systematic susceptibility testing of clinical isolates from patients with onychomycosis, who failed on therapy with terbinafine, did not reveal any correlation between the MIC of terbinafine and the clinical failure.

The guiding principles while interpreting *in vitro* MIC values are:

1. An MIC is not a physical or chemical measurement
2. Host factors are often more important than susceptibility test results in determining clinical outcome
3. Susceptibility *in vitro* does not predict successful therapy but
4. Resistance *in vitro* should often predict therapeutic failure.

Any given MIC method measures "an" MIC, not "the" MIC. This principle arises owing to the method dependence of "all" MIC measurement techniques. Changes in test format, inoculum size, time, temperature, and endpoint definition can all produce variations in the measured MIC that can be quite dramatic. In short, an MIC is meaningful only if obtained under standardized conditions for strains that are known to be susceptible or resistant on the basis of clinical information. It is more accurate to think of the MIC as a predictor of failure rather than of success.[36] Inadequate drug dosing resulting from noncompliance, inadequate absorption, or inadequate dosage and frequency that result in trivial drug concentrations, successful therapy will be impossible. Immune suppression decreases therapeutic efficacy. Coadministered agents like rifampicin induces hepatic microsomal enzymes and can dramatically lower azole blood levels. Antagonism of the action of the antimicrobial agent (e.g., although not consistently borne out by studies *in vivo*, depletion of cell-membrane ergosterol by prior azole therapy has the theoretical potential to reduce the efficacy of amphotericin B). Hence, it is understood that recovery from an infection is dependent on many patient-, drug-, and organism-related factors, of which the MIC is only one.[37]

Another important factor to be understood regarding MIC is that susceptibility *in vitro* does not predict successful therapy, but resistance *in vitro* should often predict therapeutic failure. This led to a call for the emphasis of testing *in vitro* to be changed from susceptibility testing to resistance testing. A major pitfall of clinical trials vis-à-vis MIC is that results from clinical trials will usually only be helpful if a tentative breakpoint for resistance has been set too high. On the other hand, proving that the tentative breakpoint is too low and that potentially susceptible organisms are being labeled resistant is much more difficult. This, along with the smaller number of high MIC isolates normally found in most studies, means that clinical trials provide a great deal of data on the efficacy of the antimicrobial against putatively susceptible isolates but very little data regarding isolates for which MICs are higher.[38]

Microbiologic resistance refers to nonsusceptibility of a fungus to an antifungal agent by *in vitro* susceptibility testing, in which the MICs of the drugs exceed the susceptibility breakpoint for that organism. The MIC values were placed in context by evolving interpretive breakpoints which can predict clinical response to antifungal agents. Isolates for which MICs are 8 μg/mL were found to be susceptible to fluconazole, whereas those for which MICs are more than 64 μg/mL appeared resistant. Isolates for which the MIC of fluconazole is 16–32 μg/mL are considered susceptible dependent upon dose (SDD), on the basis of data indicating clinical response when more than 100 mg of fluconazole per day is given. Tentative interpretive MIC breakpoints have been devised for itraconazole also, but with the rider that they apply only to mucosal candidal infections and are as follows: susceptible, less than 0.125 μg/mL;

SDD, 0.25–0.5 μg/mL; and resistant, more than 1 μg/mL.[39] Such interpretive breakpoints do not exist for dermatophytes. Minimum inhibitory concentration breakpoints have been evolved for voriconazole and *Candida* species: susceptible (S) less than 1 μg/mL, SDD 1–4 μg/mL, and resistant (R) more than 4 μg/mL.[40]

EMERGING ROLE OF FUNGAL BIOFILMS

Another aspect to be considered in the susceptibility to antimycotics *in vivo* is the formation of biofilms. Biofilms are differentiated masses of microbes that adhere to surfaces and are surrounded by a matrix of extracellular polymers, increasing resistance to standard antimicrobials. It is well known that *C. albicans* biofilms are highly resistant to most of the antifungals.[41] The concept of biofilm for dermatophyte was introduced by Burkhart et al. to explain dermatophytomas, a form of onychomycosis refractory to standard antifungal therapies. Dermatophytomas are characterized by a dense white mass of fungus tenaciously adherent to the surrounding nail plate, which may require surgical removal.[42] Both *T. rubrum* and *T. mentagrophytes* have been demonstrated to produce biofilms. Biofilms are known to confer resistance to both antimicrobial agents and host immunity. Hence, the antifungal resistance and recurrence of dermatophytes, along with the necessity for prolonged and high dose therapy could be attributed to the biofilms produced by this organism.[43] It has been hypothesized that a change in membrane sterol composition during biofilm formation might explain resistance to amphotericin B and the azoles.[44] In addition, the MAPK Mkc1p seems to be a regulator of azole resistance in mature biofilms. Whether steroid application increases biofilm formation in dermatophytes with resultant antifungal resistance is a matter which requires to be studied.[45] Similar biofilms have been characterized for pityriasis versicolor.[46]

MEASURES TO TACKLE ANTIFUNGAL RESISTANCE

Cellular targets for newer potential antifungal pipeline are limited because of the similarity existing between fungi and hosts, i.e., both are eukaryotic organisms. With some exceptions (e.g., griseofulvin, flucytosine, caspofungin, and ciclopiroxo lamine), the antifungal drugs in common usage are directed against the ergosterol biosynthetic pathway.[47]

Combination Therapy

Considering the wide etiology and long duration of treatment required for dermatophytosis, especially the nail and hair infection, a combination therapy involving both systemic and topical antifungal agents would provide antimicrobial synergy, wider antifungal spectrum with improved fungicidal activity, increased cure rates, suppression of resistant mutants, and enhancement of tolerability and safety. British Association of Dermatologists have given combination treatment a strength of recommendation D and level of evidence 3.[48,49] It has been suggested that combination therapies that exploit drugs with different mechanisms of action would force cells to acquire at least two simultaneous mutations to become resistant to therapy.

Efflux Pump Inhibitors

The discovery of fungal efflux pumps offers the question, can antifungal drugs be combined within efflux pump inhibitor to increase efficacy? This situation is analogous to the combination of a β-lactam antibiotic with a β-lactamase inhibitor. MC-510027 is an efflux inhibitor that has been shown to decrease the MIC values of three azoles and terbinafine by one to three orders of magnitude against several species of *Candida.*[50]

Antifungal Stewardship

Measures include: prudent use of antifungals; treatment with the appropriate antifungal (in cases where the etiological agent is known); conducting surveillance studies to determine the true frequency of antifungal resistance; and ensuring compliance by counselling and asking patient to bring back used empty tubes.

Clearing the *in vitro* Susceptibility Testing Nebulousness

Additionally, improvements to susceptibility testing methods may be helpful in reducing the use of inappropriate antifungals to which the infecting fungi are already resistant. Furthermore, standardizing protocols, such as the M38-P protocol for filamentous fungi, for other clinically important fungi will be a major advance to the field of susceptibility testing by enhancing our ability to detect resistance when it occurs.

Bolstering the Antifungal Pipeline

Calcineurin inhibitors and drugs affecting target of rapamycin pathways, and antibodies against Hsp90[51] are strategies elucidated to be fully active *in vivo* in the potentiation of fluconazole, and they also led to a dramatic decrease in fungi virulence. Such findings need to be pursued and harnessed into viable therapeutic ladder. High throughput screening of the legacy Schering-Plough compound collection has recently lead to the discovery of a new glucan synthase inhibitor effective again *C. albicans* and *C. glabrata.*[52] Luliconazole and lanoconazole in a recent study revealed potent activity against all dermatophyte isolates. Anidulafungin, caspofungin, and luliconazole showed the best activity in the said study.[53] Sertaconazole is a newer once-a-day antifungal which has demonstrated good levels of antifungal activity.[54]

Increasing Dosage of Current Antifungals and Administration for Longer Duration

In Germany, fluconazole is licensed in adults for up to 800 mg/day. As summarized by Duswald et al., even higher doses may be more effective. But the rider exists that higher doses may cause higher incidence of toxicity.[55,56] The author has consistently utilized this strategy in clinically recalcitrant dermatophytosis with good benefit. Higher dosages are recommended both continuously and in pulse mode in onychomycosis. Similar research is lacking for use of high dose terbinafine and itraconazole, either alone or in combination, for extended periods in dermatophytes of the glabrous skin. Safety studies to condone this strategy is the need of the hour.

Genome-wide Studies to Detect Potential New Antifungal Targets[57]

An important difficulty for antifungal therapy is to develop drugs that exploit factors unique to fungi, which can be challenging considering that organism are eukaryotic and share many conserved biological pathways. Studies must aim at a better understanding of the modifications occurring in the fungi submitted to antifungal treatments or of the relationship developed between the fungus and its host all along the infectious process. Such knowledge might improve the actual therapy to avoid resistance development or might allow playing on the host-fungus equilibrium to improve recovery of patients. Other studies are geared to better understand the biology of fungal species. For this purpose, mutant collections were subjected to a wide range of environmental conditions. The recent application of genome-wide studies to pathogenic fungi for both host-pathogen interactions and the biological study will hopefully encourage and facilitate the development of new, effective therapeutic strategies. Such improvements in antifungal treatment may lead to a better clinical outcome. The inclusion of five dermatophytes in the sequencing project by the Fungal Genome Initiative (The Broad Institute of Harvard and Massachusetts Institute of Technology/National Institute of Health) and the recent release of a transcription profile of *T. rubrum* developmental phases will render possible the *in silico* search for molecular targets in a near future.[58,59,60]

CONCLUSION

Thus, the effective control of dermatophytes will necessarily involve the development of a new generation of potent broad-spectrum antifungals with selective action against new targets in the fungal cells. However, to search for new molecular targets, it is essential to have a full understanding about the biology of pathogenic fungi and about the mechanisms of fungal-host interactions. In addition, knowledge of the antifungal resistance mechanisms is also essential, since the development of resistant strains to any new drug is inevitable. The complete sequencing of dermatophyte genomes and the analysis of the promoters of the genes involved in this adaptive response will allow the discovery of new genes, providing new functional information through the study of their expression, and perhaps identifying molecular targets for the design of new antifungals. The large number of already existing possibilities for potential drug targets encoded in fungal genomes (cell wall, virulence factors, proteins involved in fungal-host interactions, proteins that modulate deoxyribonucleic acid (DNA) topology, gene transcription, messenger ribonucleic acid (mRNA) translational, and post-transcriptional modifications) should be explored and validated for the successful production of new fungal inhibitors. The recent efforts in dermatophyte genome sequencing, transcriptome and proteome analysis provide effective ways to find new possibilities to cure and prevent diseases caused by fungi. Although the results of research have substantially increased our understanding of fungal resistance, especially at the molecular level, more remain to be addressed. Newer agents like tavaborole and efinaconazole offer a ray of hope. Ciclopiroxolamine through its multiple levels of action can be a potential value addition. In absence of newer systemic agents, strategies like combination therapy and off label extension in therapy duration and surveillance of susceptibility breakpoints by regional studies in tertiary institutions using standardized testing methods and correlation with *in vivo* resistance are viable strategies to tackle this menace. In the meantime, the clinical dermatologist has to play a cardinal role in identifying clinical resistance, conducting clinical research which compares *in vivo* with *ex vivo* resistance, ensuring patient compliance and adequate therapy duration, patient education against corticosteroid antifungal combinations, and thereby, decreasing the community burden of dermatomycoses. Several treatment options, including duration of treatment, drug dose, and dose administration schedule (intermittent versus continuous) will need to be evaluated for their effect on resistance development. It is a pertinent need of the hour to increase our understanding on the molecular mechanisms of antifungal drug resistance and the genetic and host factors that make us more susceptible to recurrent and recalcitrant infections.

Editor's Comment

The author has written an exhaustive review on anti-fungal resistance with apparent emphasis on the mechanisms, the contributing factors and the methods to combat the resistance. All the recent literature has been quoted appropriately, though quite lengthy yet would be very useful for those who need to understand the science of anti-fungal resistance and how to combat it. Dr Brijesh Nair has added good reading material for the dermatologist and dermato-mycologist.

Rashmi Sarkar, Seemal R Desai

REFERENCES

1. Poikonen E, Lyytikäinen O, Anttila VJ, Koivula I, Lumio J, Kotilainen P, et al. Secular trend in candidemia and the use of fluconazole in Finland, 2004-2007. *BMC Infect Dis.* 2010;10:312.
2. Dogra S, Uprety S. The menace of chronic and recurrent dermatophytosis in India: Is the problem deeper than we perceive? *Indian Dermatol Online J.* 2016;7:73-6.
3. Sentamilselvi G, Kamalam A, Ajithadas K, Janaki C, Thambiah AS. Scenario of chronic dermatophytosis: an Indian study. *Mycopathologia.* 1997-1998;140:129-35.
4. Piñeiro L, Larruskain J, Idigoras P, Perez-Trallero E. Trichophyton rubrum syndrome: the tip of the iceberg and a preventable outcome. *Mycoses.* 2010;53:186.
5. Turnidge J, Paterson DL. Setting and revising antibacterial susceptibility breakpoints. *Clin Microbiol Rev.* 2007;20:391-408.
6. White TC, Marr KA, Bowden RA. Clinical, cellular, and molecular factors that contribute to antifungal drug resistance. *Clin Microbiol Rev.* 1998;11:382-402.
7. Ellis D, Marriott D, Hajjeh RA, Warnock D, Meyer W, Barton R. Epidemiology: surveillance of fungal infections. *Med Mycol.* 2000;38 Suppl 1:173-82.
8. Dahl MV, Grando SA. Chronic dermatophytosis: What is special about Trichophyton rubrum? *Adv Dermatol.* 1994;9:97-109.
9. Ferreira-Nozawa MS, Silveira HC, Ono CJ, Fachin AL, Rossi A, Martinez-Rossi NM. The pH signaling transcription factor PacC mediates the growth of Trichophyton rubrum on human nail in vitro. *Med Mycol.* 2006;44:641-5.
10. Hay RJ. Chronic dermatophyte infections. I. Clinical and mycological features. *Br J Dermatol.* 1982;106:1-7.
11. Ranganathan S, Menon T, Selvi SG, Kamalam A. Effect of socio-economic status on the prevalence of dermatophytosis in Madras. *Indian J Dermatol Venereol Leprol.* 1995;61:16-8.
12. Hryncewicz-Gwozdz A, Kalinowska K, Plomer-Niezgoda E, Bielecki J, Jagielski T. Increase in resistance to fluconazole and itraconazole in Trichophyton rubrum clinical isolates by sequential passages in vitro under drug pressure. *Mycopathologia.* 2013;176:49-55.
13. Faria Ramos I, Farinha S, Neves-Maia J, Tavares PR, Mirannda IM, Silva RM et al. Environmental azole fungicide, prochloraz, can induce cross-resistance to medical triazoles in Candida glabrata. *FEMS Yeast Res.* 2014;14:1119-23.
14. Mukherjee PK, Leidich SD, Isham N, Leitner I, Ryder NS, Ghannoum MA. Clinical Trichophyton rubrum strain exhibiting primary resistance to terbinafine. *Antimicrob Agents Chemother.* 2003;47:82-6.
15. Sarifakioglu E, Seçkin D, Demirbilek M, Can F. In vitro antifungal susceptibility patterns of dermatophyte strains causing tinea unguium. *Clin Exp Dermatol.* 2007;32:675-9.
16. Azambuja CV, Pimmel LA, Klafke GB, Xavier MO. Onychomycosis: Clinical, mycological and in vitro susceptibility testing of isolates of Trichophyton rubrum. *An Bras Dermatol.* 2014;89:581-6.

17. Singal A, Rawat S, Bhattacharya SN, Mohanty S, Baruah MC. Clinico-mycological profile of tinea capitis in North India and response to griseofulvin. *J Dermatol.* 2001;28:22-6.
18. Goldman M, Cloud GA, Smedema M, LeMonte A, Connolly P, McKinsey DS, et al. Does long-term itraconazole prophylaxis result in in vitro azole resistance in mucosal Candida albicans isolates from persons with advanced human immunodeficiency virus infection? The National Institute of Allergy and Infectious Diseases Mycoses study group. *Antimicrob Agents Chemother.* 2000;44:1585-7.
19. Law D, Moore CB, Wardle HM, Ganguli LA, Keaney MG, Denning DW. High prevalence of antifungal resistance in Candida spp. from patients with AIDS. *J Antimicrob Chemother.* 1994;34:659-68.
20. Albertson GD, Niimi M, Cannon RD, Jenkinson HF. Multiple efflux mechanisms are involved in Candida albicans fluconazole resistance. *Antimicrob Agents Chemother.* 1996;40:2835-41.
21. Loffler J, Kelly SL, Hebart H, Schumacher U, Lass-Florl C, Einsele H. Molecular analysis of cyp51 from fluconazole-resistant Candida albicans strains. *FEMS Microbiol Lett.* 1997;151:263-8.
22. Lopez-Ribot JL, McAtee RK, Lee LN, Kirkpatrick WR, White TC, Sanglard D, et al. Distinct patterns of gene expression associated with development of fluconazole resistance in serial Candida albicans isolates from human immunodeficiency virus-infected patients with oropharyngeal candidiasis. *Antimicrob Agents Chemother.* 1998; 42:2932–7.
23. Kelly SL, Lamb DC, Kelly DE, Manning NJ, Loeffler J, Hebart H, et al. Resistance to fluconazole and cross-resistance to amphotericin B in Candida albicans from AIDS patients caused by defective sterol delta5,6-desaturation. *FEBS Lett.* 1997;400:80-2.
24. Pfaller MA, Messer SA, Hollis RJ. Strain delineation and antifungal susceptibilities of epidemiologically related and unrelated isolates of Candida lusitaniae. *Diagn Microbiol Infect Dis.* 1994;20:127-33.
25. Bhatia VK, Sharma PC. Determination of minimum inhibitory concentrations of itraconazole, terbinafine, and ketoconazole against dermatophyte species by broth microdilution method. *Indian J Med Microbiol.* 2015;33:533-7.
26. Hu Y, Hu Y, Lu Y, Huang S, Liu K, Han X, et al. A case report of penile infection caused by fluconazole and terbinafine resistant candida albicans. *Mycopathologia.* 2016. (Epub ahead of print)
27. Ashworth J, Booker J, Breathnach SM. Effects of topical steroid therapy on Langerhans cell antigen presenting function in human skin. *Br J Dermatol.* 1988;118:457-69.
28. Ali MA, Thrower SL, Hanna SJ, Coulman SA, Birchall JC, Wong FS, et al. Topical steroid therapy induces pro-tolerogenic changes in Langerhans cells in human skin. *Immunology.* 2015;146:411-22.
29. Romani L. Immunity to fungal infections. *Nat Rev Immunol.* 2011;11:275-88.
30. Blank F, Mann SJ, Reale RA. Distribution of dermatophytosis according to age, ethnic group and sex. *Sabouraudia.* 1974;12:352-61.
31. Lanternier F, Pathan S, Vincent QB, Liu L, Cypowyj S, Prando C, et al. Deep dermatophytosis and inherited CARD9 deficiency. *N Engl J Med.* 2013;369:1704-14.
32. Ghannoum MA, Rex JH, Galgiani J N. Susceptibility testing of fungi: current status of correlation of *in vitro* data with clinical outcome. *J Clin Microbiol.* 1996;34:489-95.
33. National Committee for Clinical Laboratory Standards. Reference method for broth dilution antifungal susceptibility testing of yeasts; approved standard vol. 17. M27-A. Wayne (PA): NCCLS; 1997. pp. 1-29.
34. Ghannoum MA, Arthington-Skaggs B, Chaturvedi V, Espinel-Ingroff A, Pfaller MA, Rennie R, et al. Interlaboratory study of quality control isolates for a broth microdilution method (modified CLSI M38-A) for testing susceptibilities of dermatophytes to antifungals. *J Clin Microbiol.* 2006;44:4353-6.
35. Rex JH, Pfaller MA, Rinaldi MG, Polak A, Galgiani JN. Antifungal susceptibility testing. *Clin Microbiol Rev.* 1993;6:367-81.
36. Sanders WE Jr, Sanders CC. Do in vitro antimicrobial susceptibility tests accurately predict therapeutic responsiveness in infected patients? In: Lorian V, editor. Significance of Medical Microbiology in the Care of Patients. 2nd ed. Baltimore: Williams & Wilkins; 1982. pp. 325-40.
37. Sugar AM. Use of amphotericin B with azole antifungal drugs: what are we doing? *Antimicrob Agents Chemother.* 1995;39:1907-12.
38. Sanders CC. ARTs versus ASTs: where are we going? *J Antimicrob Chemother.* 1991;28:621-3.
39. Rex JH, Pfaller MA, Galgiani JN, Bartlett MS, Espinel-Ingroff A, Ghannoum MA, et al. Development of interpretive breakpoints for antifungal susceptibility testing: conceptual framework and analysis of in

vitro-in vivo correlation data for fluconazole, itraconazole, and Candida infections. Subcommittee on Antifungal Susceptibility Testing of the National Committee for Clinical Laboratory Standards. *Clin Infect Dis.* 1997;24:235-47.
40. Pfaller MA, Andes D, Arendrup MC, Diekema DJ, Espinel-Ingroff A, Alexander BD, et al. Clinical breakpoints for voriconazole and Candida species. revisited: review of microbiologic, molecular, pharmacodynamic, and clinical data as they pertain to the development of species-specific interpretive criteria. *Diagn Microbiol Infect Dis.* 2011;70:330-43.
41. Peltroche-Llacsahuanga H, Goyard S, d'Enfert C, Prill SK, Ernst JF. Protein O-mannosyltransferase isoforms regulate biofilm formation in Candida albicans. *Antimicrob Agents Chemother.* 2006;50:3488-91.
42. Burkhart CN, Burkhart CG, Gupta AK. Dermatophytoma: recalcitrance to treatment because of existence of fungal biofilm. *J Am Acad Dermatol.* 2002;47:629-31.
43. Costa-Orlandi CB, Sardi JC, Santos CT, Fusco-Almeida AM, Mendes-Giannini MJ. In vitro characterization of Trichophyton rubrum and T. mentagrophytes biofilms. *Biofouling.* 2014;30:719-27.
44. Mateus C, Crow SA, Jr, Ahearn DG. Adherence of Candida albicans to silicone induces immediate enhanced tolerance to fluconazole. *Antimicrob Agents Chemother.* 2004;48:3358-66.
45. Kumamoto CA. A contact-activated kinase signals Candida albicans invasive growth and biofilm development. *Proc Natl Acad Sci USA.* 2005;102:5576-81.
46. Allen HB, Goyal K, Ogrich L, Joshi S. Biofilm Formation by Malassezia Furfur/Ovale as a Possible Mechanism of Pathogenesis in Tinea Versicolor. *J Clin Exp Dermatol Res.* 2015;6:311.
47. Martinez-Rossi NM, Peres NT, Rossi A. Antifungal resistance mechanisms in dermatophytes. *Mycopathologia.* 2008;166:369-83.
48. Polak A. The past, present and future of antimycotic combination therapy. *Mycoses.* 1999;42:355-70.
49. Ameen M, Lear JT, Madan V, Mohd Mustapa MF, Richardson M. British Association of Dermatologists' guidelines for the management of onychomycosis 2014. *Br J Dermatol.* 2014;171:937-58.
50. Chamberland S, Blais J, Cotter DP, Hoang MK, Galazzo J, Staley A, et al. Impact of MC- 510,027, a fungal efflux pump inhibitor, on the susceptibility of clinical isolates of Candida spp. to antifungal agents [abstract no. 1270]. Proceedings of the 39th Interscience Conference on Antimicrobial Agents and Chemotherapy; 1999 Sept 26-29; San Francisco.
51. Pachl J, Svoboda P, Jacobs F, Vandewoude K, van der Hoven B, Spronk P, et al. A randomized, blinded, multicenter trial of lipid-associated amphotericin B aloneversus in combination with an antibody-based inhibitor of heat shock protein 90 in patients with invasive candidiasis. *Clin Infect Dis.* 2016;42:1404-13.
52. Walker SS, Xu Y, Triantafyllou I, Waldman MF, Mendrick C, Brown N, et al. Discovery of a novel class of orally active antifungal beta-1,3-D-glucan synthase inhibitors. *Antimicrob Agents Chemother.* 2011;55:5099-106.
53. Baghi M, Shokohi T, Badali H, Makimura K, Rezaei-Matehkolaei A, Abdollahi M, et al. In vitro activity of new azoles luliconazole and lanoconazole compared with ten other antifungal drugs againstclinical dermatophyte isolates. *Med Mycol.* 2016;54:757-63.
54. Carrillo-Muñoz AJ, Tur-Tur C, Cárdenes DC, Estivill D, Giusiano G. Sertaconazole nitrate shows fungicidal and fungistatic activities against Trichophyton rubrum, Trichophyton mentagrophytes, and Epidermophyton floccosum, causative agents of tinea pedis. *Antimicrob Agents Chemother.* 2011;55:4420-1.
55. Duswald KH, Penk A, Pittrow L. High-dose therapy with fluconazole > or = 800 mg day-1. *Mycoses.* 1997;40:267-77.
56. Crane JK, Shih HT. Syncope and cardiac arrhythmia due to an interaction between itraconazole and terfenadine. *Am J Med.* 1993;95:445-6.
57. Vandeputte P, Ferrari S, Coste AT. Antifungal resistance and new strategies to control fungal infections. *Int J Microbiol.* 2012;2012:713687.
58. Hui X, Baker SJ, Wester RC, Barbadillo S, Cashmore AK, Sanders V, et al. In vitro penetration of a novel oxaborole antifungal (AN2690) into the human nail plate. *J Pharm Sci.* 2007;96:2622-31.
59. Odds FC. Genomics, molecular targets and the discovery of antifungal drugs. *Rev Iberoam Micol.* 2005;22:229-37.
60. Jiang B, Bussey H, Roemer T. Novel strategies in antifungal drug discovery. *Curr Opin Microbiol.* 2002;5:466-71.

World Clin Dermatol. 2016;3(1):207-19.

Tinea Incognito and Topical Corticosteroid Abuse in Dermatology

*Yogesh S Marfatia MD, Sheethal K Jose MBBS

Department of Skin-VD, Medical College Baroda
Vadodara, Gujarat, India

ABSTRACT

Tinea incognito was first described by Ive and Marks in 1968 for dermatophytic infection which has been modified by various drugs. Most common cause of tinea incognito is corticosteroids, both topical and oral, followed by topical calcineurin inhibitors. Because of its potent antiallergic and anti-inflammatory effect, many, a times corticosteroids are prescribed for skin conditions of diverse etiology without establishing a definite cause. Topical corticosteroids are available in various combinations with antifungal, antibiotics, skin-lightening agents. Many of these combinations contain potent to very potent corticosteroids. More potent the steroid, more will be the anti-inflammatory effect and chances of cutaneous adverse effects. Commonly occurring side effects include cutaneous striae, acneiform eruption, telangiectasia, purpura, hypopigmentation, folliculitis, perioral dermatitis, hypertrichosis, delayed wound healing, etc. Long-term use of potent corticosteroids leads to altered immunity, masking of inflammation, and spread of infection. Clinically, lesions of tinea incognito are polymorphic with scattered papules, pustules, and hyperpigmentation with diffuse blanching erythema and telangiectasia. In contrast to lesions of classic tinea, margins are not raised and there is less scaling and itching. Mycological examination including potassium hydroxide and culture in Sabouraud's dextrose agar must be performed in doubtful lesions of contact dermatitis, atopic dermatitis, folliculitis, rosacea, seborrheic dermatitis, lupus erythematosus, pemphigus foliaceus, etc. Once diagnosed, all steroid medication must be stopped immediately. Alternately, a low-potency corticosteroid may be used briefly to avoid the flare up after stopping steroids. Topical and/or systemic antifungal regimen should be started.

*Corresponding author
Email: ym11256@gmail.com

© 2016 Jaypee Brothers Medical Publishers. All rights reserved.

Therefore, before starting corticosteroids in a patient, any foci of fungal infection must be ruled out through proper examination. In any atypical lesions like intractable eczema, psoriasis, and also in cases of aggravation of existing dermatosis, we must look for occult foci of dermatophytoses like web spaces and nails and suspect tinea incognito.

INTRODUCTION

Tinea incognita is a dermatophyte infection of the skin where clinical presentation has been modified by the misuse of topical or systemic corticosteroids. The term tinea incognito was originally described in 1968 by Ive and Marks in 14 patients with dermatophytic infection who had an atypical clinical presentation due to previous treatment with topical corticosteroids (TCs) with one-third of cases also having typical ringworm lesions.[1] Such cases started presenting in the 1960s after the introduction of TC for treatment of diverse dermatologic diseases.[2]

Topical or systemic corticosteroids continue to be the most common cause of tinea incognito used in various combinations like skin-lightening agents, antipsoriatic creams, etc. Because of its potent antiinflammatory property, currently corticosteroids of different potency in combinations with antifungal, antimicrobial, and other ingredients are being rampantly prescribed without diagnosing the skin condition or often used as self-medication (Figure 1). They are also prescribed by family physicians and practitioners of alternate medicine considering corticosteroids as a "panacea" or "cure-all drug". For many suffering

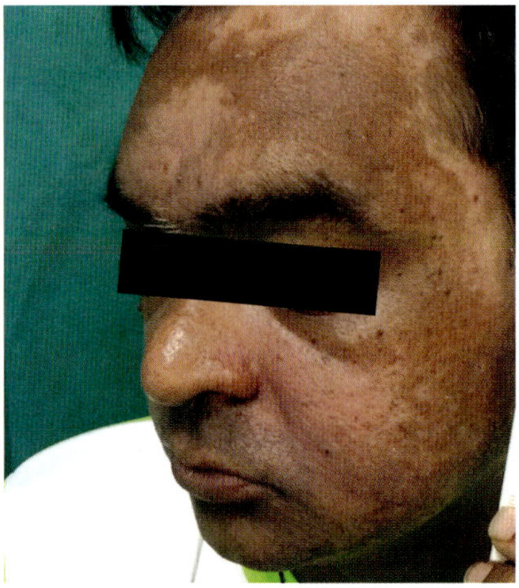

Figure 1: Well-defined nonscaly lesion of long duration due to application of triple combination—corticosteroid, antibiotic, and antifungal.

from skin diseases in India, the most accessible healthcare provider is the chemist who readily provides them corticosteroid-containing topical combinations giving prompt symptomatic relief. Hitherto TC was not included in the Drugs and Cosmetics Act of India, but now it is included in schedule H and cannot be dispensed without a prescription. Systemic steroids and other immunosuppressive agents, like cyclophosphamide, azathioprine, biologics, are widely prescribed by dermatologists and such medications while suppressing inflammatory component of tinea may perpetuate proliferation of dermatophytes with atypical presentation.

Now, cases of tinea incognito with topical tacrolimus and pimecrolimus have also been described. These immunomodulators inhibit the release of inflammatory cytokines and the activation of T cells, by inhibiting calcineurin activity. These drugs suppress the normal cutaneous immune response to dermatophytes, thus enhancing the development of atypical superficial fungal infections.

Thus, topical and systemic corticosteroids, topical immunomodulators, and systemic immunosuppressives can modify clinical features of dermatophytosis making them difficult to identify. High index of suspicion and careful enquiry about use of such medications can clench the diagnosis of tinea incognito.

CUTANEOUS RESPONSE TO DERMATOPHYTIC INFECTION

During a superficial fungal infection, the degradation of keratin (via the release of keratinases and the liberation of other pathogenic factors by the fungus) induces a first-line immune response and the subsequent release of proinflammatory cytokines. This causes the typical inflammatory symptoms, such as pruritus, erythema, swelling, and burning at the site of infection. Not only can these symptoms cause considerable discomfort and decrease patient adherence to treatment, but the induced scratching can increase the spread of infection and also leave the skin damaged and vulnerable to bacterial superinfections.[3]

PHARMACOLOGIC ACTIONS OF TOPICAL CORTICOSTEROIDS

Corticosteroids are amongst the twenty most important discoveries in the field of Medicine in the last century. In 1953, Sulzberger and Witten used topical hydrocortisone for the first time to treat dermatitis. It has antiallergic, antiproliferative, antiinflammatory, immunosuppressive, and vasoconstrictive actions (Table 1). Steroids act through glucocorticoid intranuclear receptors. Generalized distribution of these receptors is responsible for both its action and adverse drug reactions. It decreases cellular, vascular, and immunologic response at the site of application. Oral corticosteroids lead to altered inflammatory response

Table 1: Pharmacologic Actions of Corticosteroids	
Action	**Mechanism**
Antiproliferative	• Thickness of stratum corneum is reduced • Reduction of granular layer • Basal layer becomes flattened • Melanocyte pigment is inhibited
Vasoconstriction	
Anti-inflammatory	Decreases cellular, vascular, and immunologic response at the site of application
Antiallergic	
Immunosuppression	

Table 2: Potency of Topical Corticosteroids (United Kingdom Classification)		
Class	**Potency**	**Generic name and strength**
Class I	Very potent	• Clobetasol propionate 0.05% cream/ointment/scalp application • Diflucortolone valerate 0.3% cream/ointment
Class II	Potent	• Beclomethasone dipropionate 0.025% cream/ointment • Betamethasone valerate 0.1% cream/ointment/lotion • Betamethasone dipropionate 0.05% cream/ointment/lotion • Diflucortolone valerate 0.1% cream/oily cream/ointment • Fluocinolone acetonide 0.025% cream/ointment/gel • Fluocinonide 0.05% cream/ointment • Fluticasone propionate 0.05% cream • Fluticasone propionate 0.005% ointment • Hydrocortisone butyrate 0.1% cream/ointment/scalp lotion/ emulsion • Mometasone furoate 0.1% cream/ointment/scalp lotion • Triamcinolone acetonide 0.1% ointment
Class III	Moderate	• Betamethasone valerate 0.025% cream/ointment • Clobetasone butyrate 0.05% cream/ointment • Fluocinolone acetonide 0.00625% cream/ointment
Class IV	Mild	• Hydrocortisone 0.1–2.5% cream/ointment • Fluocinolone acetonide 0.0025% cream

and a disseminated infection. Topical corticosteroids are available in different potency (Table 2), and more potent the steroid more will be the antiinflammatory effect and chances of cutaneous adverse effects (Table 3). Application of potent to very potent steroid in body folds (most common site of tinea) results in atrophic striae (Figure 2).

Table 3: Adverse Drug Reactions of Topical Corticosteroids

- Local side effects like skin atrophy (striae, telangiectasia, purpura fragility, stellate pseudoscars)
- Suppression of the hypothalamic-pituitary-adrenal axis
- Hypopigmentation
- Acneiform eruption
- Contact allergy
- Rebound/addiction
- Tachyphylaxis
- Rise in intraocular pressure
- Infection
- Delayed wound healing
- Facial hypertrichosis
- Folliculitis
- Miliaria
- Granuloma gluteale infantum
- Perioral dermatitis
- Rosacea

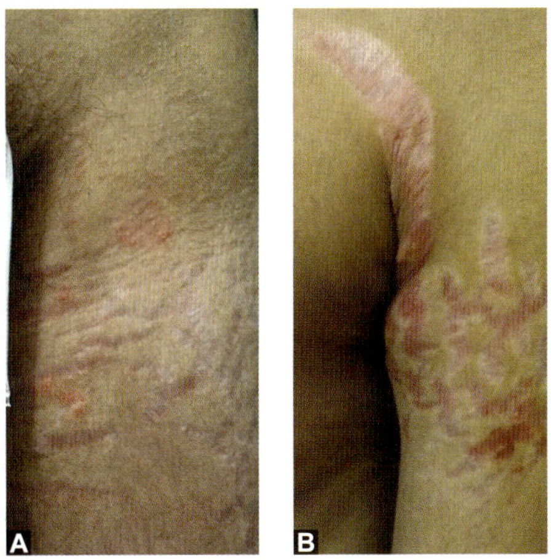

Figure 2: Topical steroid-induced striae.

TOPICAL STEROID ABUSE: INDIAN SCENARIO

According to the multicentric study in India by Saraswat et al. about TC abuse on 2,926 patients with facial dermatoses, steroid combinations were used by 258 (59.6%) patients. Potent and superpotent TCs were significantly more frequently used by the rural/suburban population. The younger age groups used more potent formulations. A nonphysician recommendation for TC use was obtainable in 59.3% patients. Of these, 90.3% were for potent/superpotent steroids.[4]

RATIONALE FOR TOPICAL STEROID-ANTIFUNGAL COMBINATION

Due to their anti-inflammatory, immunosuppressive, antimitotic, and vaso-constrictive actions, TCs play an important role in the treatment of various inflammatory skin diseases. In particular, combination therapy of mild-to-moderately potent corticosteroid with antifungal is a treatment option for superficial fungal infections with an inflammatory component. It is recommended that an antifungal-corticosteroid combination be administered at the initiation of therapy for 1–2 weeks, followed by antifungal monotherapy. By reducing inflammation and pruritus, TCs can reduce the risk of secondary bacterial superinfections, and reduce the spread of infection. They also reduce the risk of irritation and contact dermatitis that can sometimes be associated with the use of topical antifungal agents. However, corticosteroids may interfere with the therapeutic action of the antifungal agent, or increase fungal growth as a result of decreased localized immune response.[3]

IMPACT OF CORTICOSTEROID ON TINEA

Topical corticosteroids have a more profound disease modifying ability than systemic steroids. They suppress the fungus-induced local immunity, both innate, i.e., β-defensins, and acquired, including T cell-mediated immune mechanisms.[5] It has been demonstrated that potent topical steroids can increase the numbers of hyphae present on the surface of the skin in fungal infections and change the appearance of the lesions. Tinea incognito is more commonly caused by potent fluorinated steroids, like clobetasol and betamethasone, more so if applied under occlusion. Consequently, clotrimazole-betamethasone like combinations are not recommended for use in children less than 17 years of age, in immunosuppressed patients, or lesions at occluded areas.[3]

When potent topical steroid-containing antifungal combinations are applied, there is temporary resolution of inflammation with alleviation of itching and redness but without effectively eliminating the dermatophyte. This combined with other factors like tight fitting clothing, high humidity, and daily commuting for work or studies causes the dermatophyte continues to spread. In tinea cruris, the infection spreads from the inguinal region to the neighboring unaffected areas, namely the penis and the scrotum (Figure 3).[6] Because of the dramatic symptomatic improvement initially, patient may discontinue the treatment and present with a flare up. Self-medication and prolonged use is also very common.

TINEA INCOGNITO (STEROID-MODIFIED TINEA)

Common causative agents of tinea incognito reported are *Trichophyton rubrum*, *T. mentagrophytes*, *Microsporum gypseum*, *T. violaceum*, *Epidermophyton floccosum*, and *M. canis*, etc.

In tinea incognito, the classical well-defined lesions become modified (Table 4). They become ill defined with reduced itching and inflammation with spread of

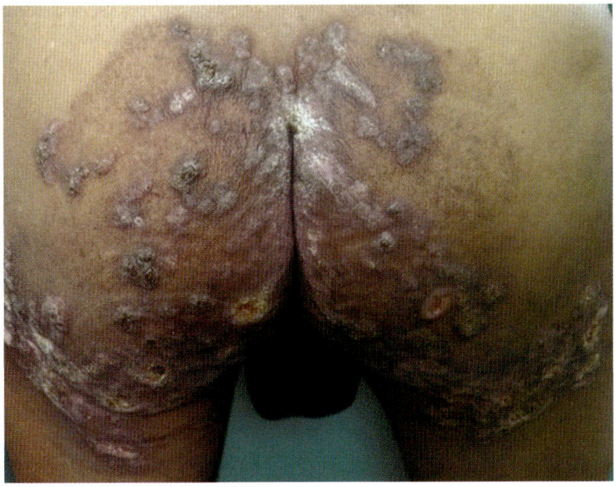

Figure 3: Chronic lichenified papules with erosions on gluteal region.

Table 4: Clinical Features—Classic versus Steroid-modified Tinea

Classic tinea	Tinea incognito
Itching present	Minimal itching until steroid is applied; if steroid withdrawn, irritation/itching
Oval or circular plaque with sharply defined borders and central clearing, erythema Peripheral vesiculation may be present	Polymorphic with scattered papules, pustules, and hyperpigmentation with diffuse blanching erythema with telangiectasis
Margins are raised	Margins are less raised
Scaly lesions	Less scaly
Less irritable	Irritable
Less chance of recurrence and dissemination	More chances of recurrence and dissemination

lesion. In many dermatoses like melasma, psoriasis, pemphigus, etc., which are steroid responsive, there can be superimposed tinea especially at occlusive sites. Therefore, before initiation of steroid, any occult foci of fungal infection like onychomycosis, tinea pedis must be ruled out.

Review of Literature

Diverse presentations of tinea incognito as reported in different literature have been shown in table 5.

Starace et al. reported a case of 17-year-old male with pustular psoriasis on nail bed of toe treated with an antipsoriatic cream, composed of topical steroids

Table 5: Diverse Presentations of Tinea Incognito as Reported in Different Literature

Author	Presentation	Age/ gender	Site	Previous treatment
Şatana et al.[7]	Allergic reaction	17/F	Face	• Topical corticosteroids
Rallis et al.[8]	Intertriginous psoriasis	58/M	Groin fold	• Pimecrolimus
Yu et al.[9]	Psoriasis vulgaris, systemic lupus erythematosus, facial dermatitis	41/F	Face	• Acitretin, prednisone • Topical corticosteroid-antifungal combination
Kim et al.[10]	Contact dermatitis	70/F	Face, scalp	• Topical corticosteroids
Hwang et al.[11]	Eczema like	15/F	Leg	• Topical corticosteroid and calcineurin inhibitor • Topical corticosteroid and calcineurin inhibitor

M, male; F, female.

and a vitamin D3 derivative, which gave rise to a tinea incognita on dorsum of foot.[12] Lecamwasam et al. reported a case of 22-year-old pregnant woman with tinea incognito on face following application over-the-counter medication for skin lightening.[13] Guenova et al. reported a case of 68-year-old female earlier diagnosed as pemphigus foliaceus for 13 years, on long-term oral and topical steroids with worsening of lesions mainly in facial, lower torso, and buttock areas. Periodic acid-Schiff (PAS) stain, fungal culture, and polymerase chain reaction (PCR) analysis showed abundant *T. rubrum*.[14]

An immune-mediated phenomenon called "tinea pseudoimbricata" is a particular type of tinea incognito which has been described. *T. mentagrophytes*, instead of *T. concentricum*, is usually isolated from these lesions (Figure 4).[5]

A case of Majocchi's granuloma of the face and the scalp has been described in a 55-year-old female who had been diagnosed with eczema and received systemic (intramuscular and oral) as well as TCs over a period of 7 months. On PAS staining, spores and hyphae were seen. Enzyme-linked immunosorbent assay-PCR of the biopsy identified *T. rubrum*, which was also grown on culture of the biopsy tissue. The patient was treated with systemic itraconazole (200 mg once daily) and topical terbinafine (twice daily) for 8 weeks.[15]

Differential Diagnosis

Corticosteroids not only modify the annular lesions of tinea but also masquerade as a number of other dermatoses (Figure 5). The main differential diagnosis depends on the affected area. In the face, the lesions may resemble neurodermatitis, atopic dermatitis, folliculitis, rosacea, seborrheic dermatitis, lupus erythematosus, or

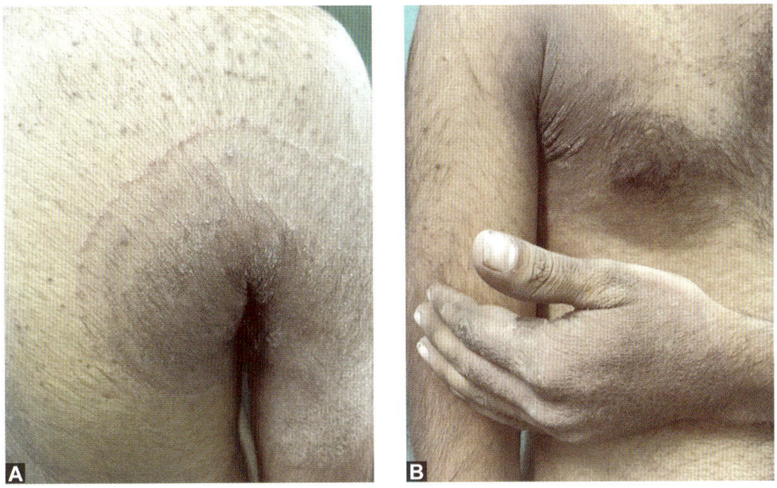

Figure 4: A and B, Tinea pseudoimbricata with acneiform eruption.

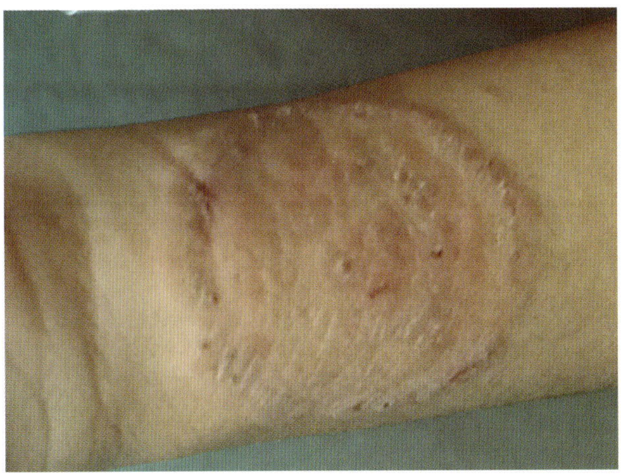

Figure 5: Long-standing annular lesion modified by application of corticosteroid-fusidic acid combination.

contact dermatitis. Facial tinea incognito can also be associated with tinea pedis or onychomycosis in toenails, or both. In the glabrous skin, the main differential diagnosis is impetigo, purpura, lichen planus, psoriasis, erythema migrans, drug eruptions, sweet neutrophilic dermatosis, contact dermatitis, discoid lupus, and tuberculoid leprosy.

Diagnosis

Clinical clues to tinea incognito have been mentioned in table 6.

Table 6: Clinical Clues to Tinea Incognito

- Ill-defined skin lesion with diffuse scaling of long duration
- Lesions occurring at sites like face, trunk, genitalia
- Unresponsiveness to topical corticosteroids (including combination therapy)
- Unresponsiveness to topical calcineurin inhibitor
- Presence of occult tinea like interdigital space, onychomycosis
- Patient on immunosuppressive treatment for conditions like autoimmune dermatological and medical condition

Laboratory Diagnosis

Mycological examination should be performed in every atypical presentation of the above-mentioned diseases. It is better to perform mycology to rule out tinea pedis in any disease of the feet that requires topical application of steroids. Microscopic examination by potassium hydroxide (KOH) preparations of skin scrapings shows branching hyphae and spores and culture in Sabouraud's dextrose agar must be performed. Culture with sensitivity is crucial in picking up resistant fungal infection (Figure 6). Scrapings may be difficult to take if steroids were used recently. Stoppage of corticosteroids will lead to re-emergence of inflammation and scaling facilitating scraping.

Treatment

There should be immediate cessation of all steroid medication. Patients should be warned for transient flaring of the lesion by use of steroid. Also, a low-potency corticosteroid may be used briefly to avoid the flare often associated with abrupt cessation of a potent steroid.

Topical and/or systemic antifungal regimen should be started. Patients with few skin lesions which are not recurrent can be treated with topical antifungals alone. However, in majority of cases, oral antifungals are required and preferred drugs are itraconazole, terbinafine, and griseofulvin. Physician should enquire the medications taken by the patient previously and their response. Medication should be continued for 4–6 weeks or till complete clearance of lesions followed by maintenance for 1 week or so. Patients are instructed to maintain proper hygiene and also treat occult foci of infection like nails.

CONCLUSION

Because of its potent antiallergic and anti-inflammatory effect, corticosteroids are prescribed for skin conditions of diverse etiology without establishing a definite

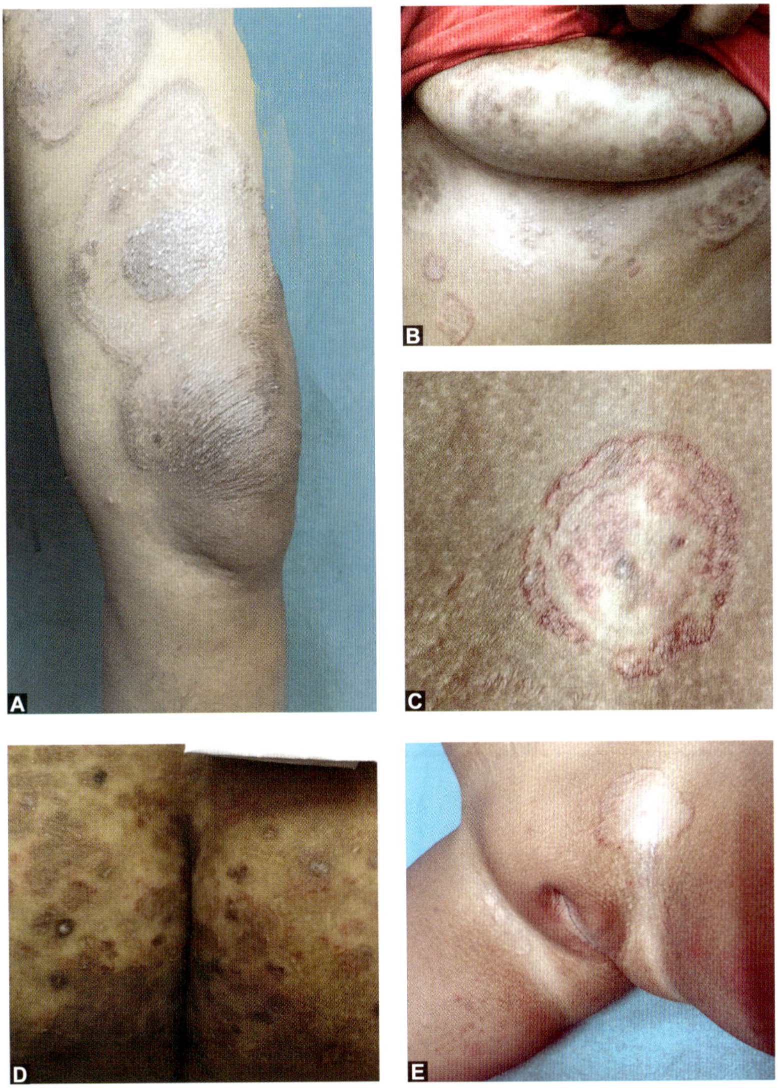

Figure 6: Three generations of the same family suffering from resistant tinea. **A,** Resistant tinea in grandmother; **B to D,** mother with resistant tinea; **E,** resistant tinea in daughter.

cause. In tinea incognito, skin lesions become ill-defined with reduced itching and inflammation with spread of lesion. There is also more chance of recurrence and dissemination.

Proper examination of patient with investigations to rule out of foci of fungal infection should be done before initiation of oral and topical steroids.

Patients on systemic steroids must be evaluated periodically for any aggravation of existing dermatosis or presence of atypical lesions. In patients with atypical lesions like intractable eczema, psoriasis, look for occult foci of fungal infection like web spaces and nails and history of topical corticosteroid application.

Mycological examination like KOH preparations and culture in Sabouraud's dextrose agar must be performed in suspicious lesions.

Systemic antifungals should be started after diagnosis. Patients must be instructed to maintain proper hygiene.

Editor's Comment

Authors, Dr Yogesh Marfatia and Dr Sheethal Jose correctly point out the pertinent point of rising Tinea incognito due to rampant and indiscriminate use of topical corticosteroid containing combination creams and OTC products. They also rightly stress that atypical lesions of eczema or psoriasis not responding to treatment,occult foci of fungal infection must be looked for.In India,under the Indian Association of Dermatologists,Venereologists and Leprologists(IADVL), a task force called ITATSA which stands for IADVL Task Force against Topical Steroid Abuse has been working continuously at local and national levels to curb this menace. The article delineates well the important features of this special form of tinea infections.

Rashmi Sarkar, Seemal R Desai

REFERENCES

1. Ive FA, Marks R. Tinea incognito. *Br Med J.* 1968;3:149-52.
2. Arenas R, Moreno-Coutiño G, Vera L, Welsh O. Tinea incognito. *Clin Dermatol.* 2010;28:137-9.
3. Schaller M, Friedrich M, Papini M, Pujol RM, Veraldi S. Topical antifungal-corticosteroid combination therapy for the treatment of superficial mycoses: conclusions of an expert panel meeting. *Mycoses.* 2016;59:365-73.
4. Saraswat A, Lahiri K, Chatterjee M, Barua S, Coondoo A, Mittal A, et al. Topical corticosteroid abuse on the face: a prospective, multicenter study of dermatology outpatients. *Indian J Dermatol Venereol Leprol.* 2011;77:160-6.
5. Verma SB, Hay R. Topical steroid-induced tinea pseudoimbricata: a striking form of tinea incognito. *Int J Dermatol.* 2015;54:192-3.
6. Verma SB, Vasani R. Male genital dermatophytosis—clinical features and the effects of the misuse of topical steroids and steroid combinations—an alarming problem in India. *Mycoses.* 2016;59(10):606-14.
7. Şatana D, Yeğenoğlu Y, Uzun M, Erturan Z, Gürler N, Özarmağan G. A case of tinea incognito diagnosed coincidentally. *J Microbiol Infect Dis.* 2011;1(2):84-6.
8. Rallis E, Koumantaki-Mathioudaki E. Pimecrolimus induced tinea incognito masquerading as intertriginous psoriasis. *Mycoses.* 2008;51:71-3.
9. Yu C, Zhou J, Liu J. Tinea incognito due to microsporum gypseum. *J Biomed Res.* 2010;24(1):81-3.
10. Kim KJ, Jee MS, Choi JH, Sung KJ, Moon KC, Koh JK. A case of tinea incognito presented as folliculitis. *Korean J Dermatol.* 2001;39:1328-30.

11. Hwang SM, Kim DM, Suh MK, Ha GY, Kim JR. Eczema-like tinea incognito occurring leg. *Korean J Med Mycol.* 2011;16:51-5.
12. Starace M, Alessandrini A, Piraccini BM. Tinea incognita following the use of an antipsoriatic gel. *Skin Appendage Disord.* 2016;1(3):123-5.
13. Lecamwasam KL, Lim TM, Fuller LC. Tinea incognito caused by skin-lightening products. *J Eur Acad Dermatol Venereol.* 2016;30(3):480-1.
14. Guenova E, Hoetzenecker W, Schaller M, Röcken M, Fierlbeck G. Tinea incognito hidden under apparently treatment-resistant pemphigus foliaceus. *Acta Derm Venereol.* 2007;88:276.
15. Liu C, Landeck L, Cai SQ, Zheng M. Majocchi's granuloma over the face. *Indian J Dermatol Venereol Leprol.* 2012;78:113-4.

World Clin Dermatol. 2016;3(1):220-50.

Changing and Rising Scenario of Dermatophytosis in India: Causes and Solutions

*R Madhu MD DCH, Janaki Chellam MD DD MAMS, Sentamilselvi Ganapati MD DD PhD FAMS

Department of Dermatology, Madras Medical College, Billroth Hospitals
Chennai, Tamil Nadu, India

ABSTRACT

Dermatophytosis is the most common superficial fungal infection caused by keratinophilic molds which have an affinity for the keratin in skin, hair, and nails. Lifetime risk of acquiring dermatophytosis is said to be 10–15%. Hot and humid weather in India, a tropical country favors the prevalence of dermatophytosis. Literature search on clinico-mycological study of superficial mycoses and dermatophytosis revealed that there is an increase in the prevalence of dermatophytosis over the last 4 years. Males were found to be more affected. However, the sex ratio has changed from 3:1 in the yester-years to 2.64:1–1.05:1. Among the clinical types, tinea corporis is the most common type observed. Multiple site involvement and tinea incognito have been observed in increased frequency compared to the previous studies. *Trichophyton rubrum* which is the most common causative organism of dermatophytosis worldwide, was found to be predominant in India also. *Trichophyton mentagrophytes*, which emerged as the second common pathogen, showed an increase in the prevalence compared to the earlier studies. Causes for this changing and rising scenario could be due to the various factors that include environment, host, agent, and drug therapy. These causative factors and the solutions have been discussed.

*Corresponding author
Email: renmadhu08@gmail.com

© 2016 Jaypee Brothers Medical Publishers. All rights reserved.

INTRODUCTION

Fungal infections are classified as superficial and deep fungal infections. Deep fungal infections which comprise the subcutaneous mycoses and the systemic mycoses have been on the rise since last three to four decades, understandably due to the increase in the incidence of solid organ transplantation, immunosuppressive states, and advent of higher antibiotics. Superficial fungal infections include the common skin infections seen in daily practice namely dermatophytosis, pityriasis versicolor, candidiasis, and the rare infections such as tinea nigra and piedra. It has been estimated that about 20–25% of the world population is affected by superficial mycoses, of which dermatophytosis is the predominant infection.[1] Lifetime risk of acquiring dermatophytosis is said to be 10–15%.[2] Dermatophytosis is more common in the tropical and subtropical countries, due to the hot and humid climate that is prevalent in these regions. Climatic conditions that prevail across India which is a tropical country, be it the hot summer in the western region or hot and humid weather in the southern states or the relatively humid weather with high rainfall in the northeastern states, predispose Indians to acquire dermatophytosis. This infection which is readily diagnosed by the clinical morphology and easily amenable to antifungal agents, has been on the rise since 3–4 years in India with increasing incidence of treatment failures.[3] Literature search by the authors revealed 85 out of 107 articles on clinico-mycological studies on superficial mycoses and dermatophytosis undertaken across India, published between 2012 and 2016. Dermatophytosis being communicable and associated with intense pruritus is a big social stigma and has evolved as a serious public health problem in our country.

RISING SCENARIO OF DERMATOPHYTOSIS

Various studies done across the country have shown the increase of prevalence of dermatophytosis from 58.5% during 1995–96 to 91.2% in 2016.[4-19] Different studies done in cities like Kolkata, Ahmedabad, and Chennai during various time periods reveal a definite increase in the occurrence of dermatophytosis.[5-8,10,11] (Table 1). Contrastingly, studies done at Mangalore and Jaipur reported a prevalence of 49.95% and 53.8% for dermatophytosis and 31.3% and 34.6% of pityriasis versicolor, respectively.[14,15] This could be due to the effect of various factors like temperature, humidity, geographic location, and sociocultural factors on dermatophytosis.

CHANGING SCENARIO OF DERMATOPHYTES

Dermatophytosis is caused by keratinophilic molds namely dermatophytes which belong to the three genera *Trichophyton, Microsporum*, and *Epidermophyton* with a special affinity for the nonliving keratinized cells of the skin, nails, and hair.[20]

Table 1: Rising Scenario of Dermatophytosis[4-19]

Study, year	Period	Place	Dermatophytosis (%)	Pityriasis versicolor (%)	Candidiasis (%)
Mishra et al.[4] 1998	1995–96	Burla, Orissa	58.5	33.8	7.7
Grover and Roy[5] 2003	1999–2001	Kolkata	70.5	9	20.5
Das et al.[6] 2009	2008	Kolkata	84.8	15.17	–
Nawal et al.[7] 2012	2007–08	Ahmedabad	68.37	22.32	9.30
Chudasama et al.[8] 2014	2010–11	Ahmedabad	88.5	11.5	–
Patel HK et al.[9] 2016	2014–15	Valsad, Gujarat	95.89	4.1	–
Kannan et al.[10] 2006	2001–02	Chennai	52.3	25.5	18.9
Narasimhalu et al.[11] 2016	–	Chennai	74	22	4
Sridevi et al.[12] 2016	2009	Tirupati	70	26	4
Surekha et al.[13] 2015	2011	Tirupati	69.7	26.3	4
Sharma and Sharma[14] 2012	2008	Jaipur	53.8	34.6	3.1
Prabhu et al.[15] 2013	–	Mangalore	49.95	31.3	18.75
Parameswari and Prasad Babu[16] 2015	2013–14	Vijayawada	95.3	4.6	–
Khan and Khan[17] 2016 Jan	2015	Lucknow	95.8	4.2	–
Gupta[18] 2016 Apr	2014–15	Ludhiana	82	8	10
Magdum et al.[19] 2016 Oct	2014–15	Satara, Maharashtra	91.2	8.8	–

While some of the dermatophytes are found worldwide (*Trichophyton rubrum, T. mentagrophytes var. interdigitale, Microsporum canis,* and *Epidermophyton floccosum*), few have a specific geographic predilection [*T. schoenleinii* (Eurasia, Africa), *T. soudanense* (Africa), *T. violaceum* (Asia, Africa, and Europe), and *T. concentricum* (Pacific Islands, Far East, and India)]. Prevalence of dermatophytosis tends to change with time and geographic location as it is influenced by multiple factors such as migration, industrialization, global travel, socioeconomic conditions, cultural practices, environment, host immunity, and the clinical type of dermatophytosis.[1,21] Dermatophytes are grouped based on their ecological niche into anthropophilic (human origin), zoophilic (animal), and geophilic (soil origin) species.[22] While the infections caused by anthropophilic species are characterized by chronic course and minimal inflammation, zoophilic and geophilic organisms produce lesions with severe inflammation which may go for self-resolution.[23] Most common causative organisms vary according to the site of involvement namely the glabrous skin of various body parts, hair, and nail.[21] Transmission of the organisms to human beings occurs through either direct contact with an infected person, animal and soil or with infected desquamated keratinocytes or shed hair-containing fungal spores present on the floor in houses, swimming pools, locker rooms, hotel rugs, clothes, towels, bed linens, pillow covers, furniture, theater seats, farm fences, combs, hair brushes, caps, and infected toys too in case of children with tinea capitis.[22,24] Spores may remain viable in the presence of a suitable environment for a period of 12–20 months. Jain and Sharma reported 89.86% prevalence of dermatophytic and related fungal flora in their study done from soil samples from different habitats of Jaipur city. They found 100% positivity of isolates from hostel, playground, factory, and farmhouse followed by 97.3% in the roadside, 88.8% in nursery, 85.7% in PG study center, and 83.3% in vegetable market.[25]

Most of the studies done across India have shown that *T. rubrum* continues to be the most common organism followed by *T. mentagrophytes* as the codominant species (Tables 2 to 5). However, the prevalence of *T. rubrum* has reduced compared to the yester-years, with a simultaneous rise in the prevalence of *T. mentagrophytes* (Figure 1). This has been documented in the various studies done in different cities all over the country including Amritsar, Patiala, and Lucknow in north India,[17,30-33,38] Kolkata in the east,[5,40] Ahmedabad in the west,[8,51] and Tirupati and Chennai in south India.[13,55,63,64] Further, few studies have also reported *T. mentagrophytes* to be the most common organism followed by *T. rubrum*.[17,29,33,37,49,57] whereas some studies have also observed *T. tonsurans* to be the most common isolate followed by *T. rubrum*.[5,9] Figures 2 to 4 depict the potassium hydroxide wet mount pictures of dermatophytes. Figures 5 to 14 show the macroscopic and microscopic pictures of *T. rubrum*, *T. mentagrophytes*, *T. tonsurans*, and *T. violaceum*.

Table 2: Changing Scenario of Dermatophytes in North India[17,26-38]

State/city	Study, year	Period	T. rubr	T. ment	T. viol	T. tons	E. floc	Others
Jammu & Kashmir								
Kashmir[26]	Munir et al. 2014	2010–11	52.94	29.42	–	–	–	–
Samba[27]	Najotra et al. 2015	2011–12	41.8	10.5	7.5	22.4	2.9	*T. sch* 5.9
Himachal Pradesh								
Shimla[28]	Bhagra et al. 2014	2008–09	66.17	19.11	7.35	1.47	–	*T. verr* 2.94
Tanda[29]	Kaur et al. 2016	2013	32	48.2	3.6	10.7	–	NDM 39
Punjab								
Patiala[30]	Rani et al. 1983	–	80	–	–	–	–	–
Patiala[31]	Singla et al. 2013	–	61.2	26.6	–	4.1	6.1	–
Amritsar[32]	Aggarwal et al. 2002	1999–2001	62.3	23.41	0.79	5.5	0.4	NDM 3.9, C 2.7
Amritsar[33]	Kansra et al. 2016	2013–15	24.29	46.43	3.57	–	–	*T. verr* 12.14, *T. sch* 11.43
Delhi[34]	Sharma et al.	2012	22.33	D 63.3, *T.* spp. 10; NDM 36.6				*M. aud* 26.6
Bihar								
East[35]	Maity et al. 2014	2010–11	31.9	21.27	–	25.5	4.2	*M. gyps* 12.7
Ranchi[36]	Singh et al. 2016	2012–15	63.2	26.4	–	2.94	5.8	–
Uttarakhand[37]	Kainthola et al. 2014	2013	28.15	42.85	–	–	42.85	*T. verr* 28.57
Uttar Pradesh								
Lucknow[38]	Singh et al. 1981	–	39.21	7.76	2.94	6.37	2.45	26.47
Lucknow[17]	Khan et al. 2016	2015	5.6	37	–	27.8	–	*M. aud* 5.6. NDM 14.8

T. rubr, Trichophyton rubrum; T. ment, T. mentagrophytes; T. viol, T. violaceum; T. tons, T. tonsurans; T. verr, T. verrucosum; E. floc, Epidermophyton floccosum; M.aud, Microsporum audouinii; T. sch, T. schoenleinii; M. gyps, Microsporum gypseum; NDM, non-dermatophyte molds.

Prevalence of organisms is given in percentage.

Table 3: Changing Scenario of Dermatophytes in Eastern and Central India[5,39-47]

State/city	Study et al., year	Period	T. rubr	T. ment	T. viol	T. tons	E. floc	Others
Odisha (Orissa)								
Cuttack[39]	Prasad et al. 2013	2009–11	48.2	26.3	–	8.7	1.7	*M. aud* 2.6 *T. sch* 11.4
West Bengal								
Kolkata[5]	Grover et al. 2003	1999–2001	21.9	7.3	–	58.5	–	*M. ferr* 14.6
Kolkata[40]	Ghosh et al. 2014	2011–14	22.2	21.16	2.11	–	–	*T. verr* 23.8 *T. sch* 6.34
Assam								
Guwahati[41]	Sen et al. 2005	–	68.6	23.5	–	–	3.92	–
Tezpur[42]	Naglot et al. 2015	2012–14	50.1	29.2	–	–	9.8	–
Manipur								
Imphal[43]	Singh et al. 2015	2010–12	60	32.72	3.63	–	3.63	–
Meghalaya								
Shillong[44]	Lyngdoh et al. 2013	2011–12	30.3	28.9	–	26.3	2.6	*T. verr* 7.9
Madhya Pradesh								
Jabalpur[45]	Shukla et al. 1983	1978–79	65.6	6.02	2.8	1.06	0.3	9.9
Gwalior[46]	Pandey et al. 2013	–	42.3	12.7	9.8	5.7	–	*M. gyp* 9.8 *T. sch* 7
Bhopal[47]	Gupta et al. 2014	2014	41.3	28.3	–	15.2	6.5	*T. verr* 8.7

T. rubr, Trichophyton rubrum; T. ment, T. mentagrophytes; T. viol, T. violaceum; T. tons, T. tonsurans; T. verr, T. verrucosum; E. floc, Epidermophyton floccosum; M. aud, Microsporum audouinii; T. sch, T. schoenleinii; M. gyp, Microsporum gypseum; M. ferr, Microsporum ferrugineum.

Prevalence of organisms is given in percentage.

Table 4: Changing Scenario of Dermatophytes in Western India[8,9,48-54]

State/city	Study, year	Period	T. rubr	T. ment	T. viol	T. tons	E. floc	Others
Rajasthan								
Udaipur[48]	Mandia 1987	–	67.38	23.01	7.69	–	2.15	1.84
Jaipur[49]	Agarwal et al. 2014	2011–12	34.2	37.9	11.3	8.3	–	*M. aud* 6.2
Rajkot[50]	Mistry et al. 2014	2011–14	53.1	27.98	3.2	5.3	1.23	*M. gyp* 5.76
Gujarat								
Ahmedabad[51]	Mankodi et al. 1969	–	84.5	1.5	8.5	3	3	–
Ahmedabad[8]	Chudasama et al. 2014	2010–11	52.1	26.05	1.68	0.84	–	*M. gyp* 3.3 *Cand* 15.9
Valsad[9]	Patel et al. 2016	2014–15	3	18	–	21.2	3	*Mic.* spp. 6 *Cand* 21.2
Maharashtra								
Mumbai[52]	Mehta et al. 1977	–	87	3.2	2	1.5	5.5	–
Loni[53]	Bose et al. 2013	–	33.3	21.3	–	–	2	*M. gyp* 1.3
Pune[54]	Sharma et al. 2016	2013–14	40	36	8	10.66	–	NDM 25

T. rubr, Trichophyton rubrum; T. ment, T. mentagrophytes; T. viol, T. violaceum; T. tons, T. tonsurans; E. floc, Epidermophyton floccosum; M. aud, Microsporum audouinii; M. gyp, Microsporum gypseum; Cand, Candida; Mic spp., *Microsporum* species, NDM, non-dermatophyte molds.

Prevalence of organisms is given in percentage.

Table 5: Changing Scenario of Dermatophytes in Southern India[13,16,55-64]

State/city	Study, year	Period	T. rubr	T. ment	T. viol	T. tons	E. floc	Others
Andhra Pradesh								
Tirupati[55]	Bhaskaran 1977	–	49.15	5.08	16.94	–	22.8	5.93
Tirupati[13]	Sureka 2015	2011	64	20	–	4		*T. verr* 12
Kakinada[16]	Parameswari and Prasad Babu 2015	–	50	35.7	8.6	–	1.4	*M. gyp* 4.3
Karnataka								
Mysore[56]	Lalithamma 1978	–	76.5	14.2	7.65	–	1.3	–
Hubli[57]	Noronha et al. 2008	2007–08	38.3	48.3	5	–		*T. verr* 8.3
Shimoga[58]	Manjunath 2016	–	38.57	22.85	4.28	–	1.4	*M. aud* 21.4
Kerala								
Calicut[59]	Maheshwariamma et al. 1978	1970–75	47.90	27.06	3.34	1.67	2.23	*M. ferr* 9.85
Calicut[60]	Bindu and Pavithran 2002	–	66.2	25	–	5.9	2.9	–
Mallapuram[61]	Sivakumar et al. 2008	2008	41.5	33.96	1.88	–	5.66	NDM 11.3
Tamil Nadu								
Chennai[62]	Pankajalakshmi et al. 1974	–	54.17	32.9	1.2	–	9.2	–
Chennai[63]	Kumar et al. 2007	2004	67.5	18	–	–	2.9	*T. sch* 5.9
Chennai[64]	Ramaraj et al. 2016	2011–14	48.9	44.75	3.49	–	0.7	*M. gyp* 1.4

T. rubr, Trichophyton rubrum; T. ment, T. mentagrophytes; T. viol, T. violaceum; T. tons, T. tonsurans; T. verr, T. verrucosum; E. floc, Epidermophyton floccosum; M. aud, Microsporum audouinii; M. gyp, Microsporum gypseum; M. ferr, M ferrugineum; T. sch, T. schoenleinii; NDM, non-dermatophyte molds.

Prevalence of organisms is given in percentage.

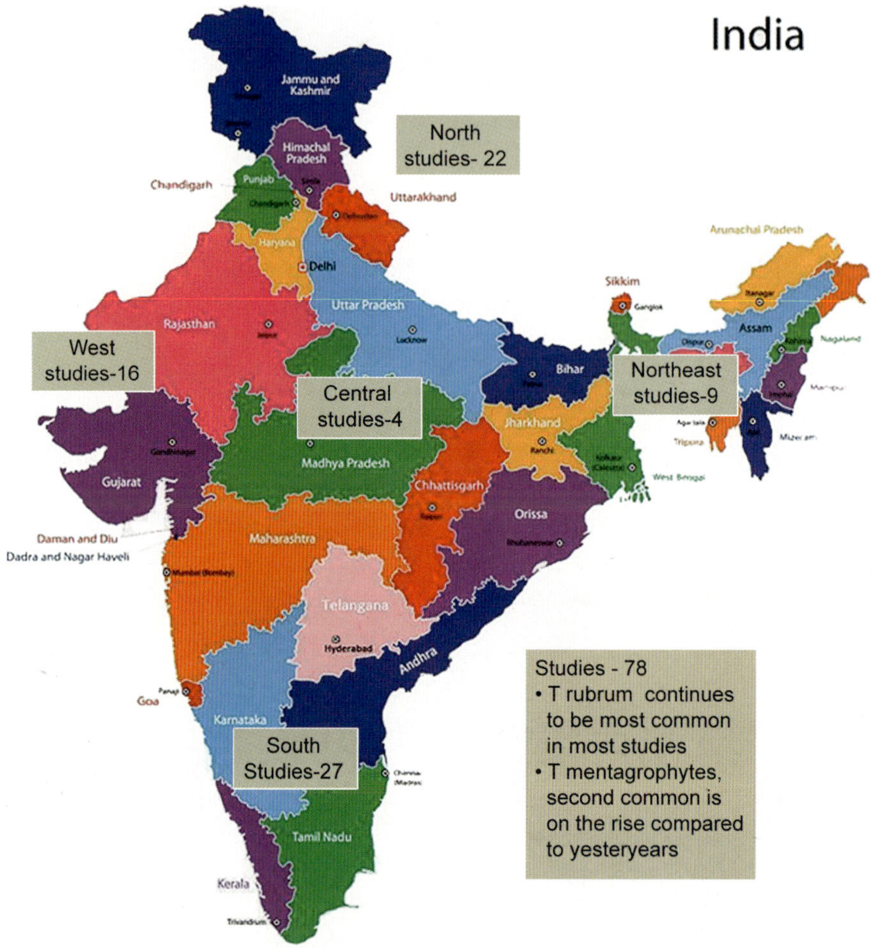

Figure 1: Clinico-mycological studies on dermatophytosis done across India.

CHANGING SCENARIO IN CLINICAL PRESENTATION OF DERMATOPHYTOSIS

Sex Ratio and Age Group

Clinical presentation of dermatophytosis depends on the etiological agent, size of the inoculum, virulence of the organism, site of involvement, and host immunity.[2,65] Indian studies done in the past decade have shown dermatophytosis to be more common in males and most of the times, the sex ratio has been around 3:1. This male preponderance was attributed to the increased time spent outdoor, exposed to hot, humid weather, and increased physical activity.

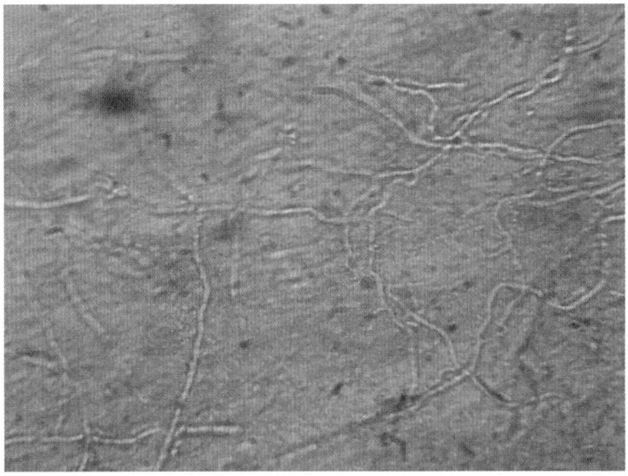

Figure 2: Potassium hydroxide (KOH) wet mount of dermatophytes showing hyaline, long, branching septate hyphae.

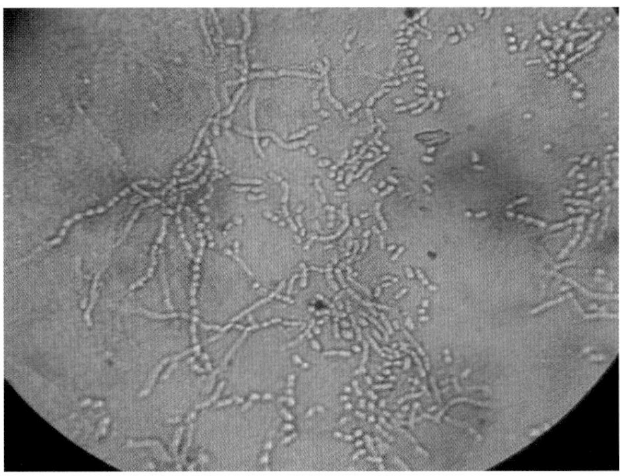

Figure 3: Potassium hydroxide (KOH) wet mount of dermatophytes showing chains of arthrospores.

Studies done across the country since 2008 have shown sex ratio to range from 2.64:1 to 1.05:1 (Tables 6 to 8). This change in the sex ratio implies that more number of women are being affected by dermatophytosis. Though estrogen was thought to be protective against dermatophytes, the increasing prevalence in dermatophytosis in females could be explained by the fact that there are more women working outdoors. Women who wear tight clothing or synthetic garments for prolonged period are more prone to be infected. In addition, it could also be due to the increased health awareness in the urban population.

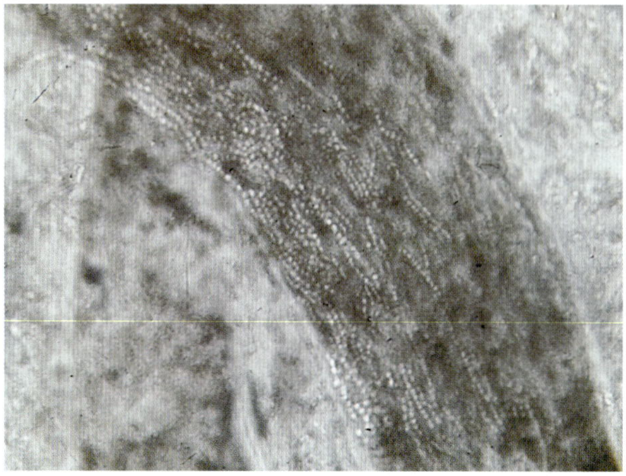

Figure 4: Potassium hydroxide (KOH) wet mount of hair in 40% KOH showing endothrix type of hair invasion—hyaline, uniform sized spores in mosaic pattern and chains of arthrospores seen.

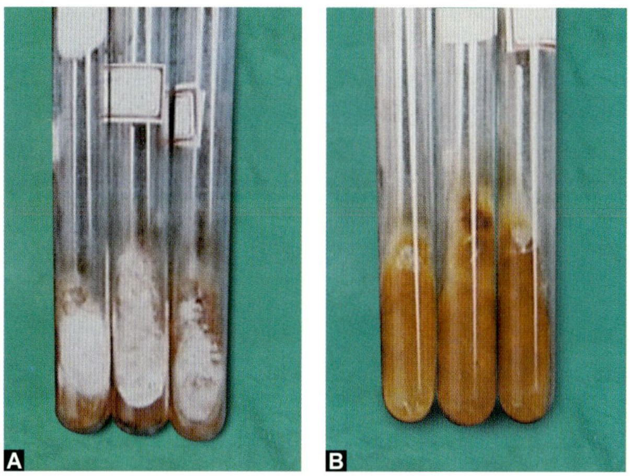

Figure 5: *Trichophyton rubrum*. White cottony dome-shaped colony with reddish brown pigmentation on the reverse.

Sivakumar et al. from Malappuram, Kerala reported a sex ratio of 1:1.8.[61] With regard to the age group involved, there has been no change, as this infection continues to be more common in the third and fourth decade.

Urban versus Rural Status and Socioeconomic Status

Multiple recent studies published over last few years have shown that dermatophytosis has evolved into an important public health problem, both in

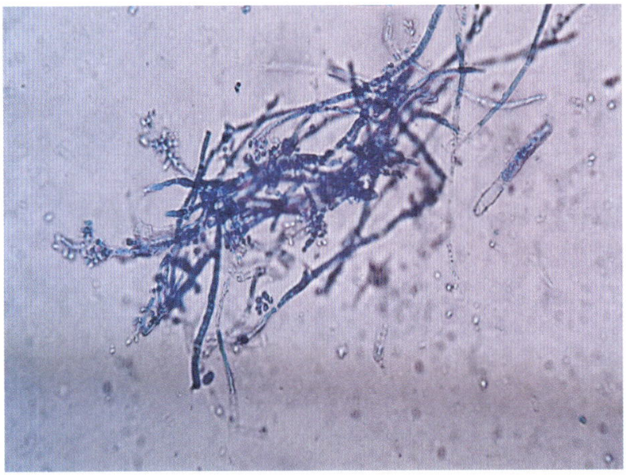

Figure 6: Microscopic picture of *T. rubrum* in lactophenol cotton blue showing microconidia in enthyrse and engreppe pattern.

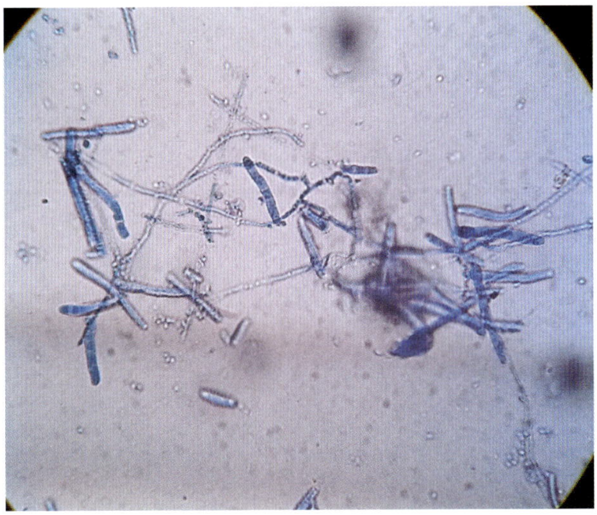

Figure 7: Microscopic picture of *T. rubrum* in lactophenol cotton blue showing the smooth walled multicellular macroconidia along with microconidia.

the urban and rural population.[17,29,69,82] Ranganathan et al. in 1995, Sivakumar et al. in 2008, and Sahai and Mishra in 2011 reported that dermatophytosis was more common in people belonging to lower socioeconomic status.[24,61,67] But, now the scenario having changed, studies done in 2015 and 2016 state that it is prevalent among people of middle and higher socioeconomic status also.[16,36,74,78]

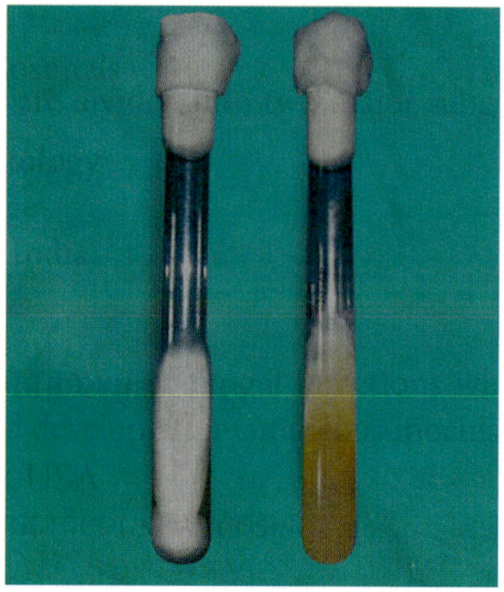

Figure 8: *Trichophyton mentagrophytes*. Fluffy white colony with reverse yellow pigmentation.

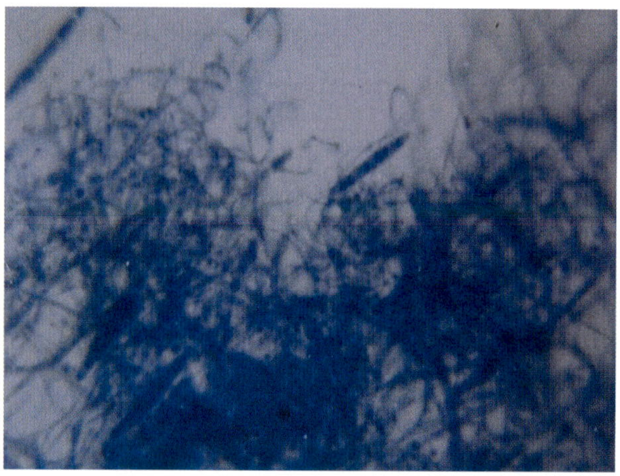

Figure 9: Microscopic picture of *T. mentagrophytes* in lactophenol cotton blue showing clavate shaped microconidia in engreppe and enthyrse pattern, thin walled pencil shaped multicellular macroconidia and spiral hyphae.

Occupation

Dermatophytosis is understandably more common in skilled and unskilled laborers. However, recent studies have found that this infection has become more common in students and is also seen in professionals and business men.[29,37,83]

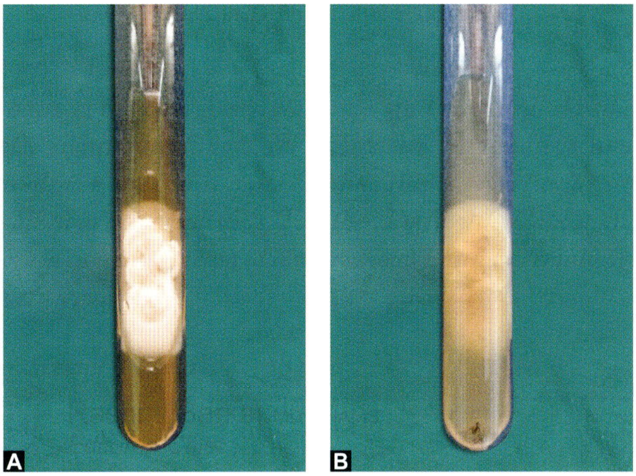

Figure 10: *Trichophyton tonsurans*. Creamy white powdery colony with yellowish brown reverse.

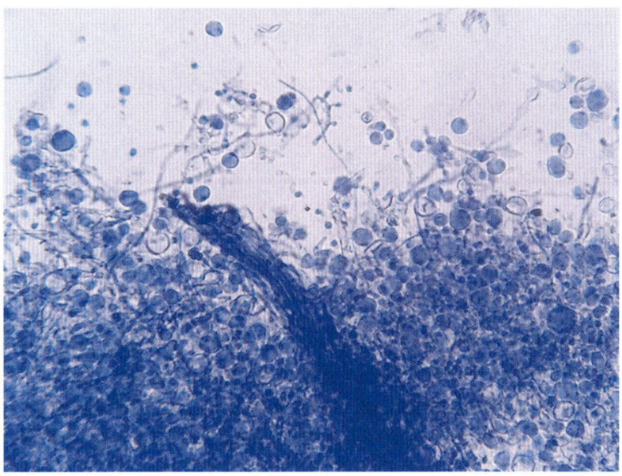

Figure 11: Microscopic picture of *T. tonsurans* in lactophenol cotton blue (LPCB) shows swollen, balloon microconidia, match-shaped microconidia and numerous chlamydoconidia which may be intercalary, lateral, or terminal.

Intrafamilial Infection and Recurrence

Intrafamilial infection is on the rise in the current scenario of increased prevalence of chronic and recurrent dermatophytosis. Sharma et al. in 2012 and Kucheria et al. in 2016 reported 26.6% and 33% of patients with history of contact with infected

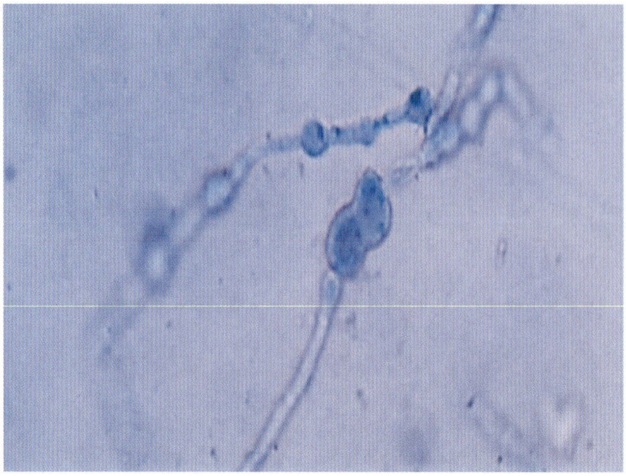

Figure 12: Intercalary and terminal chlamydoconidia of *T. tonsurans.*

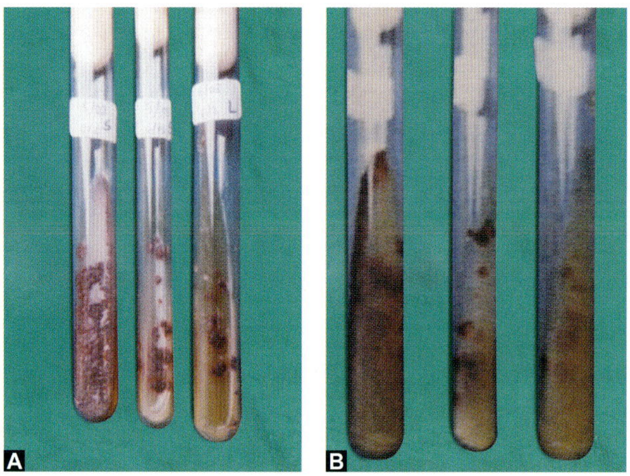

Figure 13: *Trichophyton violaceum.* Waxy, glabrous colony deep violet in color with reverse violet.

family members.[34,69] Surekha et al. in 2015 found contact history in 21.7% patients.[13] Recurrence rate of 16.6%, 31.3%, and 36.7% was observed by Sharma et al. in 2012, Surekha et al. in 2015, and Kaur et al. in 2016, respectively.[13,29,34]

Clinical Type

Clinical type of dermatophytosis depends on various factors such as occupation, sex, obesity, tight clothing, steroid abuse, etc. Most of the studies done across the

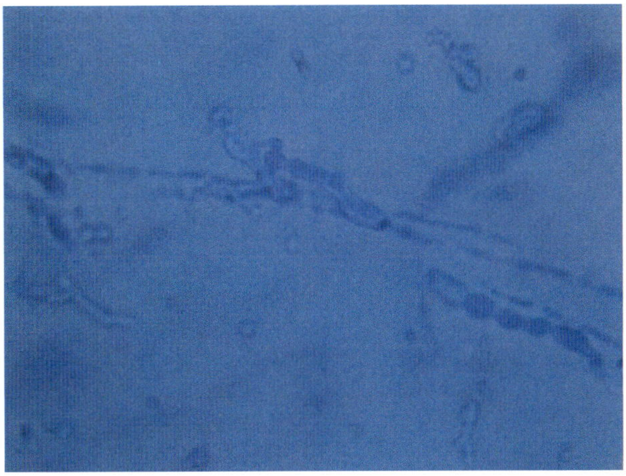

Figure 14: Microscopic picture of *T. violaceum* in lactophenol cotton blue shows chlamydoconidia and distorted hyphae. Microconidia and macroconidia are usually absent.

country have found tinea corporis to be the most common clinical presentation of dermatophytosis followed by tinea cruris, as has been in the past (Tables 6 to 8). Tinea cruris was found to be more common than tinea corporis by Chaudhary and Kumar and Sharma et al.[65,66] Tinea pedis was found to be the most common clinical type in studies from Shimla, Uttarakhand, Kolkata, and Shillong.[5,37,44,66] Increasing occurrence of combination of various clinical types has been reported at Jaipur (14.7%), Mysore (16%), Kolkata (17.3%), Ludhiana (21%), Visakhapatnam (25.4%), and Mangalore (46%).[5,49,69,75,79,84] Tinea incognito has become more common than ever before due to the rampant use of topical steroid antifungal combination creams. Anuradha and Thilak and Mitruka et al. observed tinea incognito in 12.87% and 21.15% of their patients.[85,86]

CAUSES FOR THE CHANGING AND RISING SCENARIO OF DERMATOPHYTOSIS

Current literature is indeed suggestive of an increasing prevalence of dermatophytosis across the country. Chronicity, recurrence and treatment failures of this infection are of serious concern to the dermatologists and the patients, as it causes emotional stress and affects the quality of life due to the persistent itching and cosmetic concern. Causes for this change of dermatophytosis could be attributed to various factors such as environment, host, etiological organisms, and drug therapy.

Table 6: Clinical Scenario—North, East, and Central India[5,27,29,37,40,42-44,65-71]

State/city	Year	Study	Sex ratio	Age group	T. cor	T. cru	T. fac	T. man	T. ped	Comb	T. cap	T. ung
Himachal Pradesh												
Simla[66]	2003	Sharma et al.	3:1	31–40	22.8	28.1	–	2.6	38.6	–	4.3	23.7
Tanda[29]	2016	Kaur et al.	1.6:1	21–30	40.7	4.3	2.5	13	10	7.5	7	21.6
Uttar Pradesh												
Lucknow[67]	2011	Sahai et al.	2:1	21–30	45	3	–	5	2	–	34	11
Bareilly[68]	2015	Goyal et al.	1.5:1	21–40	51.3	26.2	4.75	–	3.55		8.75	4.75
Jammu												
Samba[27]	2015	Najotra et al.	2.5:1	21–30	45.7	12.9	3.6	9.3	7.1	–	9.3	12.1
Punjab												
Ludhiana[69]	2016	Kucheria et al.	1.3:1	21–30	31	10	5	2	4	21	7	20
Uttarakhand[37]	2014	Kainthola et al.	1.84:1	20–40	28.4	9.5	–	–	18.9	–	43.2	–
Bihar[65]	2016	Chaudhary and Kumar	2.1:1	21–40	21.5	31	3.5	6.5	8.5	–	10.5	12.5
West Bengal												
Kolkata[5]	2003	Grover et al.	4.26:1	21–30	15.5	26.2	2.9	13.6	29.2	17.3	3.9	8.7
Kolkata[40]	2014	Ghosh et al.	1.1:1	31–40	8.65	3.0	0.5	0.8	3.5	–	8.9	74.58
Assam												
Dibrugarh[70]	2004	Sarma and Borthakur	3:1	21–30	42	11	–	–	–	–	–	–
Assam[42]	2015	Naglot et al.	4.38:1	21–30	34.8	21.5	3.7	0.85	11.1	–	–	27.8
Meghalaya												
Shillong[44]	2013	Lyngdoh et al.	2.64:1	21–30	18.9	14.3	6.2	7.7	26.6		4.3	13.1 Ony 2.7
Manipur												
Imphal[43]	2015	Singh et al.	2.57:1	21–30	36.8	24.2	5.2	5.2	6.3	–	–	15.78
Chhattisgarh												
Bhilai[71]	2014	Dutta et al.	1.57:1	Mean 37.5	32	4	–	–	6	42	2	2

T. cor, tinea corporis; T. cru, tinea cruris; T. fac, tinea faciei; T. man, tinea manuum; T. ped, tinea pedis; T. cap, tinea capitis; T. ung, tinea unguium; Comb, combination of various clinical types; Ony, onychomycosis.

Distribution of various clinical types is given in percentage.

Table 7: Clinical Scenario—Western India[8,9,49,50,53,72-74]

State/city	Year	Study	Sex ratio	Age group	T. cor	T. cru	T. fac	T. man	T. ped	Comb	T. cap	T. ung
Rajasthan												
Jaipur[49]	2014	Agarwal et al.	2.1:1	21–30	37.3	13.7	3	2	3.7	14.7	13	11
Rajkot[50]	2015	Mistry et al.	1.05:1	21–30	58.4	9.7	1.7	0.76	0.95	3.81	2.28	22.8
Gujarat												
Baroda[72]	2003	Singh et al.	1.57:1	16–30	58.8	12.3	1.5	6.1	11.5	–	6.92	1.9
Ahmedbad[73]	2010	Patel et al.	1.78:1	21–30	56.5	5.5	1	9	6	–	11	9
Ahmedbad[8]	2014	Chudasama et al.	2.17:1	19–59	48	8.5	1	5	6	–	5	15
Valsad[9]	2016	Patel et al.	2.17:1	19–59	41	5.4	9.5	2.7	5.4	2.7	9.5	19
Maharashtra												
Loni[53]	2013	Bose et al.	4:1	21–30	42	28	–	3.3	3.5	6.6	4	7
Solapur[74]	2016	Rathod et al.	1.81:1	21–30	52	22.6	3.3	3.3	3.3	8	2.67	2.67

T. cor, tinea corporis; T. cru, tinea cruris; T. fac, tinea faciei; T. man, tinea manuum; T. ped, tinea pedis; T. cap, tinea capitis; T. ung, tinea unguium; Comb, combination of various clinical types; Ony, onychomycosis.

Distribution of various clinical types is given in percentage.

Table 8: Clinical Scenario—Southern India12,58,61,64,75-81

State/City	Year	Study	Sex ratio	Age group	T. cor	T. cru	T. fac	T. man	T. ped	Comb	T. cap	T. ung
Karnataka												
Mysore[75]	2012	Hanumanthappa et al.	1.94:1	21–30	33.3	23.3	2.6	1.3	2	16	11.3	–
Mysore[76]	2014	Mahale et al.	1.6:1	21–30	31.6	14.6	–	1.1	3.3	–	18.6	29.3
Vijayapur[77]	2016	Khadri et al.	1.22:1	21–30	57.5	15	12.5	1.25	-		7.5	1.25
Shimoga[58]	2016	Manjunath et al.	1.4:1	20–30	50.76	19.2	–	–	5.38	–	7.69	13.8
Kerala												
Malappuram[61]	2008	Sivakumar et al.	1:1.8	20–30	*T cor>T ped>T fac> T ung>T man>T cap*							
Calicut[78]	2015	Lavanya and Solabannavar	2.38:1	31–40	44.8	18	3.8	1.9	3.8	5.7	7.6	15.2
Visakhapatnam[79]	2015	Poluri et al.	2:1	21–30	40	9.09	6.3	5.4	4.5	25.4	8.1	
Tirupati[12]	2016	Sridevi et al.	1.27:1	21–30	51.4	22.8	–	–	–	–	–	11.4
Tamil Nadu												
Tiruchi[80]	2012	Balakumar et al.	2.03:1	11–30	35.4	16.7	7.32	1.9	4.62		16.5	10.5
Chennai[81]	2014	Kumaran et al.	1.5:1	>21	23	18	–	9	4	–	21	7
Chennai[64]	2016	Ramaraj V	1.3:1	21–40	63.2	13.8	2.3	4.3	3.8	–	2.86	9.04

T. cor, tinea corporis; T. cru, tinea cruris; T. fac, tinea faciei; T. man, tinea manuum; T. ped, tinea pedis; T. cap, tinea capitis; T. ung, tinea unguium; Comb, combination of various clinical types.

Distribution of various clinical types is given in percentage.

ENVIRONMENT

Global warming which is a hot topic in the recent times, is indeed an immense environmental crisis. Scientific reports point out that the average temperature of the earth has risen between 0.4 and 0.8°C over the past 100 years. This has resulted in increased maximum temperatures, scarcity of water, less but intense rainfall, and extremes of weather conditions across India as a result of which people have become more predisposed to develop dermatophytosis. Kamalam observed a biannual peak during May and October over many years.[87] But now, in authors' institution, there is a continuous surge of patients with dermatophytosis throughout the year with a lesser frequency during January and February (unpublished data). Interstate migration of laborers to work in construction sites, metro rail work, and hotel industry have increased in large proportions in the recent years. This along with the migration of rural population to cities has led to overcrowding, poor living conditions, water scarcity and poor personal hygiene. This population by virtue of their illiteracy and ignorance are more prone to seek treatment late or use over-the-counter (OTC) topical steroid and antifungal combination creams. Agarwal et al. reported that 62.5% of patients came 3 months after the onset of infection.[49]

HOST FACTORS

Urban life in the present days is marked by sedentary lifestyle with inappropriate eating habits resulting in obesity and metabolic syndrome. Study on obesity by Pradeepa et al. stated that there is an increased prevalence of obesity, both in the urban and rural population in India, compared to the earlier reports. Abdominal obesity was more prevalent than generalized obesity in the urban population.[88] Obesity predisposes to increased sweating and maceration in the flexures which will facilitate the growth of dermatophytes. Jeans and leggings are the most popular dresses among the college students and working population. These garments do not suit the hot and humid weather conditions in our country. In addition, there is always a habit of sharing clothes among college students. Mitruka et al. observed that 36.5% and 17.3% of patients with dermatophytosis gave history of wearing occlusive clothing and footwear respectively.[86]

Daily bathing is not practiced in pockets of the country either due to water scarcity, cold weather, or as a customary practice. Many a times, people bathe, but do not wipe for lack of time while getting ready for work or college. In a study done by Das et al., it was found the about 50% of the patients did not wipe the wet parts after bath.[6] Sharing of clothes and bed linen with infected family members leads to intrafamilial infections, persistence, or reinfection. Nails and hair act as reservoirs of infection, which are many a times missed as patients do not bother to mention about the nail changes.

There is an increasing trend of chronic and recurrent dermatophytosis across the country in the recent years. Kaaman considered dermatophytosis as chronic when it was present for more than 1 year with several relapses or for a total duration of more than 1 year.[89] An individual is considered to have recurrent dermatophytosis, if the infection recurs within few weeks after completion of therapy.[3] There is also an increase in the prevalence of steroid-modified tinea—"tinea incognito" in the recent times. This is mainly due to the fact there is a rampant use of OTC topical steroid or steroid antifungal combination creams for prolonged intermittent periods which result in local immunosuppression and persistence of dermatophytosis (Figures 15 to 17).

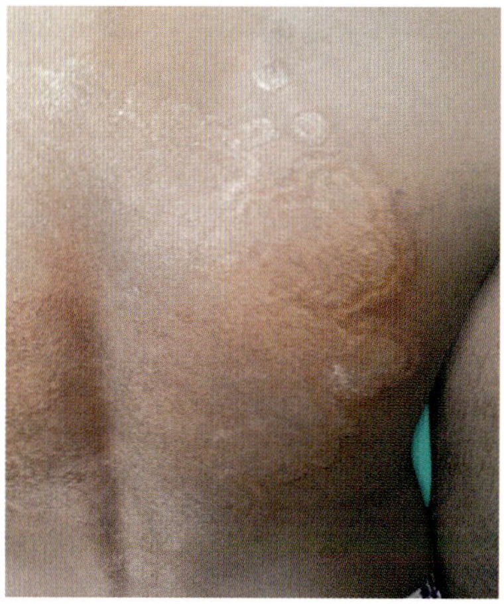

Figure 15: Tinea incognito showing ring within ring appearance and atrophy of skin.

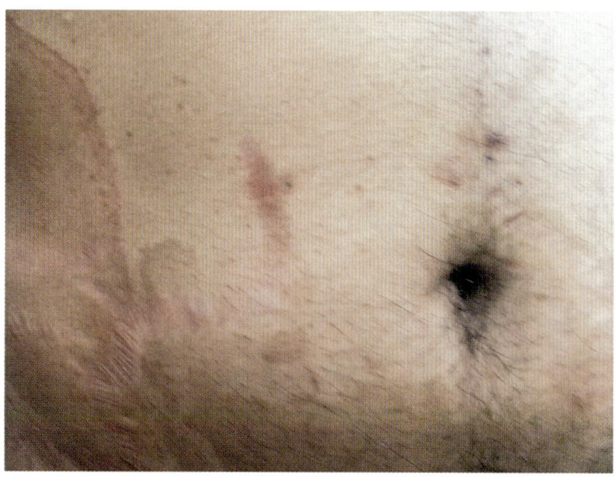

Figure 16: Tinea incognito with striae.

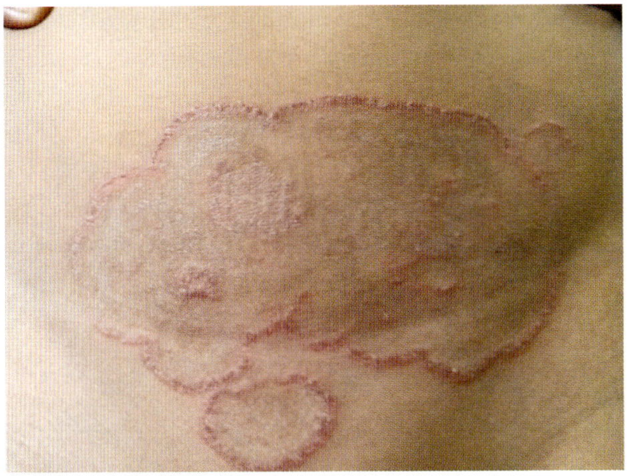

Figure 17: Tinea incognito in a child.

Poor compliance on the part of the patient and lack of counseling from the physician can result in treatment failures. Poor compliance could be due to the partial improvement or there could be an economic constraint. Presence of other associated disorders such as atopic dermatitis, ichthyosis, diabetes, bronchial asthma, Cushing's syndrome, human immunodeficiency virus, and other immunosuppressive states will affect the course of dermatophytosis.[90]

ETIOLOGICAL AGENTS

Studies done across the country have revealed that *T. rubrum* is the most prevalent organism causing dermatophytosis of the glabrous skin and that there is a definite rise in the prevalence of *T. mentagrophytes* compared to the previous studies. As far as onychomycosis is concerned, most studies have shown *T. rubrum* to be the most common etiological agent, while few have reported *T. mentagrophytes* to be the commonest organism.[91-95] However, there are emerging reports which have shown nondermatophytes to be the predominant cause of onychomycosis.[96]

Probable causes for higher prevalence and chronicity of *T. rubrum* and *T. mentagrophytes* are as follows:

Survival

Both these organisms are characterized by long survival of spores in nature. Dvorak et al. observed the survival of *T. rubrum* up to 7 months and that of *T. mentagrophytes* to range from 9 to 15 months.[97] *T. mentagrophytes* and *M. gypseum* were found to survive on towel for more than 25 weeks and in swimming pool water for 1 week by Khanjanasthiti and Srisawat. *T. rubrum* was viable on towel for a period less than 12 weeks.[98] Shimmura observed a higher occurrence of *T. mentagrophytes* in the house dust of infected persons.[99]

Dimorphism

T. rubrum and *T. mentagrophytes* exhibit dimorphism and could be induced to form germination tubes at pH 7.[98]

Keratinocyte Stimulation

In vitro studies have shown that on stimulation with *Trichophyton* antigen namely *Trichophytin*, keratinocytes produce interleukin-8 (IL-8) and leukotriene B4 which cause the inflammatory response. When filtrate from culture of *T. rubrum* or *T. mentagrophytes* was added to the keratinocyte culture, there was increased secretion of basic fibroblast growth factor and IL-1 alpha. It was found that *T. mentagrophytes* produced higher levels of IL-1 alpha than *T. rubrum*. This explains the accumulation of neutrophils seen in the epidermis of acute lesions caused by *T. mentagrophytes* in contrast to the mononuclear cells seen in chronic lesions of *T. rubrum*. Studies have also shown that there is a difference in the profile of cytokine production by these two organisms.[100]

High Parasitism of *T. rubrum*

This could be probably attributed to different enzymatic component in its negative anamorphic state compared to the positive strains which were considered extinct.[101] Mannan moiety present in the cell wall of *T. rubrum* is produced in larger amounts which result in intense inhibition of lymphocyte proliferation. It reduces the keratinocyte proliferation with resultant slow turnover of cells, thus explaining the chronicity of infection. It also causes defective antigen killing by depression of lymphoblast tansformation and by modification of polymorphonuclear cells and monocytes.[100]

Racial and Genetic Factors Implicated in Dermatophytosis

Tinea imbricata caused by *T. concentricum* is acquired through autosomal recessive inheritance. Ahmed et al. showed significant association of human leukocyte antigen (HLA)-A26 and HLA AW33 in association with chronic tinea pedis.[102] Glycoprotein from the cell wall of *T. mentagrophytes* was assessed for its cross reactivity with human blood group isoantigen leading to the possibility of cross-reacting antigens causing chronicity and wide spread infection.[103] Dermatoglyphic study by Sentamilselvi in 100 patients with chronic dermatophytosis and 100 normal subjects showed increased ulnar loop and whorl pattern along with increased ridge count in patients with chronic dermatophytosis.[104]

Antifungal Resistance

Antifungal resistance has become an increasingly discussed topic in this era of chronic and recurrent dermatophytosis associated with treatment failure. It is classified as microbiological resistance which may be primary or secondary and clinical resistance. Clinical resistance may be due to a combination of factors related to the host, pathogen, and the antifungal drug. Fungal factors responsible for causing clinical resistance are increased burden of the fungus, virulence, biofilms, and mannan. *T. rubrum* and *T. mentagrophytes* have been shown to produce biofilms which protects these organisms from the host defense mechanism and the antifungal agents. It is stated that clinical resistance does not always correlate with *in vitro* resistance, which is measured as an increase in minimum inhibitory concentration of a drug. This discordance between the *in vitro* and *in vivo* resistance has been explained by the "90-60" rule. This means that when there is infection due to a susceptible strain, 90% of patients will respond to treatment. In case of infection due to a resistant strain, 60% patients respond.[105] Mechanisms of antifungal resistance are beyond the scope of this article.

Arthroconidia versus Microconidia

Arthroconidia, the dormant forms of dermatophytes which are produced *in vivo* are responsible for the adherence and germination of dermatophytes and are resistant to adverse environmental conditions. Coelho, observed that arthroconidia were more resistant to antifungal drugs than microconidia which are produced *in vitro* and this difference in the susceptibility of arthroconidia and microconidia could be one of the causes for treatment failure.[106]

DRUG THERAPY

Suboptimal dose and duration of treatment often predicts clinical failure. Inappropriate use of systemic antifungal agents and topical steroid antifungal combinations by the general practitioners paves way for resistance and clinical failure. Other factors that have to be considered with regard to the drug are fungistatic or fungicidal nature of drug, administration, pharmacokinetics, pharmacodynamics, bioavailability, cost factor which may result in poor compliance and polypharmacy. Drug-drug interactions may reduce the level of antifungal drug and result in poor clinical response.

SOLUTIONS TO COMBAT CLINICAL FAILURE

First and foremost, it is the duty of every responsible citizen to take steps to prevent global warming. Afforestation would be the best solution as trees would suck the CO_2 from the atmosphere and reverse global warming. Health authorities should provide health education to the high-risk population such as slum residents and roadside dwellers, with special attention to the migratory population about personal hygiene and create an awareness about dermatophytosis, a serious public health problem. Corporation authorities should take measures to combat water scarcity.

The most important step taken to tackle clinical failure would be to counsel the patient regarding the general measures and to explain the nature of infection with emphasis on compliance.

General measures are as follows:

- Lifestyle modification is the need of the day. People should be sensitized about the morbidities associated with obesity and encouraged to lose weight. They should be advised to bathe twice in hot and humid climate and to wipe dry and only then wear clothes. They should be advised to wear cotton garments and avoid tight clothes. Patients with tinea cruris should be instructed to wear box-type inner garments, remove the waistband and change under garments everyday. They should also be advised to regularly remove the hair on genitalia. People who have to constantly wear shoes, should be encouraged to use only cotton socks. Patients with tinea pedis should be advised to use open foot wear
- Measures to minimize exposure to fomites by avoidance of sharing soaps, towels, clothes, combs, towels, bed linen, and toys should be practiced
- Towels, bed linen, caps, and socks should be washed regularly. Studies have shown that washing clothes at 60°C has eliminated dermatophytes.[107] Infected clothes and socks to be washed separately. Sunlight is said to be the best and hot water washed clothes should be turned inside out while drying in sunlight.[108] Those who stay in the hostel could be instructed to iron the clothes. If that is not possible, well-dried inner garments at least 3–4 days after washing could be worn
- Mechanical removal of any material containing keratin, such as shed skin and hairs, facilitates disinfection. Vacuuming is considered to be the best method in the western world and could be practiced if feasible. Wet mopping may be ideal in our country. After mechanical removal, washable surfaces should be cleaned thoroughly with detergent and hot water. All bedding, brushes, combs, caps, towels, etc. should be scrubbed, and washed with hot water and detergent. Cleaning and disinfection of the environment should be repeated at least once in every 4–6 weeks (the more often, the better) until all affected persons have eliminated the fungal infection

- Patients should be explained about the side effects of steroids and instructed to strictly avoid using OTC preparations.

Points for Consideration by the Dermatologist

- History of dermatophytosis in family members is very important as this will be one of the important causes for reinfection. History of pet animals should be enquired
- Treatment history should be probed for use of topical steroids and other concomitant morbidities
- Should be well versed with drug-drug interactions
- Nails and hair act as reservoir of infection
- Tinea of vellus hair warrants systemic therapy
- Treatment of the underlying condition or a wrong diagnosis should be considered in patients with treatment failure
- After initiation of treatment, patient could be asked to come after 2–3 weeks, if there are new lesions or if there is itching. In the first review, if there is a partial response with intense itching, we can increase the dosage. If there is no response or there are new lesions, one should consider changing the drug
- Combination therapy should be reserved for patients with chronic/recurrent/refractory infection
- Both systemic and topical antifungals should be continued for at least 2 weeks after complete resolution. Topical antifungals should be applied 2 cm beyond the active border of the lesion
- Duration of the treatment is best individualized according to the clinical response.

CONCLUSION

There is definitely an increase in the prevalence of dermatophytosis in India, which has emerged as a serious public health problem. Though dermatophytosis is more common in males, there is an increasing prevalence among the females which has been well depicted by the change in the sex ratio. Tinea corporis continues to be the most common clinical type. However, multiple site involvement has become more common. Tinea incognito has increased in prevalence due to the rampant use of OTC topical steroid antifungal combinations. *T. rubrum* continues to be the most common causative organism followed by *T. mentagrophytes* which is on the rise as a codominant pathogen. Most important of all, it is very important to offer counseling to patients with dermatophytosis and ensure that all the above-mentioned measures are practiced, so that we could bring this infection under control. Health education to create an awareness about dermatophytosis and abuse of topical steroids is the need of the hour.

Editor's Comment

We are indeed fortunate to bring the three eminent dermato-mycologists of India, Dr R Madhu, Dr Janaki Chellam and Dr Sentamilselvi Ganapati on this very relevant article addressing the problem of changing and rising trends of dermatological fungal infections in clinical practice. The role of global warming, overcrowding, fomites and incomplete treatment is highlighted. This is a problem we are living with at present and this article will provide immense knowledge to all. It also discussed the pattern of superficial fungal infections from relevant studies in India while also giving the global perspective.

Rashmi Sarkar, Seemal R Desai

REFERENCES

1. Ameen M. Epidemiology of superficial fungal infections. *Clin Dermatol.* 2010;28:197-201.
2. Pires CA, Cruz NF, Lobato AM, Sousa PO, Carneiro FR, Mendes AM. Clinical, epidemiological, and therapeutic profile of dermatophytosis. *An Bras Dermatol.* 2014;89(2):259-64.
3. Dogra S, Uprety S. The menace of chronic and recurrent dermatophytosis in India: Is the problem deeper than we perceive? *Indian Dermatol Online J.* 2016;7:73-6.
4. Mishra M, Mishra S, Singh PC, Mishra BC. Clinico-mycological profile of superficial mycoses. *Indian J Dermatol Venereol Leprol.* 1998;64:283-5.
5. Grover WC, Roy CP. Clinico-mycological profile of superficial mycosis in a hospital in North-East India. *Med J Armed Forces India.* 2003;59(2):114-6.
6. Das K, Basak S, Ray S. A study on superficial fungal infection from West Bengal: a brief report. *J Life Sci.* 2009;1(1):51-5.
7. Nawal P, Patel S, Patel M, Soni S, Khandelwal N. A study of superficial mycosis in tertiary care hospital. *NJIRM.* 2012;3(1):95-9.
8. Chudasama V, Solanki H, Vadasmiya M, Javadekar T. A study of superficial mycosis in tertiary care hospital. *IJSR.* 2014;3(3):222-4.
9. Patel HK, Patel PH, Nerurkar AB. A study of superficial mycoses with its clinical correlation at GMERS Medical College & Hospital Valsad, Gujarat. *Indian J Microbiol Res.* 2016;3(1):69-73.
10. Kannan P, Janaki C, Selvi GS. Prevalence of dermatophytes and other fungal agents isolated from clinical samples. *Indian J Med Microbiol.* 2006;24(3):212-5.
11. Narasimhalu CR, Kalyani M, Somendar S. A cross-sectional, clinico-mycological research study of prevalence, aetiology, speciation and sensitivity of superficial fungal infection in Indian patients. *J Clin Exp Dermatol Res.* 2016;7(1):324.
12. Sridevi K, Venkataramana P, Surekha A. A study on dermatomycoses. *IOSR-JDMS.* 2016;15(4):56-9.
13. Surekha A, Kumar R, Sridevi K, Murty DS, Usha G, Bharathi G. Superficial dermatomycoses: a prospective clinicomycological study. *J Clin Sci Res.* 2015;4:7-15.
14. Sharma M, Sharma R. Profile of dermatophytic and other fungal infections in Jaipur. *Indian J Microbiol.* 2012;52(2):270-4.
15. Prabhu SR, Shetty VH, Shetty NJ, Girish PN, Keshava Rao BP, Oommen RA, et al. Clinico-mycological study of superficial fungal infections in coastal Karnataka, India. *J Evolution Med Dent Sci.* 2013;2(44):8638-46.
16. Parameswari K, Prasad Babu KP. Clinico-mycological study of dermatophytosis in and around Kakinada. *Int J Med Dent Sci.* 2015;4(2):833.

17. Khan MS, Khan N. A study of fungal isolates from superficial mycoses cases attending IIMS & R, Lucknow. *Int J Life Sci Scienti Res.* 2016;2(1):37-42.
18. Monika, Gupta SK, Deepinder K Chhina, Gupta V, Deepika. Clinico-mycological correlation of superficial fungal infections. *Gulf J Dermatol Venereol.* 2016;23(1):6-13.
19. Magdum RJ, Gadgil SA, Kulkarni SA, Rajmane VS, Patil SS. Clinico-mycological study of superficial mycoses. *JKIMSU.* 2016;5(4):37-44.
20. Dermatophytosis. In: Reiss E, Shadomy HJ, Lyon GM, editors. Fundamental Medical Mycology. 1st ed. New Jersey: Wiley-Blackwell; 2012. pp. 527-66.
21. Havlickova B, Czaika VA, Friedrich M. Epidemiological trends in skin mycoses worldwide. *Mycoses.* 2008;51(4):2-15.
22. Hay RJ, Ashbee HR. Fungal infections. In: Griffiths CE, Barker J, Bleiker T, Chalmers R, Creamer D, editors. Rook's Textbook of Dermatology. 9th ed. West Sussex: Wiley-Blackwell; 2016. pp. 923-1018.
23. Gopi A, Harindranath D, Kaushik R. Mycological profile of dermatophytes isolated from clinical samples in KIMS Hospital, Bangalore. *J Evolution Med Dent Sci.* 2015;4(5):835-42.
24. Ranganathan S, Menon T, Selvi SG. Effect of socio-economic status on the prevalence of dermatophytosis in Madras. *Indian J Dermatol Venereol Leprol.* 1995;61:16-8.
25. Jain N, Sharma M. Distribution of dermatophytes and other related fungi in Jaipur city, with particular reference to soil pH. *Mycoses.* 2009;54:52-8.
26. Munir S, Ganaie F, Kumar B, Tewari R, Badakshaan S. Epidemiologic, clinico-mycological aspects of fungal infections of skin and its appendages. *J Evolution Med Dent Sci.* 2014;3(16):4212-9.
27. Najotra D, Choudhary V, Sahni B, Choudhary A. Cinico-epidemiological profile of dermatophytosis in district Samba: a cross-sectional study from the state of Jammu and Kashmir, India. *Med Sci.* 2015;3(1):183-9.
28. Bhagra S, Ganju SA, Kanga A, Sharma NL, Guleria RC. Mycological pattern of dermatophytosis in and around Shimla hills. *Indian J Dermatol.* 2014;59:268-70.
29. Kaur I, Thakur K, Sood A, Mahajan VK, Gupta PK, Chauhan S, et al. Clinico-mycological profile of clinically diagnosed cases of dermatophytosis in North India: a prospective cross-sectional study. *Int J Health Sci Res.* 2016;6(8):54-60.
30. Rani U, Saigal RK, Kanta S, Krishnan R. Study of dermatophytosis in Punjabi population. *Indian J Pathol Microbiol.* 1983;26(4):243-7.
31. Singla B, Malhotra R, Walia G. Mycological study of dermatophytosis in 100 clinical samples of skin hair and nail. *Int J Pharm Pharm Sci.* 2013;5:763-5.
32. Aggarwal A, Arora U, Khanna S. Clinical and mycological study of superficial mycoses in Amritsar. *Indian J Dermatol.* 2002;47(4):218-20.
33. Kansra S, Pushpa Devi, Sidhu S, Malhotra A. Prevalence of dermatophytoses and their antifungal susceptibility in a tertiary care hospital of North India. *IJSR.* 2016;5(3):450-3.
34. Sharma Y, Jain S, Chandra K, Khuraana VK, Kudesia M. Clinico-mycological evaluation of dermatophytes and non-dermatophytes isolated from various clinical samples: a study from North India. *J Res Med Sci.* 2012;17(8):817-8.
35. Maity MM, Nandan K, Dey S. Clinico-mycological profile of dermatophytosis in patients attending a tertiary care hospital in Eastern Bihar, India. *J Evolution Med Dent Sci.* 2014;3(29):8263-9.
36. Singh S, Kumar A, Agrawal A, Singh R. Study of dermatophytes and incidence of different clinical types of tinea in skin OPD. *Eastern J Med Sci.* 2016;1(1):24-30.
37. Kainthola A, Gaur P, Dobhal A, Sundriyal S. Prevalence of dermatophytoses in rural population of Garhwal Himalayan Region, Uttarakhand, India. *Int Res J Med Sci.* 2014;2(8):9-12.
38. Singh UK, Nath P. Fungal flora in the superficial infections of the skin and nails at Lucknow. *Indian J Pathol Microbiol.* 1981;24(3):189-93.
39. Prasad N, Mahapatra A, Chayani N, Changing trends in the fungal isolates from clinical specimens of suspected superficial mycosis. *Ind Med Gaz.* 2013;60-4.
40. Ghosh RR, Ray R, Ghosh TK, Ghosh AP. Clinico-mycological profile of dermatophytosis in a tertiary care hospital in West Bengal, an Indian scenario. *Int J Curr Microbiol App Sci.* 2014;3(9):655-66.

41. Sen SS, Rasul ES. Dermatophytosis in Assam. *Indian J Med Microbiol.* 2005;24(1):77-8.
42. Naglot A, Shrimali DD, Nath BK, Gogoi HK, Veer V, Chander J, et al. Recent trends of dermatophytosis in Northeast India (Assam) and interpretation with published studies. *Int J Curr Microbiol App Sci.* 2015;4(11):111-20.
43. Singh TN, Zamzachin G, Singh NB. Dermatophytosis: clinico-mycological study on patients attending the Department of Dermatology Rims Hospital, Imphal, Manipur. *Int J Curr Microbiol App Sci.* 2015;4(6):1066-75.
44. Lyngdoh CJ, Lyngdoh WV, Choudhury B, Sangma KA, Bora I, Khyriem AB. Clinico-mycological profile of dermatophytosis in Meghalaya. *Int J Med Public Health.* 2013;3:254-6.
45. Shukla NP, Agarwal GP, Gupta DK. Prevalence of dermatophytosis in Jabalpur. *Indian J Pathol Microbiol.* 1983;26(1):31-9.
46. Pandey A, Pandey M. Isolation and characterization of dermatophytes with tinea infections at Gwalior (MP), India. *Int J Pharm Sci Invent.* 2013;2(2):5-8.
47. Gupta CM, Tripathi K, Tiwari S, Rathore Y, Nema S, Dhanvijay AG. Current trends of clinicomycological profile of dermatophytosis in central India. *J Dent Med Sci.* 2014;13(10):23-6.
48. Mandia P. Dermatomycosis in Udaipur region, Rajasthan. *Int J Dermatol.* 1987;32(1):5-10.
49. Agarwal US, Saran J, Agarwal P. Clinico-mycological study of dermatophytes in a tertiary care centre in northwest India. *Indian J Dermatol Venereol Leprol.* 2014;80:194.
50. Mistry MA, Goswami YS, Rathod B, Dalwadi PH. Clinico-mycological studies of dermatophytosis at tertiary care centre, west India. *Int J Biol Med Res.* 2014;5(4):4556-61.
51. Mankodi RC, Kanvinde MS. Incidence of dermatophytosis in Ahmedabad, Gujarat. *Indian J Pathol Bacteriol.* 1969;12(3):114-7.
52. Mehta JP, Deodhar KP, Mehta VR, Chaphekar PM. A study of dermatophytosis in Bombay. *Indian J Pathol Microbiol.* 1977;20(1):23-31.
53. Bose S, Barapatre R, Ghosh AK. Clinico-mycological profiles of dermatophytoses in a tertiary care rural hospital. *Int J Biomed Adv Res.* 2013;4(1):31-4.
54. Sharma N, Sharma A. To study the species profile in dermatomycoses patients in a tertiary care hospital of western Maharashtra. *IJSR.* 2016;5(2):579-91.
55. Bhaskaran CS, Rao PS, Krishnamurthy T, Tarachand P. Dermatophytosis in Tirupati, Andhra Pradesh. *Indian J Pathol Microbiol.* 1977;20(4):251-9.
56. Lalithamma BP, Jayaram US, Prabhu T. A study of dermatomycosis in Mysore. *Indian J Pathol Microbiol.* 1978;21(4):329-36.
57. Noronha TM, Tophakhane RS, Nadiger S. Clinico-microbiological study of dermatophytosis in a tertiary-care hospital in north Karnataka. *Indian Dermatol Online J.* 2016;7:264-7.
58. Manjunath M, Koppad M, Dadapeer S. Clinicomycological study of dermatomycosis in a tertiary care hospital. *Indian J Microbiol Res.* 2016;3(2):190-3.
59. Maheshwariamma SM, Paniker CK, Gopinathan T. Studies on dermatomycosis in Calicut. *Indian J Pathol Microbiol.* 1982;25:11-7.
60. Bindu V, Pavithran K. Clinico-mycological study of dermatophytosis in Calicut. *Indian J Dermatol Venereol Leprol.* 2002;68:259-61.
61. Sivakumar N, Karthikeyan A, Vivek A, Santhamani M. Prevalence of etiological agents in superficial mycoses with reference to dermatophytoses and pityriasis versicolor. *Internet J Microbiol.* 2008;7(2).
62. Pankajalakshmi VV, Subramanian S. Mycoses in Madras (superficial). *Indian J Dermatol Venereol Leprol.* 1974;40(2):66-72.
63. Kumar K, Kindo AJ, Kalyani J, Anandan S. Clinico-mycological profile of dermatophytic skin infections in a tertiary care center: a cross-sectional study. *Sri Ramachandra J Med.* 2007;1(2):12-5.
64. Ramaraj V, Vijayaraman RS, Rangarajan S, Kindo AJ. Incidence and prevalence of dermatophytosis in and around Chennai, Tamil Nadu, India. *Int J Res Med Sci.* 2016;4:695-700.
65. Chaudhary JK, Kumar A. A clinico-mycological profile of dermatophytosis at a tertiary care hospital in Bihar. *Int J Curr Microbiol App Sci.* 2016;5(2):181-9.

66. Sharma NL, Gupta ML, Sharma RC, Singh P, Gupta N. Superficial mycoses in Simla. *Indian J Dermatol Venereol Leprol.* 1983;49(6):266-9.
67. Sahai S, Mishra D. Change in spectrum of dermatophytes isolated from superficial mycoses cases: first report from central India. *Indian J Dermatol Venereol Leprol.* 2011;77(3):335-6.
68. Goyal S, Mishra PP, Prakash V. A study of prevalence of etiological agents of dermatophytosis in a tertiary care hospital. *Ann Int Med Den Res.* 2015;1(3):205-8.
69. Kucheria M, Gupta SK, Chhina DK, Gupta V, Hans D, Singh K. Clinico-mycological profile of dermatophytic infections at a tertiary care hospital in north India. *Int J Com Health Med Res.* 2016;2(2):17-22.
70. Sarma S, Borthakur AK. A clinic-epidemiological study of dermatophytosis in northeast India. *Indian J Dermatol Venereol Leprol.* 2007;73(6):427-8.
71. Dutta AK, Maharana J, Sinha H. A clinico-mycological study of superficial dermatophytes. *Int J Pharm Res Scholars.* 2014;3(1):138-42.
72. Singh S, Beena PM. Profile of dermatophyte infections in Baroda. *Indian J Dermatol Venereol Leprol.* 2003;69:281-3.
73. Patel P, Mulla S, Patel D, Shrimali GA. Study of superficial mycosis in south Gujarat region. *Natl J Community Med.* 2010;1(2):85-8.
74. Rathod PG, Shaikh NK, Ingole KV, Mundhada SG, Chakote SM. Prevalence of dermatophytes in a tertiary care center of Solapur, Maharashtra. *JKIMSU.* 2016;5(3):26-34.
75. Hanumanthappa H, Sarojini K, Shilpashree P, Muddapur SB. Clinicomycological study of 150 cases of dermatophytosis in a tertiary care hospital in South India. *Indian J Dermatol.* 2012;57(4):322-3.
76. Mahale RP, Rao R, Tejashree A, Deepashree R, Kulkarni M. Clinicomycological profile of dermatophytosis in a teaching hospital. *Int J Pharm Sci Invent.* 2014;3(8):43-6.
77. Khadri SY, Koregol S, Khadri YS, Patil BS. Clinico-mycological profile of dermatophytes in Vijayapur, Karnataka. *Int J Med Microbiol Trop Dis.* 2016;2(2):75-8.
78. Lavanya V, Solabannavar SS. Prevalence and socio-economic correlation of dermatophytes isolated from clinical samples in a tertiary care centre in south India. *Asian J Adv Basic Sci.* 2015;4(1):1-4.
79. Poluri LV, Indugula JP, Kondapaneni SL. Clinicomycological study of dermatophytosis in south India. *J Lab Physicians.* 2015;7(2):84-9.
80. Balakumar S, Rajan S, Thirunalasundari T, Jeeva S. Epidemiology of dermatophytosis in and around Tiruchirappalli, Tamil Nadu, India. *Asian Pac J Trop Dis.* 2012;2:286-9.
81. Kumaran G, Jeya M. Clinico-mycological profile of dermatophytic infections. *Int J Pharm Bio Sci.* 2014;5(2):1-5.
82. Indira G. Epidemiological studies on dermatophytoses in Warangal district, Telangana state, India. *GJMR: C Microbiol Pathol.* 2015;15(2):Version 1.0.
83. Walke HR, Gaikwad AA, Paleka SS. Clinico-mycological profile of dermatophytosis in patients attending dermatology OPD in tertiary care hospital, India. *Int J Curr Microbiol App Sci.* 2014;3(10):432-40.
84. Surendran K, Bhat RM, Boloor R, Nandakishore B, Sukumar D. A clinical and mycological study of dermatophytic infections. *Indian J Dermatol.* 2014;59:262-7.
85. Anuradha M, Thilak S. Clinicomycological study of various dermatophytic infections attending dermatology op in a tertiary care hospital, Kanchipuram, with special mention on significance of proper sample collection for their definitive laboratory diagnosis. *Int J Pharm Bio Sci.* 2016;7(1):175-82.
86. Mitruka B, Kaur A, Kaur N, Mittal RK, Mahajan A, Kaur A. Study of hospital-based epidemiology and clinical types of cases of dermatophytosis presenting in outpatient department of skin and venereology. *Sch J App Med Sci.* 2016;4(5C):1603-16.
87. Kamalam A. Observations on the Gamut/Galaxy of the fungal infections in Tamil Nadu State. *Kavaka.* 1984;12(1):15-36.
88. Pradeepa R, Anjana RM, Joshi SR, Bhansali A, Deepa M, Mohan V, et al. Prevalence of generalized and abdominal obesity in urban and rural India—the ICMR-INDIAB Study (Phase-I) [ICMR-INDIAB-3]. *Indian J Med Res.* 2015;142(2):139-50.

89. Sentamilselvi G, Kamalam A, Ajithadas K, Janaki C, Thambiah AS. Scenario of chronic dermatophytosis: an Indian study. *Mycopathologia.* 1997;140:129-35.
90. Sentamilselvi G, Janaki C, Ajitha Dos K, Kamalam A. Chronic dermatophytosis. *Indian J dermatol.* 2000;45(4):168-73.
91. Lone R, Bashir D, Ahmad S, Syed A, Khurshid S. A study on clinic-mycological profile, aetiological agents and diagnosis of onychomycosis at a government medical college hospital in Kashmir. *J Clin Diagn Res.* 2013;7:1983-5.
92. Das NK, Ghosh P, Das S, Bhattacharya S, Dutta RN, Sengupta SR. A study on the etiological agent and clinico-mycological correlation of fingernail onychomycosis in eastern India. *Indian J Dermatol.* 2008;53(2):75-9.
93. Reddy KN, Srikanth BA, Ram Sharan T. Epidemiological, clinical and cultural study of onychomycosis. *Am J Dermatol Venereol.* 2012;1(3):35-40.
94. Niranjan HP, Padmaja N, Priyanka BV. Study of onychomycosis at a tertiary care hospital in south India. *J Evolution Med Dent Sci.* 2012;1(5):823-9.
95. Yadav P, Singal A, Pandhi D, Das S. Clinicomycological study of dermatophyte toenail onychomycosis in New Delhi, India. *Indian J Dermatol.* 2015;60:153-8.
96. Sharma P, Sharma S. Non-dermatophytes emerging as predominant cause of onychomycosis in a tertiary care centre in rural part of Punjab, India. *J Acad Clin Microbiol.* 2016;18:36-9.
97. Dvorak J, Hubalek Z, Otcenasek M. Survival of dermatophytes in human skin scales. *Arch Dermatol.* 1968;98(5):540-2.
98. Khanjanasthiti P, Srisawat P. Germination and survival of dermatophyte spores in various environmental conditions. *Chiang Mai Med.* 1984;23:83-98.
99. Shimmura Y. Isolation of dermatophytes from human cases of dermatophytosis and from house dust. *Jap J Med Mycol.* 1985;26:74-80.
100. Peres NT, Maranhao FC, Rossi A, Martinez-Rossi NM. Dermatophytes: host-pathogen interaction and antifungal resistance. *An Bras Dermatol.* 2010;85(5):657-67.
101. Dahl MV. Dermatophytosis and the immune response. *J Am Acad Dermatol.* 1994;31(3 Pt 2):S34-41.
102. Ahmed AR, Schreiber P, Ajello J, Tiwari L, Terasalei PI. A preliminary report on the role of some immunological factors in persistence of chronic tinea pedis. *Clin Exp Dermatol.* 1985;10:45-50.
103. Young E, Roth FJ. Immunological cross reactivity between a glycoprotein isolated from *Trichophyton mentagrophytes* and human isoantigen A. *J Invest Dermatol.* 1979;72:46-51.
104. Sentamilselvi G. Study of clinical features and isolates in nonchronic and chronic dermatophytosis in a pilot study of 200 cases in chronic dermatophytosis: a clinical and aetiopathological study. (PhD thesis) Chennai, Madras University; 1995. pp. 97-109.
105. Kanafani ZA, Perfect JR. Resistance to antifungal agents: mechanisms and clinical impact. *Clin Infect Dis.* 2008;46:120-8.
106. Coelho LM, Aquino-Ferreira RA, Maffei CM, Martinez-Rossi NM. In vitro antifungal drug susceptibilities of dermatophytes microconidia and arthroconidia. *J Antimicrob Chemother.* 2008;62:758-61.
107. Hammer TR, Mucha H, Hoefer D. Infection risk by dermatophytes during storage and after domestic laundry and their temperature-dependent inactivation. *Mycopathologia.* 2011;171(1):43-9.
108. Amichai B, Grunwald MH, Davidovici B, Shemer A. Sunlight is said to be the best of disinfectants: the efficacy of sun exposure for reducing fungal contamination in used clothes. *Isr Med Assoc J.* 2014;16:431-3.

WORLD CLINICS
Statement of Purpose

The streams of medicine and surgery are evolving constantly at a rapid pace, creating a need for the healthcare professionals to continuously update their knowledge base and skills. This is necessary to offer their patients the best 'real world' treatment options based on current concepts, status, and trends, reflecting the achievements of evidence-based medicine. This pace of advances in medicine is a compelling reason for the physicians and surgeons to seek information through multiple resources such as journals, workshops and conferences.

WORLD CLINICS are periodicals of evidence-based reviews proposed as a source of comprehensive, state-of-the art reviews written by experts representing the global academia under the mentorship of an Editor-in-Chief. The comments by the 'Guest Editor' (or Editor-in-Chief) given at the end of each article/chapter would be representative of their clinical experience. Each issue of "WORLD CLINICS Dermatology" would focus on a single theme covering topics that are relevant to clinical understanding and decision-making. Each topic would be developed to reflect the current evidence, research, existing guidelines and recommendations as well the clinical experience of experts.

Objectives

- Provide up-to-date reviews on disease management, technique, procedure, or technology.
- Help enhance knowledge and skill for application in clinical practice.
- To aid use of evidence in decision-making for improved patient care.
- To help select best treatment options and overcome treatment challenges.

Target Readers

WORLD CLINICS are meant for practicing physicians, fellows, and postgraduate students, who plan to keep abreast with the current best-evidence clinical practices that are recommended and followed by experts globally.

Periodicity

WORLD CLINICS Dermatology will be released with a frequency of two issues per year.

Themes

Each subject area of WORLD CLINICS will cover themes on any of the following:

1. A disease or a disorder (e.g., Acne) OR
2. An organ or an anatomical region (e.g., Wrist, in WORLD CLINICS Orthopedics) OR
3. A technique or a treatment approach (e.g., Various methods for the treatment of CTEV, in WORLD CLINICS Orthopedics) OR
4. A special population group (e.g., Management of HIV infected pregnant patients in WORLD CLINICS Obstetrics and Gynecology) OR
5. A technology (e.g., 3D Ultrasound in diagnosis of gynecological abnormalities in WORLD CLINICS Obstetrics and Gynecology)

WORLD CLINICS
Manuscript Guidelines for Authors

General Guidelines

- Manuscripts must be typed in double-space including all text, references, tables, and figure legends, and should be sent in a single word file.
- For any copyright work, the necessary permissions must be obtained by the author and sent along with the manuscript. These permissions apply to any borrowed, modified, or adapted text, tables, or figures.
- For any production-quality artwork (images, illustrations, etc.) please see the guidelines under images.
- Acknowledgments or disclosures, if required, should be cited before the references.

Author Credits

- Should be in the first page.
- Each author's name, degree, academic or professional affiliation, city, and state (or country).
- E-mail address, mailing address, and telephone number of each co-author.
- If more than one author, mention the corresponding author.
- Please supply 4–6 keywords which will be used to optimize search results.

Subheads

The format for article's headings and subheadings is as follows:
'A' head: All caps, bold.
'B' head: Title case (upper/lower), bold.
'C' head: Title case (upper/lower), bold, italics.
'D' head: Title case (upper lower), normal, Roman.
'E' head: Sentence case (initial letter capital), italics, run in.

References

- References must be cited sequentially only at the end of the manuscript in the order as they appear in the text.
- Follow the Vancouver style for the references, using the Index Medicus abbreviations for journals that are indexed; if a journal is not indexed, use full name.
- If there are more than six authors, cite first six and add "et al."

e.g., Lacasse Y, Selman M, Costabel U, Dalphin JC, Ando M, Morell F, et al. Clinical Diagnosis of Hypersensitivity Pneumonitis. *Am J Respir Crit Care Med.* 2003;168:952-8.

Images

- There is generally no restriction on number of boxes, tables, or images, but keep them to a minimum necessary.
- A maximum of two hand-drawn illustrations and maximum of two algorithms are allowed.
- Medium for delivery of photographs: Individual TIFF or JPEG files each at a resolution no lower than 300 dpi (118 pixels/cm) when viewed at 100 mm width.
- The images and illustrations can also be in full color.